COVID-19 AND THE CORONAVIRUS SOURCEBOOK

FIRST EDITION

Health Reference Series

COVID-19 AND THE CORONAVIRUS SOURCEBOOK

FIRST EDITION

Provides Basic Consumer Health Information about COVID-19, including Coronavirus and Its Epidemiology, Origins, Pandemic Outbreak, Variants, Symptoms, Risk Factors, Testing, Clinical Presentation in Specific Populations, Prevention and Control Measures, Treatment and Clinical Care, Vaccines, Safety Measures, the Role of Technology in Testing, and Long-Term Effects

Along with Information about the COVID-19 Impact on the Global Economy, Employment, Education, Health Care, Travel Restrictions, Transition to Endemic, a Glossary of Terms, and a Directory of Resources for Further Help and Information about COVID-19 and Other Communicable Diseases

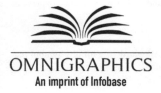

OMNIGRAPHICS
An imprint of Infobase

Bibliographic Note

Because this page cannot legibly accommodate all the copyright notices, the Bibliographic Note portion of the Preface constitutes an extension of the copyright notice.

* * *

OMNIGRAPHICS
An imprint of Infobase
132 W. 31st St.
New York, NY 10001
www.infobase.com
James Chambers, *Editorial Director*

* * *

Copyright © 2023 Infobase
ISBN 978-0-7808-2060-9
E-ISBN 978-0-7808-2061-6

Library of Congress Cataloging-in-Publication Data

Names: Chambers, James (Editor), editor.

Title: COVID-19 and the coronavirus sourcebook / edited by James Chambers.

Description: First edition. | New York, NY: Omnigraphics, an imprint of Infobase, [2023] | Series: Health reference series | "Provides Basic Consumer Health Information about COVID-19, including Coronavirus and Its Epidemiology, Origins, Pandemic Outbreak, Variants, Symptoms, Risk Factors, Testing, Clinical Presentation in Specific Populations, Prevention and Control Measures, Treatment and Clinical Care, Vaccines, Safety Measures, the Role of Technology in Testing, and Long-Term Effects" -- Title page. | Summary: "Provides basic information to help understand the coronavirus and COVID-19 infection with the facts of its origin, variants, symptoms, risks and clinical presentation, statistics of its cases and deaths, and future approaches to managing the pandemic. Includes index, glossary of related terms, and other resources"--Provided by publisher.

Identifiers: LCCN 2023000603 (print) | LCCN 2023000604 (ebook) | ISBN 9780780820609 (library binding) | ISBN 9780780820616 (ebook)

Subjects: LCSH: COVID-19 (Disease) | COVID-19 Pandemic, 2020-

Classification: LCC RA644.C67 C45228 2023 (print) | LCC RA644.C67 (ebook) | DDC 362.1962/4144--dc23/eng/20230125

LC record available at https://lccn.loc.gov/2023000603

LC ebook record available at https://lccn.loc.gov/2023000604

Electronic or mechanical reproduction, including photography, recording, or any other information storage and retrieval system for the purpose of resale is strictly prohibited without permission in writing from the publisher.

The information in this publication was compiled from the sources cited and from other sources considered reliable. While every possible effort has been made to ensure reliability, the publisher will not assume liability for damages caused by inaccuracies in the data, and makes no warranty, express or implied, on the accuracy of the information contained herein.

This book is printed on acid-free paper meeting the ANSI Z39.48 Standard. The infinity symbol that appears above indicates that the paper in this book meets that standard.

Printed in the United States

Table of Contents

Preface xiii

Part 1 | What You Need to Know about COVID-19
Chapter 1——Basics of COVID-19 3
        Section 1.1——What Is a Coronavirus? ... 5
        Section 1.2——Origins of COVID-19 8
        Section 1.3——Epidemiology and the Spread of COVID-19 Infection 12
        Section 1.4——Earlier Outbreaks Caused by the Coronavirus 17
        Section 1.5——Spread of COVID-19 across the World 22
Chapter 2——Variants of the Coronavirus 31
Chapter 3——Symptoms of Coronavirus Infection 41
        Section 3.1——Symptoms of COVID-19 43
        Section 3.2——Symptoms of Long COVID Condition 44
        Section 3.3——Similarities and Differences between Flu and COVID-19 50
Chapter 4——Testing for COVID-19 Infection 57
        Section 4.1——COVID-19 Testing: What Do You Need to Know? 59

Section 4.2—	Coronavirus Self-Test Kits 63
Section 4.3—	Community-Based Testing Sites for COVID-19 70
Section 4.4—	Waiting for Your COVID-19 Test Result 71

Chapter 5—The Immune System and COVID-19 75
Chapter 6—The Coronavirus and the Nervous System 79
Chapter 7—Understanding Your Coronavirus Risk Factors 91
Chapter 8—Clinical Presentation in Specific Population 97

Section 8.1—	COVID-19 in Pregnant and Recently Pregnant People 99
Section 8.2—	COVID-19 in People with Preexisting Medical Conditions 103
Section 8.3—	COVID-19 in People with Human Immunodeficiency Virus 111
Section 8.4—	COVID-19 in People Who Are Immunocompromised ... 115
Section 8.5—	COVID-19 in People with Asthma 121
Section 8.6—	COVID-19 Infections in Pets and Animals 124

Chapter 9—Disparities in COVID-19 129
Chapter 10—COVID-19 Statistics in United States 133

Section 10.1—	U.S. COVID-19 Cases and Deaths 135

        Section 10.2—Excess Deaths Associated with COVID-19 138
Chapter 11—Worldwide COVID-19 Cases and Deaths 151

Part 2 | Prevention and Control Measures of COVID-19

Chapter 12—How to Protect Yourself and Others from the COVID-19 Infection 159
        Section 12.1—Face Masks and Social Distancing 161
        Section 12.2—Cleaning and Disinfecting at Home... 169
Chapter 13—What to Do If You Were Exposed to COVID-19 175
Chapter 14—What to Do If You or Someone at Home Is Infected with COVID-19 179
        Section 14.1—Quarantine and Isolation 181
        Section 14.2—Breastfeeding and Caring for Newborns If You Have COVID-19 182
Chapter 15—Guidance for COVID-19 Prevention and Control in Schools 185
Chapter 16—COVID-19 Safety Considerations Related to Music, Arts, and Athletics Programs in Schools 197
Chapter 17—COVID-19 Control and Prevention at Workplaces 203
Chapter 18—COVID-19 Control Measures and Effectiveness: By Country 219

Part 3 | Clinical Care and Treatment Information for COVID-19

Chapter 19—Clinical Spectrum of SARS-CoV-2 Infection 239

Chapter 20—Interim COVID-19 Treatment in
            Outpatients 253
Chapter 21—COVID-19 Treatment in Hospital............................257
            Section 21.1—Medical Management
                          of COVID-19 259
            Section 21.2—Critical Care
                          Management of
                          COVID-19..................... 263
Chapter 22—Care of Post-COVID Conditions.............................271
Chapter 23—Managing Health-Care Operations during
            COVID-19 277
            Section 23.1—Case Investigation
                          and Contact Tracing.... 279
            Section 23.2—Surveillance and
                          Data Analytics.............. 283
            Section 23.3—Optimizing Personal
                          Protective
                          Equipment Supplies 286
            Section 23.4—Community
                          Mitigation..................... 291
            Section 23.5—CDC Strategy for Global
                          Response to
                          COVID-19
                          (2020–2023) 301
Chapter 24—Beware of Fraudulent Coronavirus
            Tests, Vaccines, and Treatments...................................313
Chapter 25—COVID-19 and Alternative Treatments....................317
Chapter 26—Spiritual and Psychosocial Support for
            People with COVID-19 at Home................................319
Chapter 27—Palliative Care and COVID-19..................................323
Chapter 28—Coronavirus and Your Health Coverage...................325
Chapter 29—Ongoing Research on COVID-19.............................329
            Section 29.1—Chronic Viral
                          Infection and Long
                          COVID......................... 331

　　　　　Section 29.2—How Breathing
　　　　　　　　　　　Activates the Lungs'
　　　　　　　　　　　Defenses against
　　　　　　　　　　　Coronavirus 332
　　　　　Section 29.3—Role of Technology
　　　　　　　　　　　during the
　　　　　　　　　　　Pandemic 334

Part 4 | Coronavirus Vaccines and Immunizations
Chapter 30—Getting Your COVID-19 Vaccine 347
　　　　　Section 30.1—How Do You Find a
　　　　　　　　　　　COVID-19 Vaccine
　　　　　　　　　　　or Booster? 349
　　　　　Section 30.2—Types of COVID-19
　　　　　　　　　　　Vaccines 350
　　　　　Section 30.3—Stay Up-to-Date
　　　　　　　　　　　with COVID-19
　　　　　　　　　　　Vaccines
　　　　　　　　　　　Including Boosters 359
　　　　　Section 30.4—COVID-19 Vaccines
　　　　　　　　　　　for Specific Groups
　　　　　　　　　　　of People 368
Chapter 31—Effectiveness and Benefits of Getting a
　　　　　　COVID-19 Vaccine 381
Chapter 32—Side Effects and COVID-19 Vaccine Safety 387
　　　　　Section 32.1—Possible Side Effects
　　　　　　　　　　　after Getting a
　　　　　　　　　　　COVID-19 Vaccine 389
　　　　　Section 32.2—COVID-19 Vaccine
　　　　　　　　　　　Safety and
　　　　　　　　　　　Monitoring 392
　　　　　Section 32.3—Vaccine Adverse
　　　　　　　　　　　Event Reporting
　　　　　　　　　　　System 394

　　　　　　Section 32.4—COVID-19 Vaccine
　　　　　　　　　　　Safety in Specific
　　　　　　　　　　　Population 399
Chapter 33—Myths and Facts about the COVID-19
　　　　　　Vaccines..403
Chapter 34—Herd Immunity against COVID-19 409

Part 5 | Long-Term Effects of COVID-19 Infection
Chapter 35—Post-COVID Health Conditions................................417
Chapter 36—Assessment and Testing for
　　　　　　Post-COVID Conditions 423
Chapter 37—Patient Tips: Health-Care Provider
　　　　　　Appointments for
　　　　　　Post-COVID Conditions 429
Chapter 38—Supporting People with Post-COVID
　　　　　　Conditions 435
Chapter 39—Supporting Employees with Long COVID...............439
Chapter 40—Long COVID as a Disability.......................................447

Part 6 | COVID-19 Pandemic and Its Social Impact
Chapter 41—Pandemics in History 455
　　　　　　Section 41.1—Endemics, Epidemics,
　　　　　　　　　　　and Pandemics:
　　　　　　　　　　　An Overview................ 457
　　　　　　Section 41.2—Pandemics of the
　　　　　　　　　　　Past 461
Chapter 42—COVID-19 Impact on the Global Economy.............483
　　　　　　Section 42.1—Pandemic Impact on
　　　　　　　　　　　Mortality and Economy
　　　　　　　　　　　Varies across Age
　　　　　　　　　　　Groups and
　　　　　　　　　　　Geographies 485
　　　　　　Section 42.2—The U.S. Economy
　　　　　　　　　　　and the Global
　　　　　　　　　　　Pandemic....................... 490

Section 42.3—Pandemic Effect on the Global Economy across Various Sectors............................ 506
Section 42.4—COVID-19 Economic Relief 519
Chapter 43—COVID-19 Impact on Well-Being............................545
Section 43.1—The Pandemic's Effects on Mental Health 547
Section 43.2—Unintended Consequences Caused by the Pandemic....................... 551
Section 43.3—Social Impact................ 556
Chapter 44—COVID-19 Impact on Education 561
Section 44.1—Education during the COVID-19 Pandemic....................... 563
Section 44.2—Distance Education during the COVID-19 Pandemic....................... 570
Chapter 45—COVID-19 Impact on Health-Care Facilities...577
Chapter 46—Impact of COVID-19 on Travel and Tourism 597
Chapter 47—Impact of the Pandemic on Population Estimates of Major Cities 601
Chapter 48—The COVID-19 Pandemic and Employment 605
Chapter 49—How to Approach a Possible Outbreak in the Future 617
Chapter 50—COVID-19: Moving from Pandemic to Endemic 623

Part 7 | Additional Help and Information
Chapter 51—Glossary of Terms Related to COVID-19
 and Other Communicable Diseases..........................631
Chapter 52—Directory of Organizations That Provide
 Information about COVID-19 and Other
 Communicable Diseases...635

Index..**643**

Preface

ABOUT THIS BOOK

Coronavirus disease 2019 (COVID-19) was caused by severe acute respiratory syndrome coronavirus 2 (SARS-CoV-2). In December 2019, this contagious virus was first identified in Wuhan, China, and rapidly spread around the world. The symptoms of coronavirus include respiratory problems similar to cold, flu, or pneumonia. The virus attacks the lungs and the respiratory system and then in most cases affects the other parts of the body. COVID-19 in people started with mild symptoms leading to severe illness—mostly for people with underlying medical conditions. Some with zero to minor symptoms suffered from post-COVID or long COVID conditions. The United States reported about a million deaths due to COVID-19 infection. According to the World Health Organization (WHO), in December 2020, just a year after the first case of COVID-19 was detected, the first COVID-19 vaccine doses were administered, which allowed the immune system to fight the virus.

COVID-19 and the Coronavirus Sourcebook, First Edition offers basic information on the coronavirus and COVID-19 infection. It provides facts about its origin, how it spreads, earlier outbreaks, variants, symptoms, risk factors, clinical presentation in specific populations and pets and animals, and the statistics of its cases and deaths. It explains the protective and control measures such as social distancing, self-isolation, face masks, and disinfecting. The guidance for COVID-19 measures in schools, workplace, and other places are discussed. Detailed information is provided on the investigation, clinical care and treatment, vaccines, management, and ongoing research. Furthermore, this book illustrates long COVID infection, mental health issues, and the impact on the global economy and social and lifestyle issues. It concludes with a glossary of terms related to COVID-19 and other infectious diseases and a list of resources for additional help and information about COVID-19 and other communicable diseases.

HOW TO USE THIS BOOK

This book is divided into parts and chapters. Parts focus on broad areas of interest. Chapters are devoted to single topics within a part.

Part 1: What You Need to Know about COVID-19 talks about the basics of coronavirus, its epidemiology, its origin, and how the infection spread. It describes earlier outbreaks such as severe acute respiratory syndrome (SARS) and Middle East respiratory syndrome (MERS). It details the variants of the coronavirus, its symptoms, risk factors, testing process, and clinical presentations. The part concludes with statistics on COVID-19 cases and deaths.

Part 2: Prevention and Control Measures of COVID-19 provides basic information about various preventive measures such as face masks and personal hygiene, cleaning and disinfecting at home, and self-isolation. This part also provides guidance for prevention and control in schools and workplaces.

Part 3: Clinical Care and Treatment Information for COVID-19 offers detailed information about the types of treatments and management processes. Individual chapters and sections explain how the research and operations took place and how the health-care industry managed the situation. It also describes the diagnostic tests and treatment techniques utilized.

Part 4: Coronavirus Vaccines and Immunizations explains the types of vaccines and their side effects. Individual chapters and sections discuss the role of vaccine safety, its benefits, its myths and facts, and herd immunity against COVID-19.

Part 5: Long-Term Effects of COVID-19 Infection describes the post-COVID-19 health condition and how it is managed. It also talks about the mental health of people with long COVID-19. It includes tips for patients and supporting people and employees with COVID-19. The part concludes with a discussion on long COVID-19 as a disability.

Part 6: COVID-19 Pandemic and Its Social Impact addresses the pandemic of the past and discusses COVID-19 impact on the U.S. economy, education, health care, and travel and tourism industries. Furthermore, it also explains the changes major cities experienced and the employment situation due to the pandemic. The part concludes with the details of how to approach a possible outbreak in the future and the transition from pandemic to endemic.

Part 7: Additional Help and Information includes a glossary of terms related to COVID-19 and a directory of agencies offering additional help and support about COVID-19 and other communicable diseases.

BIBLIOGRAPHIC NOTE

This volume contains documents and excerpts from publications issued by the following U.S. government agencies: Centers for Disease Control and Prevention (CDC); Centers for Medicare & Medicaid Services (CMS); Consumer Financial Protection Bureau (CFPB); COVID.gov; Centers for Medicare & Medicaid Services (CMS); MedlinePlus; National Center for Complementary and Integrative Health (NCCIH); National Institutes of Health (NIH); National Institute of Neurological Disorders and Stroke (NINDS); Occupational Safety and Health Administration (OSHA); Office of Inspector General (OIG); Ready.gov; U.S. Bureau of Labor Statistics (BLS); U.S. Department of Education (ED); U.S. Department of Health and Human Services (HHS); U.S. Department of Homeland Security (DHS); U.S. Department of the Treasury; U.S. Food and Drug Administration (FDA); U.S. Government Accountability Office (GAO); U.S. Senate Committee on Health, Education, Labor, and Pensions; United States Census Bureau; and White House Office of National Drug Control Policy (ONDCP).

It also contains original material produced by Infobase and reviewed by medical consultants.

ABOUT THE *HEALTH REFERENCE SERIES*

The *Health Reference Series* is designed to provide basic medical information for patients, families, caregivers, and the general public. Each volume provides comprehensive coverage on a particular topic. This is especially important for people who may be dealing with a newly diagnosed disease or a chronic disorder in themselves or in a family member. People looking for preventive guidance, information about disease warning signs, medical statistics, and risk factors for health problems will also find answers to their questions in the *Health Reference Series*. The *Series*, however, is not intended to serve as a tool for diagnosing illness, in prescribing treatments, or as a substitute for the physician–patient relationship. All people concerned about medical symptoms or the possibility of disease are encouraged to seek professional care from an appropriate health-care provider.

A NOTE ABOUT SPELLING AND STYLE

Health Reference Series editors use *Stedman's Medical Dictionary* as an authority for questions related to the spelling of medical terms and *The*

Chicago Manual of Style for questions related to grammatical structures, punctuation, and other editorial concerns. Consistent adherence is not always possible, however, because the individual volumes within the *Series* include many documents from a wide variety of different producers, and the editor's primary goal is to present material from each source as accurately as is possible. This sometimes means that information in different chapters or sections may follow other guidelines and alternate spelling authorities. For example, occasionally a copyright holder may require that eponymous terms be shown in possessive forms (Crohn's disease vs. Crohn disease) or that British spelling norms be retained (leukaemia vs. leukemia).

MEDICAL REVIEW

Infobase contracts with a team of qualified, senior medical professionals who serve as medical consultants for the *Health Reference Series*. As necessary, medical consultants review reprinted and originally written material for currency and accuracy. Citations including the phrase "Reviewed (month, year)" indicate material reviewed by this team. Medical consultation services are provided to the *Health Reference Series* editors by:

Dr. Vijayalakshmi, MBBS, DGO, MD
Dr. Senthil Selvan, MBBS, DCH, MD
Dr. K. Sivanandham, MBBS, DCH, MS (Research), PhD

HEALTH REFERENCE SERIES UPDATE POLICY

The inaugural book in the *Health Reference Series* was the first edition of *Cancer Sourcebook* published in 1989. Since then, the *Series* has been enthusiastically received by librarians and in the medical community. In order to maintain the standard of providing high-quality health information for the layperson, the editorial staff felt it was necessary to implement a policy of updating volumes when warranted.

Medical researchers have been making tremendous strides, and it is the purpose of the *Health Reference Series* to stay current with the most recent advances. Each decision to update a volume is made on an individual basis. Some of the considerations include how much new information is available and the feedback we receive from people who use the books. If there is a topic you would like to see added to the update list, or an area of medical concern you feel has not been adequately addressed, please write to: custserv@infobaselearning.com.

Part 1 | What You Need to Know about COVID-19

Chapter 1 | Basics of COVID-19

Chapter Contents
Section 1.1—What Is a Coronavirus?... 5
Section 1.2—Origins of COVID-19... 8
Section 1.3—Epidemiology and the Spread of
              COVID-19 Infection.. 12
Section 1.4—Earlier Outbreaks Caused by the
              Coronavirus 17
Section 1.5—Spread of COVID-19 across the World.................. 22

Section 1.1 | What Is a Coronavirus?

Severe acute respiratory syndrome coronavirus 2 (SARS-CoV-2) is a member of the coronavirus family and is the causative agent of coronavirus disease 2019 (COVID-19). Members of the coronavirus family cause a variety of diseases, from head or chest colds to more severe and rare diseases such as severe acute respiratory syndrome (SARS) and Middle East respiratory syndrome (MERS). Like other respiratory viruses, coronaviruses spread quickly through droplets expelled when an individual breathes, coughs, sneezes, or speaks. As SARS-CoV-2 continues to spread through populations, genetic changes can accumulate over time and form distinct evolutionary lineages or variants with differing mutation rates, transmissibility, vaccine efficacy, or pathogenicity.

KEY FINDINGS
- SARS-CoV-2 is transmitted easily between humans, primarily through close contact (either direct or within six feet) and aerosol transmission.
- Individuals are infectious 1–3 days prior to symptom onset. Presymptomatic or asymptomatic patients can transmit SARS-CoV-2. Most transmission occurs prior to and within five days of symptom onset.
- Four vaccines are approved for use in the United States to prevent COVID-19 (Moderna, Pfizer/BioNTech, Johnson & Johnson, and Novavax). Each of these vaccines provides different levels of protection.
- SARS-CoV-2 can survive on surfaces from hours to days and is stable in air for at least several hours, depending on the presence of ultraviolet (UV) light, temperature, and humidity. Transmission via contaminated surfaces is not considered to be common.
- Face masks (medical and nonmedical) are effective at reducing infections from SARS-CoV-2.

TRANSMISSIBILITY
SARS-CoV-2 is transmitted easily between humans, primarily through close contact (either direct or within six feet) and aerosol transmission. COVID-19 vaccines reduce transmission rates by approximately 54 percent (range of 38–66%). There is a substantial variation of transmission among individuals. Individuals are contagious 1–3 days prior to symptom onset. Presymptomatic or asymptomatic patients can transmit SARS-CoV-2. Most transmission occurs prior to and within five days of symptom onset.

INCUBATION PERIOD
On average, symptoms develop five days after exposure with a range of 2–14 days. Incubating individuals can transmit the disease for several days before symptom onset. Some individuals never develop symptoms but can still transmit the disease.

It is estimated that most individuals are no longer infectious beyond 10 days after symptom onset. Individuals can shed the virus for several weeks though it is not necessarily infectious.

In a small human study (n = 12 transmission pairs), the average time to symptom onset in two successive cases (i.e., the serial interval) of the Omicron variant was 2.9 days, which is faster than wild-type SARS-CoV-2.

ACUTE CLINICAL PRESENTATION
Most symptomatic COVID-19 cases are mild (81%). Fever, cough, and shortness of breath are generally the most common symptoms, followed by malaise and fatigue. Chills, muscle pain, joint pain, sore throat, gastrointestinal symptoms, neurological symptoms, and dermatological symptoms also occur.
- COVID-19 is more severe than seasonal influenza.
- Adults >60 years old and those with comorbidities are at elevated risk of hospitalization and death.
- Children are susceptible to SARS-CoV-2 though generally show milder or no symptoms.

- Minority populations are disproportionately affected by COVID-19.
- Omicron subvariants can evade antibodies produced either postvaccination or postinfection.

CHRONIC CLINICAL PRESENTATION

COVID-19 symptoms commonly persist for weeks to months after initial onset in up to 73 percent of those infected. Long-term symptoms such as fatigue, smell/taste disorders, and neurological impairment may affect the ability to return to work.

In a cohort of COVID-19 patients, 39 percent reported symptoms 7–9 months after initial infection, with fatigue, loss of taste or smell, shortness of breath, and headache as the most common chronic symptoms.

One year after intensive care unit (ICU) admission for COVID-19, lingering physical (74% of 246 ICU patients), mental (26%), and cognitive (16%) symptoms were common, with 58 percent of patients experiencing issues with returning fully to work.

CLINICAL DIAGNOSIS

Diagnosis of COVID-19 is based on symptoms consistent with COVID-19, testing based on polymerase chain reaction (PCR), and/or the presence of SARS-CoV-2 antigen in individuals (detected by enzyme-linked immunosorbent assay (ELISA)). Screening solely by temperature or other symptoms is unreliable.

The timing of diagnostic PCR tests impacts results. The false-negative rate for real-time reverse transcriptase (RT) PCR tests is lowest between seven and nine days after exposure, and PCR tests are likely to give false-negative results before symptoms begin (within four days of exposure) and more than 14 days after exposure.

Asymptomatic individuals without COVID-19 symptoms can be diagnosed with SARS-CoV-2 infection by the same tests. In children, viral loads from saliva correlated better with clinical outcomes than viral loads from nasopharyngeal swabs. This may also be true for adults, as saliva tests consistently yield fewer false-negative results.[1]

Section 1.2 | Origins of COVID-19

Over one million Americans have died from COVID-19, and tens of millions have died of this virus worldwide. In addition to the tragic loss of life, over the past three years, the world has experienced the social, educational, and economic costs of a global pandemic.

Three years after its emergence in Wuhan, exactly how severe acute respiratory syndrome coronavirus 2 (SARS-CoV-2) first emerged as a respiratory pathogen capable of sustained human-to-human transmission remains the subject of active debate. Experts have put forward two dominant theories on the origins of the virus. The first theory is that SARS-CoV-2 is the result of a natural zoonotic spillover. The second theory is that the virus infected humans as a consequence of a research-related incident.

Understanding the virus's origin is essential to understanding how this outbreak happened, to understanding why detection and reporting systems did not work as anticipated, and to better preparing for future health threats.

ANALYSIS OF NATURAL ZOONOTIC ORIGINS HYPOTHESIS

Zoonotic spillovers, in which animal diseases cross the species barrier and infect humans, are well-known, well-documented natural phenomena. By some estimations, natural zoonotic spillovers are responsible for 60–75 percent of emerging diseases in humans. Coronaviruses, to which SARS-CoV-2 belongs, are a large family of viruses that cause disease in a variety of domestic and farmed

---

[1] "Master Question List for COVID-19 (Caused by SARS-CoV-2)," U.S. Department of Homeland Security (DHS), October 22, 2022. Available online. URL: www.dhs.gov/sites/default/files/2022-11/22_1022_st_mql_sars_cov-2.pdf. Accessed December 8, 2022.

Basics of COVID-19

animals and have been responsible for previous outbreaks of new diseases in humans. All coronaviruses known to infect humans are the result of natural zoonotic spillover from animals into humans. Two prominent examples include severe acute respiratory syndrome (SARS) and Middle East respiratory syndrome (MERS), both of which are caused by a coronavirus (SARS-CoV and MERS-CoV, respectively) leading to severe respiratory disease in humans. Moreover, recent infectious disease pandemics, with the exception of the 1977 Russian flu pandemic, are believed to have natural zoonotic origins (refer to Figure 1.1).

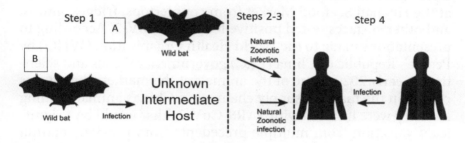

Figure 1.1. Example of a Zoonotic Spillover from Bats
U.S. Senate Committee on Health, Education, Labor, and Pensions
A: Direct spillover from a bat to humans followed by human-to-human transmission. B: Spillover from a bat to an unknown intermediate host and then to humans, followed by human-to-human transmission.

Natural zoonotic spillovers are a sequential process. In this process, an animal virus must evolve in order to become a human-adapted virus. First, a virus infects animals. Second, those infected animals come into contact with humans (known as the "human-animal interface"). Third, the virus is able to infect humans. Fourth, the virus is able to adapt to efficiently transmit between humans. Thus, a spillover event, in which disease is spread from animals to humans, can result in one of two outcomes—either the pathogen, once transmitted from animals, is then transmitted from humans to humans or the pathogen does not spread, resulting in a "dead-end" spillover. In many respects, once human-to-human transmission of SARS-CoV-2 was established, the onward human-to-human transmission of the virus would look similar regardless of whether it originated from a natural zoonotic spillover or a research-related incident. The natural zoonotic spillover hypothesis is a plausible explanation for how the COVID-19 pandemic started. There are a number of anomalies in the SARS-CoV-2 outbreak and the early COVID-19 pandemic compared to the emergence of past natural zoonotic spillovers, most notably the 2002–2004 SARS epidemic.

MISSING EVIDENCE OF A NATURAL ZOONOTIC SPILLOVER

Environmental samples collected between January and March 2020 at the Huanan Seafood Market from countertops, fridges, gloves, and other surfaces tested positive for SARS-CoV-2. According to presentations made to the World Health Organization (WHO) by People's Republic of China (PRC) government officials and scientists in early 2020, none of the animals at the market when it was closed, in the market's supply chain, or in China's animal farming industry were infected with SARS-CoV-2. That would be a significant variation from multiple precedents from previous natural zoonotic spillovers. For example, the discovery of infected palm civets during the SARS epidemic, as well as infected chickens and other farmed birds during multiple outbreaks of avian influenza, indicates a pattern where infected animals are expected to be present at the location of zoonotic spillovers and in the related supply chains.

ANALYSIS OF RESEARCH-RELATED INCIDENT HYPOTHESIS

Research-related incidents at labs in China, the United States, and elsewhere have happened and, in some instances, resulted in limited human-to-human transmission. For example, there have been at least six research-related incidents involving the escape of SARS-CoV from high-containment laboratories in China, Taiwan, and Singapore. The 1977 hemagglutinin type 1 and neuraminidase type 1–Influenza A (H1N1) pandemic is now widely accepted to have been the result of a research-related incident, most likely a vaccine trial in the Soviet Union or China. In June 2014, while investigating the unintentional exposure of one of its researchers to potentially viable anthrax during an experiment in one of its biosafety level 3 (BSL-3) laboratories, the U.S. Centers for Disease Control and Prevention (CDC) discovered that a culture of nonpathogenic avian influenza was unintentionally cross-contaminated with the highly pathogenic avian influenza A (H5N1) strain of influenza and shipped to a BSL3 U.S. Department of Agriculture (USDA) laboratory.

Nearly three years after the COVID-19 pandemic began, substantial evidence demonstrates that the COVID-19 pandemic was the result of a research-related incident. A research-related incident is consistent with the early epidemiology showing rapid spread of the virus in Wuhan, with the earliest calls for assistance being located near the original campus of the Wuhan Institute of Virology (WIV) in central Wuhan. It also explains the low genetic diversity of the earliest known SARS-CoV-2 human infections in Wuhan because the likely index case, which would be an infected researcher, is the likely primary source of the virus in Wuhan. A research-related incident also explains the failure to find an intermediate host as well as the failure to find any animal infections predating human COVID-19 cases. Although the WIV's coronavirus research is best documented because of its collaborations with western scientists, multiple institutions in Wuhan study coronaviruses including Wuhan University, Huazhong Agricultural University, Hubei Centers for Disease Control and Prevention, Hubei Animal Centers for Disease Control and Prevention, Wuhan Centers for Disease Control and Prevention, and the Wuhan Institute of Biological Products, a vaccine manufacturing subsidiary of state-owned Sinopharm.

As noted by the WHO Scientific Advisory Group for the Origins of Novel Pathogens, the COVID-19 Lancet Commission, and the U.S. Office of the Director of National Intelligence 90-Day Assessment on COVID-19 Origins, more information is needed to arrive at a more precise, if not a definitive, understanding of the origins of SARS-CoV-2 and how the COVID-19 pandemic began. Governments, leaders, public health officials, and scientists involved in addressing the COVID-19 pandemic and working to prevent future pandemics must commit to greater transparency, engagement, and responsibility in their efforts.

Based on the analysis of the publicly available information, it appears reasonable to conclude that the COVID-19 pandemic was, more likely than not, the result of a research-related incident. New information, made publicly available and independently verifiable, could change this assessment. However, the hypothesis of a natural zoonotic origin no longer deserves the benefit of the doubt or the presumption of accuracy.[2]

Section 1.3 | Epidemiology and the Spread of COVID-19 Infection

HOW DO INFECTIONS SPREAD?

Germs are a part of everyday life and are found in the air, soil, and water and in and on bodies. Some germs are helpful; others are harmful. Many germs live in and on bodies without causing harm, and some even help us stay healthy. Only a small portion of germs are known to cause infection.

HOW DO INFECTIONS OCCUR?

An infection occurs when germs enter the body, increase in number, and cause a reaction in the body.

The following are the three things that are necessary for an infection to occur:

- **Source**. Places where infectious agents (germs) live (e.g., sinks, surfaces, human skin).
- **Transmission**. A way germs are moved to the susceptible person.
- **Susceptible person**. One with increased vulnerability to germs entering the body.

---

[2] "An Analysis of the Origins of the COVID-19 Pandemic," U.S. Senate Committee on Health, Education, Labor, and Pensions, October 26, 2022. Available online. URL: www.help.senate.gov/imo/media/doc/report_an_analysis_of_the_origins_of_covid-19_102722.pdf. Accessed December 8, 2022.

Basics of COVID-19

Source

A source is an infectious agent or germ and refers to a virus, bacteria, or another microbe.

In health-care settings, germs are found in many places. People are one source of germs, including the following:
- patients
- health-care workers
- visitors and household members

People can be sick with symptoms of an infection or colonized with germs (not have symptoms of an infection but able to pass the germs to others).

Germs are also found in the health-care environment. Examples of environmental sources of germs include the following:
- dry surfaces in patient care areas (e.g., bed rails, medical equipment, countertops, and tables)
- wet surfaces, moist environments, and biofilms (e.g., cooling towers, faucets, sinks, and equipment such as ventilators)
- indwelling medical devices (e.g., catheters and intravenous (IV) lines)
- dust or decaying debris (e.g., construction dust or wet materials from water leaks)

Susceptible Person

A susceptible person is someone who is not vaccinated or otherwise immune, or a person with a weakened immune system. For an infection to occur, germs must enter a susceptible person's body and invade tissues, multiply, and cause a reaction.

Devices such as IV catheters and surgical incisions can provide an entryway, but a healthy immune system helps fight infection.

When patients are sick and receive medical treatment in health-care facilities, the following factors can increase their susceptibility to infection:
- Patients who have underlying medical conditions such as diabetes, cancer, and organ transplantation are at an

increased risk for infection because often these illnesses decrease the immune system's ability to fight infection.
- Certain medications used to treat medical conditions, such as antibiotics, steroids, and certain cancer-fighting medications, increase the risk of some types of infections.
- Lifesaving medical treatments and procedures used in health care, such as urinary catheters, tubes, and surgery, increase the risk of infection by providing additional ways that germs can enter the body.

Recognizing the factors that increase patients' susceptibility to infection allows providers to recognize risks and perform basic infection prevention measures to prevent infection from occurring.

Transmission

Transmission refers to the way germs are moved to the susceptible person.

Germs do not move themselves. Germs depend on people, the environment, and/or medical equipment to move around in health-care settings.

There are a few general ways that germs travel in health-care settings—through contact (i.e., touching), sprays and splashes, inhalation, and sharps injuries (i.e., when someone is accidentally stuck with a used needle or sharp instrument).
- Contact moves germs by touch (e.g., methicillin-resistant *Staphylococcus aureus* (MRSA) or vancomycin-resistant enterococci (VRE)). For example, health-care providers' hands become contaminated by touching germs present on medical equipment or high-touch surfaces, and then they carry the germs on their hands and spread to a susceptible person when proper hand hygiene is not performed before touching the susceptible person.
- Sprays and splashes occur when an infected person coughs or sneezes, creating droplets that carry germs short distances (within approximately six feet). These

germs can land on a susceptible person's eyes, nose, or mouth and can cause infection (e.g., pertussis or meningitis).
- Close-range inhalation occurs when a droplet containing germs is small enough to breathe in but not durable over distance.
- Inhalation occurs when germs are aerosolized in tiny particles that survive on air currents over great distances and time and reach a susceptible person. Airborne transmission can occur when infected patients cough, talk, or sneeze germs into the air (e.g., tuberculosis (TB) or measles) or when germs are aerosolized by medical equipment or by dust from a construction zone (e.g., nontuberculous mycobacteria or aspergillus).
- Sharps injuries can lead to infections (e.g., human immunodeficiency virus (HIV), hepatitis B virus (HBV), hepatitis C virus (HCV)) when blood-borne pathogens enter a person through a skin puncture by a used needle or sharp instrument.[3]

When a new infectious disease is discovered, scientists called "epidemiologists" work with other scientists to find who has it, why they have it, and what the Centers for Disease Control and Prevention (CDC) can do about it. From the beginning of the COVID-19 outbreak, scientists at the CDC and around the world have been working on the following.

IDENTIFY THE SOURCE OF THE OUTBREAK

Epidemiologists went to the area in China where the disease first appeared and conducted surveys in the community and health facilities. They collected nose and throat specimens for lab analyses. These field investigations showed them who was infected, when they became sick, and where they had been just before they got sick—and ultimately led them to a possible source.

---

[3] "How Infections Spread," Centers for Disease Control and Prevention (CDC), January 7, 2016. Available online. URL: www.cdc.gov/infectioncontrol/spread/index.html#. Accessed December 8, 2022.

MONITOR AND TRACK THE DISEASE

The CDC keeps track of the number of COVID-19 cases and collects information on the disease from surveillance systems that report different kinds of data, such as new cases, hospitalizations, deaths, demographic information (such as age, race/ethnicity, or sex), symptoms, and treatments.

STUDY THE DISEASE

The CDC scientists use surveillance data, including information from antibody testing and other kinds of studies, to find out more about the disease, such as how long someone with COVID-19 is contagious, the risk factors for severe illness, and which medical treatments are most effective.

DEVELOP GUIDANCE FOR ACTIONS TO SLOW THE SPREAD OF THE DISEASE AND LESSEN ITS IMPACT

Using study findings, case counts, and surveillance, the CDC publishes resources to help people in different risk groups (such as health-care workers or older people) stay safe in different settings (such as grocery stores, home, or school). This guidance is constantly being updated as new information becomes available.[4]

---

[4] "About COVID-19 Epidemiology," Centers for Disease Control and Prevention (CDC), July 1, 2020. Available online. URL: www.cdc.gov/coronavirus/2019-ncov/science/about-epidemiology/index.html. Accessed December 8, 2022.

Basics of COVID-19

Section 1.4 | Earlier Outbreaks Caused by the Coronavirus

WHAT IS SEVERE ACUTE RESPIRATORY SYNDROME?

Severe acute respiratory syndrome (SARS) is a viral respiratory illness caused by a coronavirus, called "SARS-associated coronavirus (SARS-CoV)." SARS was first reported in Asia in February 2003. Over the next few months, the illness spread to more than two dozen countries in North America, South America, Europe, and Asia before the SARS global outbreak of 2003 was contained. This section gives basic information about the illness and what the Centers for Disease Control and Prevention (CDC) did to control SARS in the United States.

THE SEVERE ACUTE RESPIRATORY SYNDROME OUTBREAK OF 2003

According to the World Health Organization (WHO), a total of 8,098 people worldwide became sick with SARS during the 2003 outbreak. Of these, 774 died. In the United States, only eight people had laboratory evidence of SARS-CoV infection. All of these people had traveled to other parts of the world where SARS was spreading. SARS did not spread more widely in the community in the United States.

SYMPTOMS OF SEVERE ACUTE RESPIRATORY SYNDROME

In general, SARS begins with a high fever (temperature greater than 100.4°F (>38.0°C)). Other symptoms may include headache, an overall feeling of discomfort, and body aches. Some people also have mild respiratory symptoms at the outset. About 10–20 percent of patients have diarrhea. After 2–7 days, SARS patients may develop a dry cough. Most patients develop pneumonia.

WHAT DOES "CLOSE CONTACT" MEAN?

In the context of SARS, close contact means having cared for or lived with someone with SARS or having direct contact with respiratory secretions or body fluids of a patient with SARS. Examples of close contact include kissing or hugging, sharing eating or drinking utensils, talking to someone within three feet, and touching someone directly. Close contact does not include activities such as walking by a person or briefly sitting across a waiting room or office.

THE CDC'S RESPONSE TO SARS DURING THE 2003 OUTBREAK

The CDC worked closely with the WHO and other partners in a global effort to address the SARS outbreak of 2003. For its part, the CDC took the following actions:
- It activated its Emergency Operations Center to provide round-the-clock coordination and response.
- It committed more than 800 medical experts and support staff to work on the SARS response.
- It deployed medical officers, epidemiologists, and other specialists to assist with on-site investigations around the world.
- It provided assistance to state and local health departments in investigating possible cases of SARS in the United States.
- It conducted extensive laboratory testing of clinical specimens from SARS patients to identify the cause of the disease.
- It initiated a system for distributing health alert notices to travelers who may have been exposed to cases of SARS.[5]

WHAT IS MIDDLE EAST RESPIRATORY SYNDROME?

Middle East respiratory syndrome (MERS) is an illness caused by a virus (more specifically, a coronavirus) called "Middle East respiratory syndrome coronavirus (MERS-CoV)." Most MERS patients developed severe respiratory illness with symptoms of fever, cough, and shortness of breath. About three or four out of every 10 patients reported with MERS have died.

---

[5] "SARS Basics Fact Sheet," Centers for Disease Control and Prevention (CDC), December 6, 2017. Available online. URL: www.cdc.gov/sars/about/fs-sars.html. Accessed December 9, 2022.

ALL CASES ARE LINKED TO THE ARABIAN PENINSULA

Health officials first reported the disease in Saudi Arabia in September 2012. Through retrospective (backward-looking) investigations, they later identified that the first known cases of MERS occurred in Jordan in April 2012. So far, all cases of MERS have been linked through travel to, or residence in, countries in and near the Arabian Peninsula. The largest known outbreak of MERS outside the Arabian Peninsula occurred in the Republic of Korea in 2015. The outbreak was associated with a traveler returning from the Arabian Peninsula.

PEOPLE WITH MIDDLE EAST RESPIRATORY SYNDROME CAN SPREAD IT TO OTHERS

MERS-CoV has spread from ill people to others through close contact, such as caring for or living with an infected person.

MERS can affect anyone. MERS patients have ranged in age from younger than one year old to 99 years old.

The CDC continues to closely monitor the MERS situation globally. The CDC is working with partners to better understand the risks of this virus, including the source, how it spreads, and how to prevent infections. The CDC recognizes the potential for MERS-CoV to spread further and cause more cases globally and in the United States. The CDC has provided information for travelers and is working with health departments, hospitals, and other partners to prepare for this.

Symptoms and Complications

Most people confirmed to have MERS-CoV infection have had severe respiratory illness with symptoms of the following:
- fever
- cough
- shortness of breath

Some people also had diarrhea and nausea/vomiting. For many people with MERS, more severe complications followed, such as pneumonia and kidney failure. About three or four out of every

10 people reported with MERS have died. Most of the people who died had a preexisting medical condition that weakened their immune system or an underlying medical condition that had not yet been discovered. Medical conditions sometimes weaken people's immune systems and make them likely to get sick or have severe illness.

Preexisting conditions among people who got MERS are as follows:
- diabetes
- cancer
- chronic lung disease
- chronic heart disease
- chronic kidney disease

Some infected people had mild symptoms (such as cold-like symptoms) or no symptoms at all.

The symptoms of MERS start to appear about five or six days after a person is exposed but can range from 2 to 14 days.

Transmission

MERS-CoV, like other coronaviruses, likely spreads from an infected person's respiratory secretions, such as through coughing, but the exact way COVID-19 is spread is unknown.

MERS-CoV has spread from ill people to others through close contact, such as caring for or living with an infected person. Infected people have spread MERS-CoV to others in health-care settings, such as hospitals. Researchers studying MERS have not seen any ongoing spreading of MERS-CoV in the community.

All reported cases have been linked to countries in and near the Arabian Peninsula. Most infected people either lived in the Arabian Peninsula or recently traveled from the Arabian Peninsula before they became ill. A few people have gotten MERS after having close contact with an infected person who had recently traveled from the Arabian Peninsula. The largest known outbreak of MERS outside the Arabian Peninsula occurred in the Republic of Korea in 2015 and was associated with a traveler returning from the Arabian Peninsula.

Basics of COVID-19

Public health agencies continue to investigate clusters of cases in several countries to better understand how MERS-CoV spreads from person to person.

Prevention

There is currently no vaccine to protect people against MERS. But scientists are working to develop one.

You can help reduce your risk of getting respiratory illnesses by doing the following:
- Wash your hands often with soap and water for at least 20 seconds and help young children do the same. If soap and water are not available, use an alcohol-based hand sanitizer.
- Cover your nose and mouth with a tissue when you cough or sneeze; then throw the tissue in the trash.
- Avoid touching your eyes, nose, and mouth with unwashed hands.
- Avoid personal contact, such as kissing or sharing cups or eating utensils, with sick people.
- Clean and disinfect frequently touched surfaces and objects, such as doorknobs.

Treatment

There is no specific antiviral treatment recommended for MERS-CoV infection. Individuals with MERS often receive medical care to help relieve symptoms. For severe cases, current treatment includes care to support vital organ functions.[6]

---

[6] "Middle East Respiratory Syndrome (MERS)," Centers for Disease Control and Prevention (CDC), August 2, 2019. Available online. URL: www.cdc.gov/coronavirus/mers/about/index.html. Accessed December 9, 2022.

Section 1.5 | Spread of COVID-19 across the World

The outbreak of the novel coronavirus, also known as "severe acute respiratory syndrome coronavirus 2" or "SARS-CoV-2," began in the city of Wuhan in China's Hubei province in December 2019. Rapidly spreading to other regions of China and other nations, the virus commonly known as "COVID-19" caused a worldwide health crisis and was announced as a global pandemic by the World Health Organization (WHO) in March 2020. The rapid spread of the virus resulted in widespread economic disruption, lockdowns, and other measures to contain the outbreak.

PER CAPITA CASE NUMBERS AND TIME LAGS

One way to analyze how the outbreak spread in different countries is to look at the per capita case numbers, which is the number of cases per 100,000 people in a population. In the United States, the per capita case numbers of COVID-19 have fluctuated significantly since the start of the pandemic in 2020. According to data from the Centers for Disease Control and Prevention (CDC), the per capita case numbers in the United States reached high values in January 2021, with approximately 516 weekly cases per 100,000 people, peaking at 1,696 in January 2022. As of January 2023, the per capita weekly case numbers have dropped significantly to approximately 91 cases per 100,000 people.

In order to understand the time lags that exist in different countries, we must first look at the time period between the first case and the outbreak of the virus among the populace. For example, in China, the time lag between the first case and the outbreak was about three months, which is longer than in many other countries, such as the United States (two months), Brazil (two months), and India (one month).

BEHAVIOR OF COVID-19 IN DIFFERENT COUNTRIES

Some countries, such as the United States, experienced exponential virus growth, where cases have risen sharply since the pandemic's beginning. This could be partly due to the country's large population, geographic size, and lack of early intervention measures. Other countries, such as South Korea and Taiwan, with smaller populations and geographic size, had controlled spread in cases. In Europe, countries such as Italy and Spain saw rapid growth in cases, while Germany and the United Kingdom had controlled growth. Countries that implemented strong early intervention measures and a comprehensive testing and contact-tracing system have been able to contain the spread of the virus more effectively.

LOCAL STAGE OF THE OUTBREAK

The local stage of the outbreak was a crucial factor in the spread of COVID-19. In the early stages, the virus was primarily confined to China and other nearby countries in Asia. However, as the outbreak progressed, it spread to other parts of the world, mainly Europe and North America.

The growth of the number of cases within a specific area or community characterizes the local stage of the COVID-19 outbreak. One factor is exponential growth, which means the number of cases will increase rapidly at first as individuals spread the contagion to multiple people who go on to contaminate multiple people and so on before the spread levels off as the number of available hosts decreases. This is often seen in the early stages of an outbreak, as the virus spreads rapidly through a population with little immunity.

Another factor is logistics, which recognize that the growth of cases will eventually slow down and stabilize as the number of available hosts decreases and control measures are implemented. This is often seen in the later stages of an outbreak. Statistics reported by Worldometer suggest that when the United States implemented renewed containment measures such as lockdowns and testing protocols, the growth rate dropped within a span of one month from 897,642 daily new confirmed cases on January 13, 2022, to 88,699 on February 14, 2022.

GROWTH BEHAVIORS CONCERNING COUNTRY SIZE AND DENSITY

Another way to analyze the outbreak in different countries is to look at the size (total population) and density (number of people per square mile) of each country. Countries such as India and China with larger populations (around 1.42 billion each) and higher population densities have been more susceptible to the spread of the virus, while smaller, less populated countries saw slower growth.

SHIFTING EPICENTERS OF THE PANDEMIC

The term "epicenter" is often used to describe the location where the number of COVID-19 cases is highest. At the beginning of the pandemic, the epicenter was Wuhan, China, where the virus was first identified. However, as the pandemic spread, the epicenter shifted to other countries and regions worldwide. In the first few months of the pandemic, the epicenter was in Asia, particularly China and South Korea. In the spring of 2020, the epicenter shifted to Europe, with Italy and Spain particularly hard-hit. Later in the year, the epicenter moved to the United States, where the number of cases and deaths was higher than in any other country and, at present, the epicenter of COVID-19 is said to be China. The pandemic's epicenter can change quickly. The overall number of cases and deaths can fluctuate daily, depending on factors such as testing, health-care infrastructure, and mitigation efforts.

HOW COVID-19 HAS AFFECTED DIFFERENT COUNTRIES

The COVID-19 pandemic has affected both urban and rural areas around the world and in different ways in different countries. Some of the places most impacted by COVID-19 with highest confirmed cases as of January 2023 include:

- **United States**. The United States is one of the countries most affected by COVID-19. The country has seen a high number of confirmed cases and more than 1,113,00 confirmed deaths according to the CDC as of February 24, 2023. The United States has had a higher rate of vaccination compared to other countries.
- **China**. The virus first emerged in Wuhan and quickly spread throughout the country. China implemented strict lockdown measures and travel restrictions to slow the virus's spread. Despite these efforts, China still has one of the highest COVID-19 confirmed cases of close to 98 million as of January 9, 2023*.

Basics of COVID-19

- **India**. India saw a massive surge in COVID-19 cases and more than 530,000 confirmed deaths as of January 9, 2023*, and hospitals have been overwhelmed with patients, mainly because of high population density. India initiated a comprehensive vaccination effort, resulting in a decrease in cases.
- **Brazil**. Brazil has also been hard hit by COVID-19. The country has seen a high number of confirmed cases and more than 695,236 confirmed deaths as of January 9, 2023* mainly due to insufficient containment and restriction measures to control the spread of the virus.
- **Italy**. Being one of the first European countries to experience a large outbreak of COVID-19, the country saw a high number of deaths—186,158—as of January 9, 2023* and was forced to implement strict lockdown measures. One reason for the uncontrolled outbreak is cited as the high number of travelers between China and Italy and the age of Italy's population, of whom nearly 23 percent are 65 years of age or older.

*Data were published by the WHO.

HOW THE OUTBREAK SPREAD COUNTRY BY COUNTRY

The pandemic spread country by country, with each country's response to the virus affecting the severity of the outbreak. The Chinese government initially tried to downplay the outbreak's severity but eventually implemented strict lockdown measures and widespread testing to control its spread.

As the virus continued to spread within China, it also began to spread to other countries. The first reported case outside of China was in Thailand in January 2020. The virus quickly spread to other countries in Asia, such as South Korea, Japan, and Singapore.

As the virus continued to spread globally, it reached Europe in early January 2020, with cases reported in France, Italy, and Germany. The virus spread rapidly throughout Europe, leading to widespread lockdowns and travel bans.

In January 2020, the virus reached the United States. The first case was reported in Washington state, which then quickly spread throughout the country, leading to a nationwide lockdown and widespread testing. The virus also spread throughout Latin America and the Caribbean, with Brazil and Mexico having the highest numbers of cases in the region.

GLOBAL CASES AND DEATH DETAILS

According to the WHO, there were over 750 million confirmed cases of COVID-19 and around 6.8 million deaths worldwide as of February 24, 2023. The United States, China, and India have the highest number of cases, and the United States, Brazil, and India have the highest number of deaths.

Some of the countries with the highest number of cases and deaths are listed in Table 1.1.

Various nations are initiating vaccination efforts and gradually rebounding from the pandemic. However, the pandemic continues to evolve, and the world will continue to grapple with its effects for the foreseeable future.

Table 1.1. Total COVID-19 Confirmed Cases and Deaths in Top 10 Countries as of February 24, 2023

Country	Cases	Deaths
United States	101,752,396	1,106,783
China	98,932,687	698,056
India	44,685,132	530,761
France	38,487,043	395,867
Germany	38,018,111	332,839
Brazil	36,989,373	219,344
Japan	33,097,952	206,246
South Korea	30,445,775	187,850
Italy	25,547,414	167,387
United Kingdom	24,341,615	161,083

Source: "WHO Coronavirus (COVID-19) Dashboard," World Health Organization (WHO).

References

"A Timeline of the Coronavirus Pandemic," The New York Times, December 28, 2020. Available online. URL: www.nytimes.com/article/coronavirus-timeline.html. Accessed February 3, 2023.

Achenbach, Joel; Cha, Ariana Eunjung and Sellers, Frances Stead. "A Viral Tsunami: How the Underestimated Coronavirus Took Over the World," The Washington Post, March 9, 2021. Available online. URL: www.washingtonpost.com/health/2021/03/09/coronavirus-spread-world. Accessed February 3, 2023.

Brahma, Dweepobotee; Chakraborty, Sikim and Menokee, Aradhika. "The Early Days of a Global Pandemic: A Timeline of COVID-19 Spread and Government Interventions," The Brookings Institution, April 2, 2020. Available online. URL: www.brookings.edu/2020/04/02/the-early-days-of-a-global-pandemic-a-timeline-of-covid-19-spread-and-government-interventions. Accessed February 3, 2023.

Burnett, Garrett W.; Katz, Daniel; Park, Chang H.; Hyman, Jaime B.; Dickstein, Elisha; Levin, Matthew A.; Sim, Alan; Salter, Benjamin; Owen, Robert M.; Leibowitz, Andrew B. and Hamburger, Joshua. "Managing COVID-19 from the Epicenter: Adaptations and Suggestions Based on Experience," National Library of Medicine (NLM), October 1, 2020. Available online. URL: www.ncbi.nlm.nih.gov/pmc/articles/PMC7529354. Accessed February 3, 2023.

"Coronavirus: First Brazil Death 'Earlier than Thought,'" The British Broadcasting Corporation (BBC), May 12, 2020. Available online. URL: www.bbc.com/news/world-latin-america-52638352. Accessed February 3, 2023.

"Coronavirus (COVID-19) Cases," Our World in Data, 2020. Available online. URL: https://ourworldindata.org/covid-cases#daily-confirmed-cases-per-million-people. Accessed February 3, 2023.

"Coronavirus Outbreak: The Countries Affected," PharmaceuticalTechnology, April 16, 2020. Available online. URL: www.pharmaceutical-technology.com/features/coronavirus-outbreak-the-countries-affected/. Accessed February 3, 2023.

"COVID-19: Did You Know about Italy's China Connection," Bennett, Coleman & Co. Ltd., March 19, 2020. Available online. URL: https://timesofindia.indiatimes.com/videos/international/covid-19-did-you-know-about-italys-china-connection/videoshow/74694266.cms. Accessed February 3, 2023.

"COVID-19 India Timeline: Looking Back at Pandemic-Induced Lockdown and How the Country Is Coping with the Crisis," The Indian Express [P] Ltd., March 23, 2021. Available online. URL: https://indianexpress.com/article/india/covid-19-india-timeline-looking-back-at-pandemic-induced-lockdown-7241583. Accessed February 3, 2023.

"COVID Live-Coronavirus Statistics," Worldometer, January 11, 2023. Available online. URL: www.worldometers.info/coronavirus. Accessed February 3, 2023.

Feuer, Will. "South America Is a 'New Epicenter' of the Coronavirus Pandemic, WHO Says," CNBC LLC, May 22, 2020. Available online. URL: www.cnbc.com/2020/05/22/south-america-is-a-new-epicenter-of-the-coronavirus-pandemic-who-says.html. Accessed February 3, 2023.

Hamidi, Shima; Sabouri, Sadegh and Ewing, Reid. "Does Density Aggravate the COVID-19 Pandemic?" Taylor & Francis Group, June 18, 2020. Available online. URL: www.tandfonline.com/doi/full/10.1080/01944363.2020.1777891. Accessed February 3, 2023.

"How COVID-19 Is Spreading across the World," The Straits Times, August 19, 2022. Available online. URL: www.straitstimes.com/multimedia/graphics/2020/02/coronavirus-global-numbers/index.html. Accessed February 3, 2023.

Komarova, Natalia L.; Schang, Luis M. and Wodarz, Dominik. "Patterns of the COVID-19 Pandemic Spread around the World: Exponential versus Power Laws," The Royal Society, September 30, 2020. Available online. URL: htttps://royalsocietypublishing.org/doi/10.1098/rsif.2020.0518#RSIF20200518F6. Accessed February 3, 2023.

"Listings of WHO's Response to COVID-19," World Health Organization (WHO), January 29, 2021. Available online. URL: www.who.int/news/item/29-06-2020-covidtimeline. Accessed February 3, 2023.

"Mapping the Coronavirus Outbreak across the World," Bloomberg L.P., January 3, 2022. Available online. URL: www.bloomberg.com/graphics/2020-coronavirus-cases-world-map. Accessed February 3, 2023.

Nadeau Sarah A.; Vaughan, Timothy G.; Scire, Jérémie and Stadler, Tanja. "The Origin and Early Spread of SARS-CoV-2 in Europe," National Academy of Science, February 10, 2021. Available online. URL: www.pnas.org/doi/10.1073/pnas.2012008118. Accessed February 3, 2023.

"Number of Coronavirus (COVID-19) Cases Worldwide as of January 9, 2023, by Country or Territory," Statista, January 9, 2023. Available online. URL: www.statista.com/statistics/1043366/novel-coronavirus-2019ncov-cases-worldwide-by-country. Accessed February 3, 2023.

Schnirring, Lisa. "WHO: Europe Now World's COVID-19 Epicenter," Center for Infectious Disease Research & Policy (CIDRAP), March 13, 2020. Available online. URL: www.cidrap.umn.edu/covid-19/who-europe-now-worlds-covid-19-epicenter. Accessed February 3, 2023.

Sharifi, Ayyoob and Khavarian-Garmsir, Amir. "The COVID-19 Pandemic: Impacts on Cities and Major Lessons for Urban Planning, Design, and Management," ScienceDirect, December 20, 2020. Available online. URL: www.sciencedirect.com/science/article/pii/S0048969720359209. Accessed February 3, 2023.

Sullivan, Kaitlin. "A Brief History of COVID, 1 Year In," Everyday Health, Inc., February 19, 2021. Available online. URL: www.everydayhealth.com/coronavirus/a-brief-history-of-covid-one-year-in/. Accessed February 3, 2023.

Tan, Huileng. "Coronavirus Epicenter Could 'Possibly' Shift Back to Asia, Says Public Health Expert," CNBC LLC, April 2, 2020. Available online. URL: www.cnbc.com/2020/04/02/coronavirus-epicenter-could-possibly-shift-back-to-asia-health-expert.html. Accessed February 3, 2023.

"The Territorial Impact of COVID-19: Managing the Crisis and Recovery across Levels of Government," Organisation for Economic Co-operation and Development (OECD), May 10, 2021. Available online. URL: www.oecd.org/coronavirus/policy-responses/the-territorial-impact-of-covid-19-managing-the-crisis-and-recovery-across-levels-of-government-a2c6abaf. Accessed February 3, 2023.

"Trends in Number of COVID-19 Cases and Deaths in the US Reported to CDC, by State/Territory," Centers for Disease Control and Prevention (CDC), January 27, 2023. Available online. URL: https://covid.cdc.gov/covid-data-tracker/#trends_totalcases_7daycasesper100k_00. Accessed February 3, 2023.

"United States COVID-Coronavirus Statistics," Worldometer, April 5, 2020. Available online. URL: www.worldometers.info/coronavirus/country/us. Accessed February 3, 2023.

Chapter 2 | **Variants of the Coronavirus**

Numerous variants of the virus that causes COVID-19 are being tracked in the United States and globally during this pandemic. The Centers for Disease Control and Prevention (CDC) is working with public health officials to monitor the spread of all variants and provide an estimate of how common they are in the nation and at the regional level. These data can change over time as more information is available.

VARIANTS ARE EXPECTED
Viruses constantly change through mutation, and sometimes, these mutations result in a new variant of the virus. Some variations allow the virus to spread more easily or make it resistant to treatments or vaccines. As the virus spreads, it may change and may become harder to stop.

Regardless of the Variant, a Surge in Cases Can Impact Health-Care Resources
Even if a variant causes less severe disease in general, an increase in the total number of cases could cause an increase in hospitalizations, put more strain on health-care resources, and potentially lead to more deaths.

MONITORING VARIANTS
The CDC uses viral genomic surveillance to quickly identify and track COVID-19 variants and acts upon these findings to best

protect the public's health. Some variants spread more easily and quickly than others, which may lead to more cases of COVID-19.

Scientists monitor all variants but may classify them as follows:
- **Variants being monitored.** No risk to public health; circulating at very low levels in the United States.
- **Variants of interest.** Potential impact on spread, severity, testing, treatment, and vaccinations; evidence it has caused an increased proportion of cases or unique outbreak clusters.
- **Variants of concern.** Evidence of impact on spread, severity, testing, treatment, and vaccination.
- **Variants of high consequence.** Clear evidence of significant impact on spread and severity and reduction of effectiveness of testing, treatment, and vaccination.

In the United States, the CDC uses viral genomic surveillance to track COVID-19 variants, to more quickly identify and act upon these findings to best protect the public's health. The CDC established multiple ways to connect and share viral genomic sequence data being produced by the CDC, public health laboratories, and commercial diagnostic laboratories within publicly accessible databases.[1]

WHAT IS THE DELTA VARIANT, AND WHY ARE SCIENTISTS CONCERNED?

- The Delta variant of the severe acute respiratory syndrome coronavirus 2 (SARS-CoV-2) emerged in India in September 2020, spread to 105 countries, and now accounts for more than 90 percent of new COVID-19 cases in the United States.
- The Delta variant is much more transmissible, may produce more severe illness, and is likely to cause reinfection than previous variants, particularly for the unvaccinated.

---

[1] "Variants of the Virus," Centers for Disease Control and Prevention (CDC), August 11, 2021. Available online. URL: www.cdc.gov/coronavirus/2019-ncov/variants/index.html. Accessed December 12, 2022.

Variants of the Coronavirus

- Full vaccination, mask use, and decontamination remain the major tools to combat COVID-19.

HOW DOES THE DELTA VARIANT COMPARE TO PREVIOUS SARS-COV-2 STRAINS AND VARIANTS?

- The Delta variant is a SARS-CoV-2 mutant strain with a unique set of genetic changes, including important mutations in the spike protein. One of these, L452R, has been linked to partial resistance to neutralizing antibodies and higher transmissibility.
- The Delta variant (and subvariants AY.1, AY.2, and AY.3) currently accounts for 95 percent of sequenced new cases in the United States.

HOW DOES DELTA VARIANT SPREAD FROM ONE HOST TO ANOTHER? HOW EASILY IS IT SPREAD?

- The Delta variant is highly transmissible. Its basic reproduction number (R0), defining the average number of new infections from a single infectious individual, is estimated between five and nine, compared to 2.2–3.1 for wild-type SARS-CoV-2.
- Household secondary attack rates of the Delta variant may be as high as 53 percent and may be higher in individuals younger than 10. Early evidence suggests that the Delta variant spreads rapidly in schools.
- The Delta variant produces higher virus levels for infected persons than the original SARS-CoV-2 and other variants. Also, the Delta variant virus levels in vaccinated breakthrough infections are similar to unvaccinated infections, which means that vaccinated people may spread infections as well as unvaccinated people.

ARE THERE EFFECTIVE VACCINES FOR DELTA VARIANT? HOW COMMON ARE BREAKTHROUGH INFECTIONS?

- Current vaccines in the United States are protective against the Delta variant when individuals are fully

vaccinated. The Pfizer/BioNTech vaccine provides 93–96 percent efficacy against hospitalization and 64–88 percent efficacy against symptomatic infection. Preliminary in vitro results show neutralization of the Delta variant by both the Moderna and J&J/Janssen (one-dose type) vaccines. Preliminary work suggests that vaccine efficacy in the United States was lower in July though additional research is needed.
- Partial vaccination, however, is ineffective. Receiving only one dose of a two-dose vaccine (Pfizer/BioNTech or Moderna) is only 10–30 percent effective against the Delta variant. Pfizer/BioNTech is researching Delta-specific booster vaccine doses.
- Breakthrough cases (i.e., infections after vaccination) involving the Delta variant are more common than with wild-type viruses or other variants (but are still rare overall), and vaccination drastically reduces the risk of severe disease or hospitalization.
- The Delta variant results in greater reinfection risk than wild-type SARS-CoV-2 or other SARS-CoV-2 variants (e.g., Alpha). Vaccination provides greater protection against infection with the Delta variant than prior infection with wild-type SARS-CoV-2 or other variants.

HOW LONG DOES THE IMMUNE RESPONSE PROVIDE PROTECTION FROM DELTA VARIANT REINFECTION?

- Vaccination provides greater protection from the Delta variant than prior infection with SARS-CoV-2. Convalescent plasma from those infected with Gamma or Beta variants showed reduced neutralization of the Delta variant, suggesting elevated potential for reinfection.
- Reinfection with the Delta variant was 46 percent more likely than with the Alpha variant, with the highest risk seen more than six months after the initial infection. However, reinfections in this study were rare overall (1.2%).

Variants of the Coronavirus

ARE THERE EFFECTIVE TREATMENTS FOR DELTA VARIANT?
- The Delta variant is resistant to the monoclonal antibody bamlanivimab.
- Proposed medical treatments for the SARS-CoV-2 Delta variant are the same as for other lineages and variants. The COVID-19 Master Question List (MQL) has additional details on recommended treatment guidelines.

HOW LONG DOES THE DELTA VARIANT TAKE UNTIL SYMPTOM ONSET? WHAT ARE THE INITIAL SYMPTOMS?
- There is some evidence that the Delta variant spreads faster than prior virus lineages (i.e., the time between successive cases of 2.9 versus 5.7 days, respectively) though additional studies are needed.
- Individuals infected with the Delta variant are hospitalized almost twice as often as those with the B.1.1.7 (Alpha) variant.
- The Delta variant may cause higher rates of headache and runny nose and lower rates of taste/smell dysfunction than wild-type SARS-CoV-2 and other variants.
- There is anecdotal evidence of more severe disease in younger, healthy individuals due to the Delta variant though it is unclear if the variant itself causes more severe illness or if other factors (e.g., lower vaccine prevalence) are responsible.

WHAT ELSE DO YOU NEED TO KNOW ABOUT THE DELTA VARIANT?
Other aspects of the Delta variant are either presumed or confirmed to agree with those of previously identified SARS-CoV-2 strains. Additional information can be found in the U.S. Department of Homeland Security (DHS) Science & Technology (S&T) MQL for COVID-19.[2]

---

[2] "DHS Science and Technology Supplemental Reference for SARS-CoV-2 Delta Variant," U.S. Department of Homeland Security (DHS), August 13, 2021. Available online. URL: www.dhs.gov/sites/default/files/publications/21_0816_st_delta_variant_sr_cleared_for_public_release.pdf. Accessed December 12, 2022.

WHAT IS THE OMICRON VARIANT, AND WHY ARE SCIENTISTS CONCERNED?

- The Omicron variant of the SARS-CoV-2 virus emerged in South Africa in November 2021 and has since spread to at least 27 countries and territories. On December 1, 2021, the United States confirmed its first COVID-19 case with the Omicron variant.
- Very early reports suggest that the Omicron variant is more transmissible than other variants (e.g., Delta).
- Given a high number of mutations in the viral spike protein, it is anticipated that Omicron will be resistant to existing antibodies and may lead to a higher rate of reinfection, but confirmation is needed.
- Currently, very little is known about its transmissibility, ability to evade the immune system, clinical severity, and susceptibility to vaccines and other medical therapeutics.

HOW DOES THE OMICRON VARIANT COMPARE TO PREVIOUS SARS-COV-2 STRAINS AND VARIANTS?

- Current SARS-CoV-2 polymerase chain reaction (PCR) diagnostic testing can successfully identify this variant. Several labs have reported a phenomenon termed S gene dropout. This test can thus be used to distinguish cases of Omicron from other variants. This S gene dropout is the result of a two-amino deletion at locations 69/70. These deletions are also seen in Alpha and Eta variants.
- Omicron has 30 amino acid changes, three small deletions, and one insertion in the spike protein.
- Mutations present in Omicron were previously studied in vitro and demonstrated 4–50 times greater binding affinity to ACE2 than wild-type SARS-CoV-2, which may confer increased transmissibility.
- Nucleocapsid (N) mutations in Omicron have been linked to increased ribonucleic acid (RNA) expression and increased viral loads.

Variants of the Coronavirus

HOW DOES OMICRON VARIANT SPREAD FROM ONE HOST TO ANOTHER? HOW EASILY IS IT SPREAD?

- Mutations in the spike protein furin cleavage site (H655Y, N679K, and P682H) may be linked to higher transmissibility.
- The rate of new cases in particular areas of South Africa has increased recently, consistent with a transmission advantage for the newly discovered Omicron variant. Early reports indicate that Omicron has become the dominant variant in the Gauteng province of South Africa in a short period of time, which is also consistent with elevated transmissibility compared to other circulating variants.
- As of November 25, 2021, the effective reproduction number (Re), defining the average number of new infections caused by a single infectious individual, was 1.47 for South Africa nationally, where the Delta variant is dominant, but 1.93 in the Gauteng province, which is dominated by the Omicron variant.
- The European Center for Disease Control recommends that existing nonpharmaceutical interventions, such as masks and social distancing, must be maintained or reintroduced, even in countries with high vaccination levels.

ARE THERE EFFECTIVE VACCINES FOR OMICRON VARIANT? HOW COMMON ARE BREAKTHROUGH INFECTIONS?

- The exact impact on efficacy is unknown, but the mutation profile of the spike protein, which is what the antibodies recognize, has been determined and suggests reduced antibody recognition. Tests are underway to determine vaccine effectiveness, with results expected in mid-December.
- Several sequence mutations observed in Omicron have been associated with increased transmissibility and immune escape. Scientists are concerned because a prior, synthetic variant with 20 mutations similar to Omicron

in the spike protein was almost entirely resistant to serum from previously infected and previously vaccinated individuals.
- Moderna is currently testing booster candidates against the Omicron variant, including two that were designed against Beta and Delta variants, which have some of the same mutations as Omicron. They are also designing a new booster candidate specifically against Omicron, which they anticipate will be ready in three months.

HOW LONG DOES THE IMMUNE RESPONSE PROVIDE PROTECTION FROM OMICRON VARIANT REINFECTION?

- The level of protection in previously infected individuals is unknown. However, preliminary evidence indicates Omicron may cause an increased risk of reinfection. Concern regarding the ability of the Omicron variant to escape immunity induced by the Pfizer, Moderna, and Johnson & Johnson vaccines remains high. Currently, available vaccines may offer some level of protection against hospitalization and death, potentially through memory T cells directed at nonsurface proteins.
- Convalescent patients likely will have some level of protection to neutralize the Omicron variant; however, a drop in protection is expected based on the combination of mutations.

ARE THERE EFFECTIVE TREATMENTS FOR OMICRON VARIANT?

- There are currently no data suggesting this variant is resistant to any current COVID-19 treatments. Experimental research is in progress to understand the capabilities.

HOW LONG DOES OMICRON VARIANT TAKE UNTIL SYMPTOM ONSET? WHAT ARE THE INITIAL SYMPTOMS?

- Preliminary information from South Africa reports that there are no unusual symptoms associated with Omicron and that some individuals are asymptomatic.

Variants of the Coronavirus

WHAT ELSE DO YOU NEED TO KNOW ABOUT THE OMICRON VARIANT?

- Other aspects of the Omicron variant are either presumed or confirmed to agree with those of previously identified SARS-CoV-2 strains. Additional information can be found in the DHS S&T MQL for COVID-19.
- Currently, there are key gaps in our understanding of Omicron's ability to infect previously infected and vaccinated individuals, its transmission rate in unvaccinated and vaccinated populations, and its clinical disease severity in patients of different ages and comorbidities.[3]

---

[3] "DHS Science and Technology Supplemental Reference for SARS-CoV-2 Omicron Variant," U.S. Department of Homeland Security (DHS), December 1, 2021. Available online. URL: www.dhs.gov/sites/default/files/2021-12/2021_12_01_st_sars_omicron_sr_cleared_for_public_release.pdf. Accessed December 12, 2022.

Chapter 3 | Symptoms of Coronavirus Infection

Chapter Contents
Section 3.1—Symptoms of COVID-19 43
Section 3.2—Symptoms of Long COVID Condition 44
Section 3.3—Similarities and Differences between
          Flu and COVID-19 50

Section 3.1 | **Symptoms of COVID-19**

People with COVID-19 have had a wide range of symptoms reported—ranging from mild symptoms to severe illness. Symptoms may appear 2–14 days after exposure to the virus. Anyone can have mild-to-severe symptoms.

Possible symptoms include the following:
- fever or chills
- cough
- shortness of breath or difficulty breathing
- fatigue
- muscle or body aches
- headache
- new loss of taste or smell
- sore throat
- congestion or runny nose
- nausea or vomiting
- diarrhea

This list does not include all possible symptoms. Symptoms may change with new COVID-19 variants and can vary depending on vaccination status. The Centers for Disease Control and Prevention (CDC) will continue to update this list as you learn more about COVID-19. Older adults and people who have underlying medical conditions such as heart or lung disease or diabetes are at a higher risk of getting very sick from COVID-19.

FEELING SICK?

If you are experiencing any of these symptoms, consider the following options:
- Get tested for COVID-19 (www.cdc.gov/coronavirus/2019-ncov/symptoms-testing/testing.html).
- If you have already tested positive for COVID-19, learn more about the CDC's isolation guidance (www.cdc.gov/coronavirus/2019-ncov/your-health/isolation.html).

When to Seek Emergency Medical Attention

Look for emergency warning signs* for COVID-19:
- trouble breathing
- persistent pain or pressure in the chest
- new confusion
- inability to wake or stay awake
- pale, gray, or blue-colored skin, lips, or nail beds, depending on skin tone

*This list is not all possible symptoms. Please call your medical provider for any other symptoms that are severe or concerning to you.

If someone is showing any of these signs, call 911 or call ahead to your local emergency facility. Notify the operator that you are seeking care for someone who has or may have COVID-19.[1]

Section 3.2 | Symptoms of Long COVID Condition

ABOUT LONG COVID OR POST-COVID CONDITIONS

Post-COVID conditions are a wide range of new, returning, or ongoing health problems that people experience after being infected with the virus that causes COVID-19. Most people with COVID-19 get better within a few days to a few weeks after infection, so at least four weeks after the infection is the start of when post-COVID conditions could first be identified. Anyone who was infected can experience post-COVID conditions. Most people with post-COVID conditions experienced symptoms days after first learning they had COVID-19, but some people who later experienced post-COVID conditions did not know when they got infected.

There is no test to diagnose post-COVID conditions, and people may have a wide variety of symptoms that could come from other health problems. This can make it difficult for health-care providers to recognize post-COVID conditions. Your health-care provider

---

[1] "Symptoms of COVID-19," Centers for Disease Control and Prevention (CDC), October 26, 2022. Available online. URL: www.cdc.gov/coronavirus/2019-ncov/symptoms-testing/symptoms.html. Accessed December 15, 2022.

Symptoms of Coronavirus Infection

considers a diagnosis of post-COVID conditions based on your health history, including if you had a diagnosis of COVID-19 either by a positive test or by symptoms or exposure, as well as doing a health examination.

SYMPTOMS FOR LONG COVID

People with post-COVID conditions can have a wide range of symptoms that can last more than four weeks or even months after infection. Sometimes, the symptoms can even go away or come back again.

Post-COVID conditions may not affect everyone the same way. People with post-COVID conditions may experience health problems from different types and combinations of symptoms happening over different lengths of time. Most patients' symptoms slowly improve with time. However, for some people, post-COVID conditions can last weeks, months, or longer after COVID-19 illness and can sometimes result in disability.

People who experience post-COVID conditions most commonly report the following.

General Symptoms
- tiredness or fatigue that interferes with daily life
- symptoms that get worse after physical or mental effort (also known as "post-exertional malaise")
- fever

Respiratory and Heart Symptoms
- difficulty breathing or shortness of breath
- cough
- chest pain
- fast-beating or pounding heart (also known as "heart palpitations")

Neurological Symptoms
- difficulty thinking or concentrating (sometimes referred to as "brain fog")
- headache

- sleep problems
- dizziness when you stand up (lightheadedness)
- pins-and-needles feelings
- change in smell or taste
- depression or anxiety

Digestive Symptoms
- diarrhea
- stomach pain

Other Symptoms
- joint or muscle pain
- rash
- changes in menstrual cycles

SYMPTOMS THAT ARE HARD TO EXPLAIN AND MANAGE

People with post-COVID conditions may develop or continue to have symptoms that are hard to explain and manage. Clinical evaluations and results of routine blood tests, chest x-rays, and electrocardiograms (ECGs) may be normal. The symptoms are similar to those reported by people with myalgic encephalomyelitis/chronic fatigue syndrome (ME/CFS) and other poorly understood chronic illnesses that may occur after other infections. People with these unexplained symptoms may be misunderstood by their healthcare providers, which can result in a long time for them to get a diagnosis and receive appropriate care or treatment.

HEALTH CONDITIONS

Some people, especially those who had severe COVID-19, experience multiorgan effects or autoimmune conditions with symptoms lasting weeks or months after COVID-19 illness. Multiorgan effects can involve many body systems, including the heart, lungs, kidneys, skin, and brain. As a result of these effects, people who have had COVID-19 may be more likely to develop new health conditions such as diabetes, heart conditions, or neurological conditions than people who have not had COVID-19.

PEOPLE EXPERIENCING ANY SEVERE ILLNESS MAY DEVELOP HEALTH PROBLEMS

Post-intensive care syndrome (PICS) refers to the health effects that may begin when a person is in an intensive care unit (ICU) and that may persist after a person returns home. These effects can include muscle weakness, problems with thinking and judgment, and symptoms of posttraumatic stress disorder (PTSD). PTSD involves long-term reactions to a very stressful event. For people who experience PICS following a COVID-19 diagnosis, it is difficult to determine whether these health problems are caused by a severe illness, the virus itself, or a combination of both.

WHO IS LIKELY TO DEVELOP LONG COVID?

Researchers are working to understand which people or groups of people are likely to have post-COVID conditions and why. Studies have shown that some groups of people may be affected more by post-COVID conditions. These are examples and not a comprehensive list of people or groups who might be more at risk than other groups for developing post-COVID conditions:
- people who have experienced more severe COVID-19 illness, especially those who were hospitalized or needed intensive care
- people who had underlying health conditions prior to COVID-19
- people who did not get a COVID-19 vaccine
- people who experience multisystem inflammatory syndrome (MIS) during or after COVID-19 illness

HEALTH INEQUITIES MAY AFFECT POPULATIONS AT RISK FOR LONG COVID

Some people are at an increased risk of getting sick from COVID-19 because of where they live or work or because they cannot get health care. Health inequities may put some people from racial or ethnic minority groups and some people with disabilities at a greater risk for developing post-COVID conditions. Scientists are researching some of those factors that may place these communities at a higher risk of both getting infected or developing post-COVID conditions.

PREVENTING LONG COVID
Research suggests that people who are vaccinated but experience a breakthrough infection are less likely to report post-COVID conditions than people who are unvaccinated.

LIVING WITH LONG COVID
However, people experiencing post-COVID conditions can seek care from a health-care provider to come up with a personal medical management plan that can help improve their symptoms and quality of life (QoL). Review these tips to help prepare for a health-care provider appointment for post-COVID conditions. In addition, there are many support groups being organized that can help patients and their caregivers.

Although post-COVID conditions appear to be less common in children and adolescents than in adults, long-term effects after COVID-19 do occur in children and adolescents.

DATA FOR LONG COVID
The Centers for Disease Control and Prevention (CDC) is using multiple approaches to estimate how many people experience post-COVID conditions. Each approach can provide a piece of the puzzle to give you a better picture of who is experiencing post-COVID conditions. For example, some studies look for the presence of post-COVID conditions based on self-reported symptoms, while others collect symptoms and conditions recorded in medical records. Some studies focus only on people who have been hospitalized, while others include people who were not hospitalized. The estimates for how many people experience post-COVID conditions can be quite different depending on who was included in the study, as well as how and when the study collected information.

Symptoms of Coronavirus Infection

Estimates of the proportion of people who had COVID-19 that go on to experience post-COVID conditions can vary.
- about 13.3 percent at one month or longer after infection
- 2.5 percent at three months or longer, based on self-reporting
- more than 30 percent at six months among patients who were hospitalized

Scientists are also learning more about how new variants could potentially affect post-COVID symptoms. Scientists are still learning to what extent certain groups are at a higher risk and if different groups of people tend to experience different types of post-COVID conditions. These studies, including, for example, the CDC's *INSPIRE* (www.covidinspire.org) and *RECOVER* (https://recovercovid.org)by the National Institutes of Health (NIH), will help you better understand post-COVID conditions and how health-care providers can treat or support patients with these longer-term effects. The CDC will continue to share information with health-care providers to help them evaluate and manage these conditions.

The CDC is working to:
- better identify the most frequent symptoms and diagnoses experienced by patients with post-COVID conditions
- better understand how many people are affected by post-COVID conditions and how often people who are infected with COVID-19 develop post-COVID conditions afterward
- better understand risk factors, including which groups might be more at risk and if different groups experience different symptoms
- help understand how post-COVID conditions limit or restrict people's daily activity
- help identify groups that have been more affected by post-COVID conditions, lack access to care and treatment for post-COVID conditions, or experience stigma

- better understand the role vaccination plays in preventing post-COVID conditions
- collaborate with professional medical groups to develop and offer clinical guidance and other educational materials for health-care providers, patients, and the public[2]

Section 3.3 | Similarities and Differences between Flu and COVID-19

Influenza (flu) and COVID-19 are both contagious respiratory illnesses, but they are caused by different viruses. COVID-19 is caused by infection with a coronavirus (SARS-CoV-2) first identified in 2019. Flu is caused by infection with a flu virus (influenza viruses).

From what you know, COVID-19 spreads more easily than flu. Efforts to maximize the proportion of people in the United States who are up-to-date with their COVID-19 vaccines remain critical to reducing the risk of severe COVID-19 illness and death.

Compared with flu, COVID-19 can cause more severe illness in some people. Compared to people with flu, people infected with COVID-19 may take longer to show symptoms and may be contagious for longer periods of time.

You cannot tell the difference between flu and COVID-19 by the symptoms alone because they have some of the same signs and symptoms. Specific testing is needed to tell what the illness is and to confirm a diagnosis. Having a medical professional administer a specific test that detects both flu and COVID-19 allows you to get diagnosed and treated for the specific virus you have more quickly. Getting treated early for COVID-19 and flu can reduce your risk of getting very sick. Testing can also reveal if someone has both flu and COVID-19 at the same time although this is uncommon.

---

[2] "Long COVID or Post-COVID Conditions," Centers for Disease Control and Prevention (CDC), September 1, 2022. Available online. URL: www.cdc.gov/coronavirus/2019-ncov/long-term-effects/index.html. Accessed December 15, 2022.

Symptoms of Coronavirus Infection

People with flu and COVID-19 at the same time can have more severe disease than people with either flu or COVID-19 alone. Additionally, some people with COVID-19 may also be affected by post-COVID conditions (also known as "long COVID").

SIGNS AND SYMPTOMS
Similarities
Both COVID-19 and flu can have varying degrees of symptoms, ranging from no symptoms (asymptomatic) to severe symptoms. Common symptoms that COVID-19 and flu share include the following:
- fever or feeling feverish/having chills
- cough
- shortness of breath or difficulty breathing
- fatigue (tiredness)
- sore throat
- runny or stuffy nose
- muscle pain or body aches
- headache
- vomiting
- diarrhea (more frequent in children with flu but can occur in any age with COVID-19)
- change in or loss of taste or smell although this is more frequent with COVID-19

HOW LONG AFTER EXPOSURE AND INFECTION SYMPTOMS APPEAR
Similarities
For both COVID-19 and flu, one or more days can pass from when a person becomes infected to when they start to experience symptoms of illness. It is possible to be infected with the virus that causes COVID-19 without experiencing any symptoms. It is also possible to be infected with flu viruses without having any symptoms.

Differences
If a person has COVID-19, it could take them longer from the time of infection to experience symptoms than if they have flu.

FLU
Typically, a person may experience symptoms anywhere from one to four days after infection.

COVID-19
Typically, a person may experience symptoms anywhere from two to five days and up to 14 days after infection.

HOW LONG SOMEONE CAN SPREAD THE VIRUS
Differences
If a person has COVID-19, they could be contagious for a longer time than if they have flu.

FLU
- People with flu virus infection are potentially contagious for about one day before they show symptoms. However, it is believed that flu is spread mainly by people who are symptomatic with flu virus infection.
- Older children and adults with flu appear to be most contagious during the first 3–4 days of their illness, but some people might remain contagious for slightly longer periods.
- Infants and people with weakened immune systems can be contagious for even longer.

COVID-19
- On average, people can begin spreading the virus that causes COVID-19 two to three days before their symptoms begin, but infectiousness peaks one day before their symptoms begin.
- People can also spread the virus that causes COVID-19 without experiencing any symptoms.
- On average, people are considered contagious for about eight days after their symptoms begin.

Symptoms of Coronavirus Infection

HOW IT SPREADS
Similarities
Both COVID-19 and flu can spread from person to person between people who are near or in close contact with one another. Both are spread mainly by large and small particles containing the virus that are expelled when people with the illness (COVID-19 or flu) cough, sneeze, or talk. These particles can land in the mouths or noses of people who are nearby and possibly be inhaled into the respiratory tract. In some circumstances, such as indoor settings with poor ventilation, small particles containing the virus might be spread longer distances and cause infections.

Most spread is by inhalation of large and small droplets; however, it may be possible that a person can get infected by touching another person (e.g., shaking hands with someone who has the virus on their hands) or by touching a surface or object that has the virus on it and then touching their own mouth, nose, or eyes.

Differences
While the virus that causes COVID-19 and flu viruses are thought to spread in similar ways, the virus that causes COVID-19 is generally more contagious than flu viruses. Also, COVID-19 has been observed to have more super-spreading events than flu. This means the virus that causes COVID-19 can quickly and easily spread to a lot of people and result in continual spreading among people as time progresses. The virus that causes COVID-19 can be spread to others by people before they begin showing symptoms, by people with very mild symptoms, and by people who never experience symptoms (asymptomatic people).

PEOPLE AT A HIGHER RISK FOR SEVERE ILLNESS
Similarities
Both COVID-19 and flu illness can result in severe illness and complications. Those at increased risk include the following:
- older adults
- people with certain underlying medical conditions (including infants and children)
- people who are pregnant

Differences

Overall, COVID-19 seems to cause more severe illness in some people.

Severe COVID-19 illness resulting in hospitalization and death can occur even in healthy people.

Some people who had COVID-19 can go on to develop post-COVID conditions or multisystem inflammatory syndrome (MIS).

COMPLICATIONS
Similarities

Both COVID-19 and flu can result in complications, including the following:
- pneumonia
- respiratory failure
- acute respiratory distress syndrome (fluid in the lungs)
- sepsis (a life-threatening illness caused by the body's extreme response to an infection)
- cardiac injury (e.g., heart attacks and stroke)
- multiple-organ failure (respiratory failure, kidney failure, shock)
- worsening of chronic medical conditions (involving the lungs, heart, or nervous system or diabetes)
- inflammation of the heart, brain, or muscle tissues
- secondary infections (bacterial or fungal infections that can occur in people with flu or COVID-19)

Differences
FLU

Most people who get flu will recover on their own in a few days to two weeks, but some people will experience severe complications, requiring hospitalization. Some of these complications are listed above. Secondary bacterial infections are more common with influenza than with COVID-19.

Diarrhea is more common in young children with flu than in adults with flu.

Symptoms of Coronavirus Infection

COVID-19
Additional complications associated with COVID-19 can include the following:
- blood clots in the veins and arteries of the lungs, heart, legs, or brain
- MIS in children (MIS-C) and MIS in adults (MIS-A)

Anyone who has had COVID-19, even if their illness was mild or if they had no symptoms, can experience post-COVID conditions. Post-COVID conditions are a range of symptoms that can last weeks or months after first being infected with the virus that causes COVID-19 or can appear weeks after infection.

APPROVED TREATMENTS
Similarities
People at a higher risk of complications or who have been hospitalized for COVID-19 or flu should receive recommended treatments and supportive medical care to help relieve symptoms and complications.

Differences
FLU
Prescription influenza antiviral drugs are approved by the U.S. Food and Drug Administration (FDA) to treat flu. These antiviral drugs are only for treatment of flu and not COVID-19. People who are hospitalized with flu or who are at an increased risk of complications and have flu symptoms are recommended to be treated with antiviral drugs as soon as possible after illness onset.

COVID-19
The National Institutes of Health (NIH) has developed guidance on treatment of COVID-19, which is regularly updated as new evidence on treatment options emerges. This includes antiviral treatment for nonhospitalized people at an increased risk for severe COVID-19 and antiviral treatment for people hospitalized with severe COVID-19. People who are at an increased risk of severe

COVID-19 should seek treatment within days of when their symptoms first start.

VACCINE
Similarities
Vaccines for COVID-19 and flu are approved or authorized for emergency use (EUA) by the FDA.

Differences
FLU
There are multiple FDA-licensed influenza vaccines produced annually to protect against the four flu viruses that scientists expect will circulate each year.

COVID-19
Multiple COVID-19 vaccines are authorized or approved for use in the United States to help prevent COVID-19.[3]

---

[3] "Similarities and Differences between Flu and COVID-19," Centers for Disease Control and Prevention (CDC), September 28, 2022. Available online. URL: www.cdc.gov/flu/symptoms/flu-vs-covid19.htm. Accessed December 15, 2022.

Chapter 4 | Testing for COVID-19 Infection

Chapter Contents
Section 4.1—COVID-19 Testing: What Do You
           Need to Know? 59
Section 4.2—Coronavirus Self-Test Kits 63
Section 4.3—Community-Based Testing Sites
           for COVID-19 70
Section 4.4—Waiting for Your COVID-19 Test Result 71

Section 4.1 | COVID-19 Testing: What Do You Need to Know?

WHEN TO GET TESTED FOR COVID-19
Key times to get tested are as follows:
- If you have symptoms, test immediately.
- If you were exposed to COVID-19 and do not have symptoms, wait at least five full days after your exposure before testing. If you test too early, you may be more likely to get an inaccurate result.
- If you are in certain high-risk settings, you may need to test as part of a screening testing program.
- Consider testing before contact with someone at high risk for severe COVID-19, especially if you are in an area with a medium or high COVID-19 community level.

TYPES OF TESTS
Viral tests look for a current infection with severe acute respiratory syndrome coronavirus 2 (SARS-CoV-2), the virus that causes COVID-19, by testing specimens from your nose or mouth. There are two main types of viral tests: nucleic acid amplification tests (NAATs) and antigen tests. In certain circumstances, one test type may be recommended over the other. All tests should be performed following U.S. Food and Drug Administration (FDA) requirements.
- NAATs, such as tests based on polymerase chain reaction (PCR), are most often performed in a laboratory. They are typically the most reliable tests for people with or without symptoms. These tests detect viral genetic material, which may stay in your body for up to 90 days after you test positive. Therefore, you should not use an NAAT if you have tested positive in the last 90 days.
- Antigen tests* are rapid tests that produce results in 15–30 minutes. They are less reliable than NAATs, especially for people who do not have symptoms. A single, negative antigen test result does not rule out

infection. To best detect infection, a negative antigen test should be repeated at least 48 hours apart (known as "serial testing"). Sometimes, a follow-up NAAT may be recommended to confirm an antigen test result.

*Self-tests, or at-home tests, are usually antigen tests that can be taken anywhere without having to go to a specific testing site. Follow the instructions of the FDA and the manufacturer, including for the number of times you may need to test. Multiple negative test results increase the confidence that you are not infected with the virus that causes COVID-19.

- You can order free self-test kits at COVIDtests.gov (www.covid.gov/tests) or purchase tests online, in pharmacies, and in retail stores.
- You can also visit the FDA's website (www.fda.gov/medical-devices/coronavirus-covid-19-and-medical-devices/home-otc-covid-19-diagnostic-tests?utm_medium=email&utm_source=govdelivery#list) to see a list of authorized tests.
- As noted in the labeling for authorized over-the-counter (OTC) antigen tests, negative results should be treated as presumptive (meaning that they are preliminary results). Negative results do not rule out SARS-CoV-2 infection and should not be used as the sole basis for treatment or patient management decisions, including infection control decisions.

CHOOSING A COVID-19 TEST

There are two circumstances where you should get tested and:
- You have not had COVID-19 or you have not had a positive test within the past 90 days.
  - You may choose NAAT or antigen tests.
  - If you use an antigen test and your result is negative, multiple tests may be necessary.
- If you have tested positive for COVID-19 in the last 90 days, refer to Table 4.1.

Testing for COVID-19 Infection

Table 4.1. You Tested Positive for COVID-19 in the Last 90 Days

My First Positive Test Result Was Within: 30 Days or Less	My First Positive Test Result Was Within: 31–90 Days
I have symptoms Use antigen tests. If negative, multiple tests may be necessary.	**I have symptoms** Use antigen tests. If negative, multiple tests may be necessary.
I do not have symptoms Testing is not recommended to detect a new infection.	**I do not have symptoms** Use antigen tests. If negative, multiple tests may be necessary.

After a positive test result, you may continue to test positive for some time after. You may continue to test positive on antigen tests for a few weeks after your initial positive. You may continue to test positive on NAATs for up to 90 days. Reinfections can occur within 90 days, which can make it hard to know if a positive test indicates a new infection. Consider consulting a health-care provider if you have any questions or concerns about your individual circumstances.

INTERPRETING YOUR RESULTS
If Your COVID-19 Test Is Positive

Any positive COVID-19 test means the virus was detected, and you have an infection.
- Isolate and take precautions including wearing a high-quality mask to protect others from getting infected.
- Tell people you had recent contact with that they may have been exposed to.
- Monitor your symptoms. If you have any emergency warning signs, seek emergency care immediately.
- Consider contacting a health-care provider, community health center, or pharmacy to learn about treatment options that may be available to you. Treatment must be started within several days after you first develop symptoms to be effective.
  - You are likely to get very sick if you are an older adult or have an underlying medical condition. Possible treatment may be available for you.

If Your COVID-19 Test Is Negative

A negative COVID-19 test means the test did not detect the virus, but this does not rule out that you could have an infection.
- If you have symptoms:
  - you may have COVID-19 but tested before the virus was detectable or you may have another illness
  - take general public health precautions to prevent spreading an illness to others
  - contact a health-care provider if you have any questions about your test result or if your symptoms worsen
- If you do not have symptoms but were exposed to the virus that causes COVID-19, you should continue to take recommended steps after exposure.
- If you do not have symptoms, and you have not been exposed to the virus that causes COVID-19, you may return to normal activities.
  - Continue to take steps to protect yourself and others, including monitoring for symptoms. Get tested again if symptoms appear.

TESTING FOR ANTIBODIES

Antibody or serology tests look for antibodies in your blood that fight the virus that causes COVID-19. Antibodies are proteins created by your immune system after you have been infected or have been vaccinated against an infection. They can help protect you from infection, or severe illness if you do get infected, for a period of time afterward. How long this protection lasts is different for each disease and each person.

Antibody tests should not be used to diagnose a current infection with the virus that causes COVID-19. An antibody test may not show if you have a current infection because it can take 1–3 weeks after the infection for your body to make antibodies.[1]

---

[1] "COVID-19 Testing: What You Need to Know," Centers for Disease Control and Prevention (CDC), September 28, 2022. Available online. URL: www.cdc.gov/coronavirus/2019-ncov/symptoms-testing/testing.html. Accessed December 8, 2022.

Testing for COVID-19 Infection

Section 4.2 | **Coronavirus Self-Test Kits**

WHAT IS A SELF-TEST OR AT-HOME TEST?
Self-tests for COVID-19 give rapid results and can be taken anywhere, regardless of your vaccination status or whether or not you have symptoms.
- They detect current infection and are sometimes also called "home tests," "at-home tests," or "over-the-counter (OTC) tests."
- They give your result in a few minutes and are different from laboratory-based tests that may take days to return your result.
- Self-tests along with vaccination, wearing a well-fitted mask, and physical distancing help protect you and others by reducing the chances of spreading COVID-19.
- Self-tests do not detect antibodies that would suggest a previous infection, and they do not measure your level of immunity.

WHEN AND HOW TO GET AN AT-HOME COVID-19 TEST
- Buy tests online or in pharmacies and retail stores. Private health insurance may reimburse the cost of purchasing self-tests. Visit the U.S. Food and Drug Administration (FDA) website (www.fda.gov/medical-devices/coronavirus-covid-19-and-medical-devices/home-otc-covid-19-diagnostic-tests?utm_medium=email&utm_source=govdelivery#list) for a list of authorized tests.
- Free tests may also be available through local health departments.
- If you are not able to obtain a self-test when you need it, you might also visit a community testing site or call your local health department for more options (refer to Table 4.2).

Table 4.2. How to Take the COVID-19 At-Home Test

Test Yourself If	Timing
You have any COVID-19 symptoms.	Immediately.
You were exposed to someone with COVID-19.	• At least five days after your exposure. • If you test negative for COVID-19, consider testing again 1–2 days after your first test.
You are going to an indoor event or a gathering.	• Immediately before the gathering or as close to the time of the event as possible. • This is especially important before gathering with individuals at risk of severe disease, older adults, those who are immunocompromised, or people who are not up-to-date on their COVID-19 vaccines, including children who cannot get vaccinated yet.

HOW TO USE AN AT-HOME COVID-19 TEST

Read the complete manufacturer's instructions for use before using the test.

- To use an at-home test, you will collect a nasal specimen and then test that specimen.
- If you do not follow the manufacturer's instructions, your test result may be incorrect.
- Wash your hands before and after you collect a nasal specimen for your test.

WHAT DO YOUR TEST RESULTS MEAN?

If your test is positive, do the following:

- The test detected the virus, and you have an infection.
- Stay home for at least five days and isolate from others in your home.
- Tell your close contacts.
- Wear a well-fitted mask when around others. If available, an N95 or KN95 respirator is recommended.
- Watch for symptoms. If you have any emergency warning signs, seek emergency care immediately.

Testing for COVID-19 Infection

- Tell your health-care provider. Contact them as soon as possible for the following:
    - Your symptoms get worse.
    - You are likely to get very sick because you are an older adult or have an underlying medical condition. Possible treatment may be available for you.
    - You have questions about your isolation.

If your test is negative, do the following:
- The test did not detect the virus but does not rule out an infection.
- Some self-tests are designed to be used in a series (also known as "serial testing"). Consider repeating the test 24–48 hours later. Multiple negative tests increase the confidence that you are not infected with the virus that causes COVID-19.[2]

WHEN SHOULD YOU TEST FOR COVID-19?

COVID-19 testing is important to find out if you have COVID-19 so that you can get treatment, if needed, as well as to be aware if you are infected and should stay away from people to help reduce the spread of the virus. You should test for COVID-19 in the following situations:
- If you have symptoms, test immediately.
- If you were exposed to someone who has COVID-19 and do not have symptoms, wait at least five full days after your exposure before testing. If you test too early, you may have an inaccurate result.
- If you are in certain high-risk settings, you may need to test as part of a screening testing program.
- Consider testing before coming into contact with someone who has a high risk for severe COVID-19, especially if you are in an area with a medium or high COVID-19 community level.

---

[2] "Self-Testing at Home or Anywhere," Centers for Disease Control and Prevention (CDC), September 6, 2022. Available online. URL: www.cdc.gov/coronavirus/2019-ncov/testing/self-testing.html. Accessed December 9, 2022.

WHAT DO AT-HOME COVID-19 TEST RESULTS MEAN?

If you receive a positive result on any COVID-19 test, assume you have COVID-19. Be sure to follow guidelines of the Centers for Disease Control and Prevention (CDC) for people with COVID-19, including to stay home, isolate from others, and seek follow-up care with a health-care provider to determine what steps to take next.

If you receive a negative result on your at-home COVID-19 antigen test, it means the test did not detect the virus that causes COVID-19, but it does not rule out an infection because some tests may not detect the virus early in an infection. Always do a repeat test after a negative result on an antigen test.

YOU GOT A NEGATIVE TEST RESULT ON AN AT-HOME COVID-19 ANTIGEN TEST. DO YOU NEED TO TAKE ANOTHER TEST?

Yes. The FDA recommends repeat testing following a negative COVID-19 antigen test result whether or not you have COVID-19 symptoms. COVID-19 antigen tests are less accurate than molecular tests and may not detect the severe acute respiratory syndrome coronavirus 2 (SARS-CoV-2) virus early in an infection or in people who do not have COVID-19 symptoms.

You should perform repeat testing following a negative result on a COVID-19 antigen test to reduce the risk an infection may have been missed (false-negative result) and to help prevent unknowingly spreading the SARS-CoV-2 virus to others.

- If you have COVID-19 symptoms, test again 48 hours after the first negative test, for a total of at least two tests.
- If you do not have COVID-19 symptoms, test again 48 hours after the first negative test and then 48 hours after the second negative test, for a total of at least three tests.
- If you get a positive result on any COVID-19 test, you most likely have COVID-19 and should follow the CDC guidance for people with COVID-19.

In August 2022, the FDA issued a safety communication on the need to perform repeat testing to reduce your risk of a false-negative result. In November 2022, the FDA required all manufacturers of COVID-19 antigen tests authorized by the Emergency Use Authorization (EUA) to update their labeling to reflect the need for repeat testing at least twice over three days for individuals with symptoms of COVID-19 and at least three times over five days for individuals without symptoms of COVID-19, as appropriate based on their authorized uses.

ARE AT-HOME COVID-19 TESTS SAFE TO USE? DO THEY CONTAIN TOXIC CHEMICALS?

The FDA-authorized at-home COVID-19 tests are safe to use when people follow the manufacturer's step-by-step instructions. However, incorrect use of at-home COVID-19 tests can cause harm if the parts of the test kit, such as liquid solutions in small vials that may contain chemicals such as sodium azide, are swallowed or if the liquid solutions touch a person's skin or eyes. The FDA has provided recommendations to promote the safe use of at-home COVID-19 tests in a safety communication issued on March 18, 2022, including to keep all parts of at-home COVID-19 tests out of reach of children and pets before and after use, and to follow the test's step-by-step instructions exactly, including the warning, precautions, and safety information.

CAN YOU USE AN AUTHORIZED AT-HOME COVID-19 DIAGNOSTIC TEST IF IT WAS LEFT OUTSIDE IN FREEZING TEMPERATURES OR IN THE HEAT?

Since shipping conditions may vary, test developers perform stability testing to ensure that the test performance will remain stable when tests are stored at various temperatures, including shipping during the summer in very hot regions and in the winter in very cold regions.

However, test performance may be impacted if the test is used while it is still cold, such as being used outdoors in freezing temperatures or being used immediately after being brought inside from freezing temperatures, or in a hotter-than-expected environment, such as outside in the summer. The stated performance generally assumes the test is being performed in an environment that is between 15 and 30 °C (approximately 59–86 °F). The specific conditions that were validated are included in the authorized instructions for use for each test.

In order to ensure appropriate test performance with a test that is delivered to you in below freezing temperatures or in very hot temperatures, you should bring the package inside your home and leave it unopened at room temperature for at least two hours before opening it. Once the package is at room temperature, you may open it and perform the test according to the authorized instructions for use. As long as the test line(s) appear as described in the instructions, you can be confident that the test is performing as it should. If the line(s) do not appear in the correct location(s) and within the correct time as shown in the test instructions when you perform the test, then the results may not be accurate, and a new test is needed to get an accurate result.

In addition, long exposure to high temperatures may impact the test performance. If your test has been left in a high-temperature environment beyond the normal shipping time to be delivered to you, such as being left outside in the heat for several days, the FDA recommends considering using a different test.

HOW IS THE EXPIRATION DATE DETERMINED FOR AN AT-HOME COVID-19 DIAGNOSTIC TEST?

COVID-19 test manufacturers perform studies to show how long after manufacturing COVID-19 tests perform as accurately as the day the test was manufactured. The shelf life is how long the test should perform as expected and is measured from the date the test was manufactured. The expiration date listed on the box label for at-home COVID-19 tests is set at the end of the shelf life and is the date through which the test is expected to perform as accurately as when manufactured.

The testing to determine this time period is called "stability testing" because it is confirming the time period over which the performance is expected to remain stable. There are different types of stability testing. The most accurate is real-time stability testing, where the manufacturer stores the tests for the time period of the proposed shelf life (plus a little extra time to ensure the expiration date can be relied upon) and then evaluates its ability to perform accurately. For example, for a proposed 12-month shelf life, the manufacturer would evaluate the performance after storing the test for 13 months.

In some cases, accelerated testing provides a faster way to estimate the stability of a test's performance over time by storing the test for a shorter time at a higher temperature and then evaluating its ability to perform accurately. However, since accelerated testing only estimates the test stability, it does not provide as much assurance as real-time data, especially for longer time periods. Based on experience with tests and stability testing, accelerated testing typically provides sufficient assurance to label tests with a shelf life of up to six months.

Since it takes time for test manufacturers to perform stability testing, the FDA typically authorizes at-home COVID-19 tests with a shelf life of about 4–6 months from the day the test was manufactured, based on initial study results, and it may be extended later as additional data are collected.

CAN YOU USE AN EXPIRED FDA-AUTHORIZED AT-HOME COVID-19 DIAGNOSTIC TEST?

No, the FDA does not recommend using at-home COVID-19 diagnostic tests beyond their authorized expiration dates. COVID-19 tests and the parts they are made of may degrade, or break down, over time. Because of this, expired test kits could give inaccurate or invalid test results.

However, the expiration dates for at-home COVID-19 diagnostic tests may be extended as additional stability data are collected.

CAN THE EXPIRATION DATE OF AN AT-HOME COVID-19 DIAGNOSTIC TEST BE EXTENDED?

Yes. Once the test manufacturer has more stable testing results, such as 12 or 18 months, the test manufacturer can contact the FDA to request that the FDA authorize a longer shelf life. When a longer shelf life is authorized, the expiration dates will be extended, and the test manufacturer may send a notice to customers to provide the new authorized expiration dates, so the customers know how long they can use the tests they already have. If you did not purchase your at-home COVID-19 diagnostic test directly from the test manufacturer, you may not receive such a notice.

HOW DO YOU KNOW IF THE EXPIRATION DATE OF YOUR AT-HOME COVID-19 TEST HAS BEEN EXTENDED? WHERE DO YOU FIND THE UPDATED EXPIRATION DATE?

You can check the expiration date column of the list of authorized at-home OTC COVID-19 diagnostic tests to see if the expiration date for your at-home OTC COVID-19 test has been extended and how to find any new expiration date.[3]

Section 4.3 | Community-Based Testing Sites for COVID-19

Low- or no-cost COVID-19 tests are available to everyone in the United States, including the uninsured, at health centers and select pharmacies nationwide. Additional testing sites may be available in your area. Contact your health-care provider or your state or local public health department for more information.

PHARMACIES

The U.S. Department of Health and Human Services (HHS) has partnered with pharmacies and retail companies to accelerate testing for more Americans in communities across the country. These companies are coordinating with state and local governments to:
- provide Americans with faster, less invasive, and more convenient testing
- protect health-care personnel by eliminating direct contact with symptomatic individuals

---

[3] "At-Home COVID-19 Diagnostic Tests: Frequently Asked Questions," U.S. Food and Drug Administration (FDA), December 14, 2022. Available online. URL: www.fda.gov/medical-devices/coronavirus-covid-19-and-medical-devices/home-covid-19-diagnostic-tests-frequently-asked-questions. Accessed December 19, 2022.

Testing for COVID-19 Infection

- expand testing to communities across the United States, especially those that are undertested and socially vulnerable

HEALTH CENTERS

Health centers are an important component of the national response to the COVID-19 pandemic. Find a health center near you for available COVID-19 screening and testing. Please call the health center for more information about the availability of low- or no-cost testing.

Health centers provide COVID-19 testing services to individuals who meet the criteria for COVID-19 testing, regardless of their ability to pay. Health centers will determine whether there is available reimbursement, funding, compensation sources, and any related cost sharing restrictions for COVID-19 testing prior to billing patients. If there are any out-of-pocket costs—for example, in the case of no or only partial coverage by private insurance—health centers will provide sliding fee discounts for eligible patients based on income and family size.[4]

Section 4.4 | Waiting for Your COVID-19 Test Result

To help stop the spread of COVID-19, take the following three key steps now while waiting for your test results.

STAY HOME AND MONITOR YOUR HEALTH

Stay home and monitor your health to help protect your friends, family, and others from possibly getting COVID-19 from you.

Stay home and away from others:
- If possible, stay away from others, especially people who are at a higher risk for getting very sick from

---

[4] "Community-Based Testing Sites for COVID-19," U.S. Department of Health and Human Services (HHS), September 2, 2022. Available online. URL: www.hhs.gov/coronavirus/community-based-testing-sites/index.html. Accessed December 9, 2022.

COVID-19, such as older adults and people with other medical conditions.
- If you have been in contact with someone with COVID-19, stay home and away from others for 14 days after your last contact with that person.
- If you have a fever, cough, or other symptoms of COVID-19, stay home and away from others (except to get medical care).

Monitor your health:
- Watch for fever, cough, shortness of breath, or other symptoms of COVID-19. Remember, symptoms may appear 2–14 days after exposure to COVID-19 and can include the following:
  - congestion or runny nose
  - cough
  - diarrhea
  - fever or chills
  - headache
  - muscle or body aches
  - nausea or vomiting
  - new loss of taste or smell
  - shortness of breath or difficulty breathing
  - sore throat
  - tiredness

ANSWER PHONE CALLS FROM THE HEALTH DEPARTMENT

If you are diagnosed with COVID-19, a public health worker may call you to check on your health, discuss who you have been around, and ask where you spent time while you may have been able to spread COVID-19 to others. While you wait for your COVID-19 test result, think about everyone you have been around recently. This will be important information to give health workers if your test is positive.

If a public health worker calls you, answer the call to help slow the spread of COVID-19 in your community.

Testing for COVID-19 Infection

- Discussions with health department staff are confidential. This means that your personal and medical information will be kept private and only shared with those who may need to know, such as your health-care provider.
- Your name will not be shared with those you came in contact with. The health department will only notify people you were in close contact with (within six feet for more than 15 minutes) that they might have been exposed to COVID-19.

THINK ABOUT THE PEOPLE YOU HAVE RECENTLY BEEN AROUND

If you test positive and are diagnosed with COVID-19, someone from the health department may call to check in on your health, discuss who you have been around, and ask where you spent time while you may have been able to spread COVID-19 to others. This form can help you think about people you have recently been around, so you will be ready if a public health worker calls you. The following are the things to think about:

- Have you gone to work or school?
- Have you gotten together with others (eaten out at a restaurant, gone out for drinks, exercised with others or gone to a gym, had friends or family over to your house, volunteered, or gone to a party, pool, or park)?
- Have you gone to a store in person (e.g., grocery store, mall)?
- Have you gone to in-person appointments (e.g., salon, barber, doctor's office, or dentist's office)?
- Have you ridden in a car with others (e.g., Uber or Lyft) or taken public transportation?
- Have you been inside a church, synagogue, mosque, or other places of worship?[5]

---

[5] "3 Key Steps to Take While Waiting for Your COVID-19 Test Result," Centers for Disease Control and Prevention (CDC), November 19, 2020. Available online. URL: www.cdc.gov/coronavirus/2019-ncov/downloads/3key-steps-when-waiting-for-COVID-19-results_508.pdf. Accessed December 9, 2022.

Chapter 5 | **The Immune System and COVID-19**

ANTIBODIES AND THE IMMUNE SYSTEM
- The immune system is a complex network of cells, tissues, and organs that work together to protect the body from infection.
- Antibodies are proteins that your immune system makes to help fight infection and protect you from getting sick in the future.

When you are infected with a virus or bacterium, your immune system makes antibodies specifically to fight it. Your immune system can also safely learn to make antibodies through vaccination. Once you have antibodies to a particular disease, they provide some protection from that disease. Even if you do get sick, having antibodies can protect you from getting severely ill because your body has some experience in fighting that disease. How long this protection lasts can be different for each disease and each person or influenced by other factors. Antibodies are just one part of your immune response.

ANTIBODIES AND COVID-19
Antibodies to severe acute respiratory syndrome coronavirus 2 (SARS-CoV-2), the virus that causes COVID-19, can be detected in the blood of people who have recovered from COVID-19 or people who have been vaccinated against COVID-19. Getting a vaccine is safer than getting COVID-19, and vaccination against COVID-19 is recommended for everyone five years of age and older. If

someone has already had COVID-19, vaccination against COVID-19 increases their body's antibody response, which improves their protection.

It is important to remember that some people with antibodies to SARS-CoV-2 may become infected after vaccination (vaccine breakthrough infection) or after recovering from a past infection (reinfected). Based on what you know right now, risk of reinfection is low for at least the first six months following an infection with the virus that causes COVID-19 diagnosed by a laboratory test. When someone who is fully vaccinated gets COVID-19, it is called a "vaccine breakthrough infection." No vaccine is 100 percent effective, so some breakthrough infections are expected. The risk of infection, severe illness, hospitalization, and death are all much lower for vaccinated people than those for people who are unvaccinated. When reinfections or breakthrough infections happen, having antibodies plays an important role in helping prevent severe illness, hospitalization, and death.

For many diseases, including COVID-19, antibodies are expected to decrease or "wane" over time. After a long enough period of time, your level of antibodies can decrease below a level that provides effective protection. This level is called the "threshold of protection." When antibodies decrease below the threshold of protection, you may become more vulnerable to severe illness. You do not yet know what the threshold of protection for antibodies is for the virus that causes COVID-19 or how long it takes these antibodies to wane. Even after antibodies wane, your immune system may have cells that remember the virus that can act quickly to protect you from severe illness if you become infected. These topics are being researched by scientists all over the world.

YOU HAVE COVID-19 ANTIBODIES. WHAT DOES IT MEAN?

A positive antibody test result can help identify someone who has had COVID-19 in the past or has been vaccinated against COVID-19. Antibody tests are not used if you have symptoms of COVID-19 or for diagnosing a current case of COVID-19. This is because it takes most people with a healthy immune system 1–3 weeks after getting COVID-19 to develop antibodies. A viral test is recommended to identify a current infection with the virus that causes COVID-19.

Most people who have a positive antibody test result can continue with normal activities, including work, but they should still take steps to protect themselves and others, including getting vaccinated.

A positive antibody test result alone, especially one from an infection at an unknown time or that was determined by a viral test more than six months ago, does not necessarily mean that you are immune to getting COVID-19. If you have had an antibody test, it is important to review your test results with your health-care provider.

HOW DO SCIENTISTS STUDY ANTIBODIES?

The science of antibodies is called "serology." Antibody tests, also called "serology tests," identify antibodies in blood samples. While other parts of the immune system also contribute to protection, it is easiest to test for antibodies.

As of August 2021, more than 80 antibody tests have been granted the U.S. Food and Drug Administration (FDA) Emergency Use Authorization (EUA) to detect antibodies to SARS-CoV-2. Scientists are using these antibody tests to learn more about the level of antibodies needed to protect people from COVID-19 (threshold of protection) and how long this protection lasts. Antibody tests are not currently recommended by the FDA for routine, widespread use in making individual medical decisions while this information is being gathered and evaluated. If you have questions about whether an antibody test is right for you, talk with your health-care provider or your state or local health department.

Not all antibody tests identify the same antibodies. Some antibody tests are more or less sensitive to specific sections of the antibody protein than others. This means that different antibody tests might not have the same results, even when they are both testing for antibodies to SARS-CoV-2. Scientists use these differences in tests to help answer different research questions about how immune systems respond to the virus that causes COVID-19 and to improve your understanding of COVID-19.

WHAT INFORMATION DO ANTIBODIES TO SARS-COV-2 TELL YOU ABOUT HOW TO RESPOND TO COVID-19?

As scientists learn more about the antibodies to SARS-CoV-2, we will understand a lot more about how to treat and control COVID-19.

Serological surveillance (studies that investigate antibodies in the population) provides information about how long antibody protection against COVID-19 lasts and if this protection is different among people who have antibodies from infection, compared with people who have antibodies from vaccination, or both.

You can also learn more about which groups of people might not produce as many antibodies or maintain them as long as others—for example, immunocompromised people compared with people who have healthy immune systems. This is important information for making decisions about whether or not additional vaccine doses or boosters are needed, when they would be recommended, and who would need them first.

You can also learn if antibodies to SARS-CoV-2 provide the same protection against new variants of the virus that causes COVID-19.[1]

---

[1] "Antibodies and COVID-19," Centers for Disease Control and Prevention (CDC), November 10, 2021. Available online. URL: www.cdc.gov/coronavirus/2019-ncov/your-health/about-covid-19/antibodies.html. Accessed December 9, 2022.

Chapter 6 | The Coronavirus and the Nervous System

WHAT DO WE KNOW ABOUT THE EFFECTS OF SARS-COV-2 AND COVID-19 ON THE NERVOUS SYSTEM?

Much of the research to date has focused on the acute infection and saving lives. These strategies have included preventing infection with vaccines, treating COVID-19 symptoms with medicines or antibodies, and reducing complications in infected individuals.

Research shows the many neurological symptoms of COVID-19 are likely a result of the body's widespread immune response to infection rather than the virus directly infecting the brain or nervous system. In some people, the SARS-CoV-2 infection causes an overreactive response of the immune system that can also damage body systems. Changes in the immune system have been seen in studies of the cerebrospinal fluid, which bathes the brain, in people who have been infected by SARS-CoV-2. This includes the presence of antibodies—proteins made by the immune system to fight the virus—that may also react with the nervous system. Although still under intense investigation, there is no evidence of widespread viral infection in the brain. Scientists are still learning how the virus affects the brain and other organs in the long term. Research is just beginning to focus on the role of autoimmune reactions and other changes that cause the set of symptoms that some people experience after their initial recovery. It is unknown if injury to the nervous system or other body organs causes lingering effects that will resolve over time or whether COVID-19 infection sets up a more persistent or even chronic disorder.

WHAT ARE THE IMMEDIATE (ACUTE) EFFECTS OF SARS-COV-2 AND COVID-19 ON THE BRAIN?

Most people infected with the SARS-CoV-2 will have no or mild-to-moderate symptoms associated with the brain or nervous system. However, most individuals hospitalized due to the virus do have symptoms related to the brain or nervous system, most commonly including muscle aches, headaches, dizziness, and altered taste and smell. Some people with COVID-19 either initially have or develop in the hospital a dramatic state of confusion called "delirium." Although rare, COVID-19 can cause seizures or major strokes. Muscular weakness, nerve injury, and pain syndromes are common in people who require intensive care during infections. There are also very rare reports of conditions that develop after SARS-CoV-2 infection, as they sometimes do with other types of infections. These disorders of inflammation in the nervous system include Guillain-Barré syndrome (which affects nerves), transverse myelitis (which affects the spinal cord), and acute necrotizing leukoencephalopathy (which affects the brain).

BLEEDING IN THE BRAIN, WEAKENED BLOOD VESSELS, AND BLOOD CLOTS IN ACUTE INFECTION

The SARS-CoV-2 virus attaches to a specific molecule (called a "receptor") on the surface of cells in the body. This molecule is concentrated in the lung cells but is also present in certain cells that line blood vessels in the body. The infection causes some arteries and veins—including those in the brain—to become thin, weaken, and leak. Breaks in small blood vessels have caused bleeding in the brain (so-called microbleeds) in some people with COVID-19 infection. Studies in people who have died due to COVID-19 infection show leaky blood vessels in different areas of the brain that allow water and a host of other molecules as well as blood cells that are normally excluded from the brain to move from the bloodstream into the brain. This leak, as well as the resulting inflammation around blood vessels, can cause multiple small areas of damage. COVID-19 also causes blood cells to clump and form clots in arteries and veins throughout the body. These blockages reduce or block the flow of blood, oxygen, and nutrients that cells need to function and can lead to a stroke or heart attack.

A stroke is a sudden interruption of continuous blood flow to the brain. A stroke occurs either when a blood vessel in the brain becomes blocked or narrowed or when a blood vessel bursts and spills blood into the brain. Strokes can damage brain cells and cause permanent disability. The blood clots and vascular (relating to the veins, capillaries, and arteries in the body) damage from COVID-19 can cause strokes even in young healthy adults who do not have the common risk factors for stroke.

COVID-19 can cause blood clots in other parts of the body, too. A blood clot in or near the heart can cause a heart attack. A heart attack or inflammation in the heart, called "myocarditis," can cause heart failure and reduce the flow of blood to other parts of the body. A blood clot in the lungs can impair breathing and cause pain. Blood clots also can damage the kidneys and other organs.

Low levels of oxygen in the body (called "hypoxia") can permanently damage the brain and other vital organs in the body. Some hospitalized individuals require artificial ventilation on respirators. To avoid chest movements that oppose the use of the ventilator, it may be necessary to temporarily "paralyze" the person and use anesthetic drugs to put the individual to sleep. Some individuals with severe hypoxia require artificial means of bringing oxygen into their bloodstream, a technique called "extracorporeal membrane oxygenation (ECMO)." Hypoxia combined with these intensive care unit measures generally causes cognitive disorders that show slow recovery.

Diagnostic imaging of some people who have had COVID-19 shows changes in the brain's white matter that contains the long nerve fibers, or "wires," over which information flows from one brain region to another. These changes may be due to a lack of oxygen in the brain, the inflammatory immune system response to the virus, injury to blood vessels, or leaky blood vessels. This "diffuse white matter disease" might contribute to cognitive difficulties in people with COVID-19. Diffuse white matter disease is not uncommon in individuals requiring intensive hospital care, but it is not clear if it also occurs in those with mild-to-moderate severity of COVID-19 illness.

WHAT IS THE TYPICAL RECOVERY FROM COVID-19?

Fortunately, people who have mild-to-moderate symptoms typically recover in a few days or weeks. However, some people who have had only mild or moderate symptoms of COVID-19 continue to experience dysfunction of body systems—particularly in the lungs but also possibly affecting the liver, kidneys, heart, skin, and brain and nervous system—months after their infection. In rare cases, some individuals may develop new symptoms (called "sequelae") that stem from but were not present at the time of the initial infection. People who require intensive care for acute respiratory distress syndrome (ARDS), regardless of the cause, usually have a long period of recovery. Individuals with long-term effects, whether following mild or more severe COVID-19, have in some cases self-identified as having "long COVID" or "long-haul COVID." These long-term symptoms are included in the scientific term, post-acute sequelae of SARS-CoV-2 infection (PASC).

WHAT ARE POSSIBLE LONG-TERM NEUROLOGICAL COMPLICATIONS OF COVID-19?

Researchers are following some known acute effects of the virus to determine their relationship to the post-acute complications of COVID-19 infection. These post-acute effects usually include fatigue in combination with a series of other symptoms. These may include trouble with concentration and memory, sleep disorders, fluctuating heart rate and alternating sense of feeling hot or cold, cough, shortness of breath, problems with sleep, inability to exercise to previous normal levels, feeling sick for a day or two after exercising (postexertional malaise (PEM)), and pain in the muscle, joints, and chest. It is not yet known how the infection leads to these persistent symptoms and why in some individuals and not others.

Nerve Damage, Including Peripheral Neuropathy

Some symptoms experienced by some people weeks to months after COVID infection suggest the peripheral nervous system, the vast communication network that sends signals between the central nervous system (CNS; the brain and spinal cord) and all other parts of the body, is impaired. Peripheral nerves send many types of sensory information to the CNS, such as a message that the feet are cold. They also carry signals from the CNS to the rest of the body, including those that control voluntary movement. Nerve dysfunction is also a known complication in those with critical care illness such as the ARDS.

Symptoms of peripheral neuropathy vary depending on the type of nerves—motor, sensory, or autonomic—that are damaged.

- **Motor nerves.** They control the movement of all muscles under conscious control, such as those used for walking, grasping things, or talking. Damage to the motor nerves can cause muscle weakness and cramps.
- **Sensory nerves.** They carry messages from your sense of touch, sight, hearing, taste, and smell. They transmit information such as the feeling of a light touch, temperature, or pain. The symptoms of sensory nerve damage can include loss of sense of touch, temperature, and pain or a tingling sensation.
- **Autonomic nerves.** They control organs to regulate activities that people do not control consciously, such as breathing, digestion, and heart and gland functions. Common symptoms include excess or absence of sweating, heat intolerance, and drop in blood pressure upon standing. Postural orthostatic tachycardia syndrome (also known as "POTS") can increase the heart rate when standing up and cause symptoms such as lightheadedness (or fainting) or difficulty concentrating.

Fatigue and Post-Exertional Malaise

The most common persistent symptom weeks and months after COVID-19 infection is fatigue. The fatigue is similar to what one experiences with many viral infections such as the flu. The sense of fatigue can be brought on by both physical and mental activity. Some people are unable to return to work or school after COVID-19 due to fatigue, while others find it extremely difficult to accomplish their normal level of activity. Tasks such as walking the dog or going shopping can cause extreme tiredness and fatigue; some people cannot carry out everyday activities without feeling pain or tiredness. COVID-related complications such as depressed heart, lung, or kidney function, poor sleep, or muscle deconditioning are known to cause fatigue and affect the ability to exercise. Fatigue is very common in most inflammatory conditions. The cause(s) of fatigue in many of those suffering weeks and months after COVID-19 is not known.

PEM is a condition in which otherwise usual activities are followed by a period of very severe fatigue and a sense of feeling sick. PEM can occur with a delay after the activity but can last for days thereafter.

Cognitive Impairment/Altered Mental State

People with severe acute COVID-19 illness may develop confusion, delirium, and a depressed level of consciousness. Those suffering from postacute sequelae of COVID-19 frequently have difficulty concentrating and memory problems, sometimes called "brain fog." This impairment is a common symptom in those with severe fatigue of any cause. A variety of immune, metabolic, or blood vessel abnormalities or drug effects can contribute to the dramatic effects on cognitive function in the acute infection. Whether these also underlie the problems experienced weeks or months after mild or moderate illness is not known.

Muscle, Joint, and Chest Pain

Some people continue to report pain in a muscle or group of muscles (myalgia), aching joints, and fatigue after recovering from the initial course of the virus. Persistent muscle pain and chest pain are commonly reported by persons recovering from ARDS but are now being reported by those who had a mild or moderate infectious illness. Some individuals also have a sense of shortness of breath despite testing normal on pulmonary function tests.

Prolonged/Lingering Loss of Smell (Anosmia) or Taste

Some people who have had COVID-19 may lose their sense of taste or smell or the sensation of flavor. The loss of sense of taste or smell is characteristic of COVID-19 because the SARS-CoV-2 virus infects the tissue that forms the lining of the nose. The virus has been found to target certain cells in the nose that support the nerve cells. Those nerve cells detect odors and send that information to the brain. Damage to these supporting cells can cause smell or taste loss that can continue for weeks or months as these cells repair themselves or are replaced by new cells. During the recovery period, some odors may smell different—even sometimes unpleasant or foul—than people remember prior to being infected.

Persistent Fevers and Chills

Some people who recover from their acute (short-term) infection continue to have on-and-off fever, along with chills and body aches. Some people have a high, prolonged fever after the infection is gone, which might contribute to the sense of fatigue. In some instances, people who recover from the initial infection may have temperature dysregulation, in which it is difficult for the body to keep a normal temperature.

Prolonged Respiratory Effects and Lung Damage

COVID-19 is primarily a respiratory disease that can seriously affect the lungs during and after the infection. Some people with the disease have breathing difficulties, and some require supplemental oxygen support or mechanical ventilation via a respirator. The disease can also damage the muscles that help you breathe. Lung injury can cause low blood oxygen and brain hypoxia, which occurs when the brain is not getting enough oxygen. This can lead to cognitive impairment, seizures, stroke, and permanent damage to the brain and other organs. Results from several studies show that even in people who have had mild-to-moderate infection, the effects of COVID-19 can persist in the lungs for months. Some people develop pneumonia after their acute illness has passed. Several people need pulmonary (lung) rehabilitation to rebuild their lung function. Studies show several people who had the infection, particularly those who had a more severe course of illness, also develop scarring of the lung and permanent lung dysfunction.

Headaches
Headaches are often among the many symptoms that can accompany infection from the coronavirus. Some people continue to have mild-to-serious headaches sometimes for weeks after recovery. The sensation of pressure is different from a migraine, which may be brought on by stress. The headaches may be infrequent or occur chronically (some people report having daily headaches).

Sleep Disturbances
Some people with long-term neurological effects from the SARS-CoV-2 infection report having trouble falling asleep or staying asleep (insomnia), excessive daytime sleepiness (hypersomnia), unrefreshing sleep, and changes in sleep patterns. It may be difficult for some people to wake up and fall asleep at their regular times. Depression, anxiety, and posttraumatic stress disorder (PTSD) can negatively affect sleep. Sleep disorders can contribute to fatigue and cognitive troubles. Some people report an increase in pain, headache, and stress because of a lack of sleep. Continued loss of sleep also negatively affects attention and mood.

Anxiety, Depression, and Stress after COVID
The outbreak of COVID-19 is stressful for many people. People respond to stress in different ways, and it is normal to experience a range of emotions, including fear, anxiety, and grief. Being isolated from others during the infection, the real risk of death, and the stress of hospitalization and critical care can trigger PTSD. In addition, given the contagious nature of COVID-19, the individual is often not the only affected person in the family or circle of friends, some of whom may even have died. Some people may develop a mood or anxiety disorder.

HOW DO THE LONG-TERM EFFECTS OF SARS-COV-2 INFECTION/ COVID-19 RELATE TO MYALGIC ENCEPHALOMYELITIS/CHRONIC FATIGUE SYNDROME?
Some of the symptom clusters reported by people still suffering months after their COVID-19 infection overlap with symptoms

described by individuals with myalgic encephalomyelitis/chronic fatigue syndrome (ME/CFS). People with a diagnosis of ME/CFS have wide-ranging and debilitating effects including fatigue, PEM, unrefreshing sleep, cognitive difficulties, postural orthostatic tachycardia, and joint and muscle pain. Unfortunately, many people with ME/CFS do not return to predisease levels of activity. The cause of ME/CFS is unknown, but many people report its onset after an infectious-like illness. Rest, conserving energy, and pacing activities are important to feeling better but do not cure the disease. Although the long-term symptoms of COVID-19 may share features with it, ME/CFS is defined by symptom-based criteria, and there are no tests that confirm an ME/CFS diagnosis.

ME/CFS is not diagnosed until the key features, especially severe fatigue, PEM, and unrefreshing sleep, are present for greater than six months. It is now becoming more apparent that following infection with SARS-CoV-2/COVID-19, some individuals may continue to exhibit these symptoms beyond six months and qualify for an ME/CFS diagnosis. It is unknown how many people will develop ME/CFS after SARS-CoV-2 infection. It is possible that many individuals with ME/CFS, as well as other disorders impacting the nervous system, may benefit greatly if research on the long-term effects of COVID-19 uncovers the cause of debilitating symptoms including intense fatigue, problems with memory and concentration, and pain.

ARE YOU AT A HIGHER RISK IF YOU CURRENTLY HAVE A NEUROLOGICAL DISORDER?

Much is still unknown about the coronavirus, but people having one of several underlying medical conditions may have an increased risk of illness. However, not everyone with an underlying condition will be at risk of developing severe illness. People who have a neurological disorder may want to discuss their concerns with their doctors.

Because COVID-19 is a new virus, there is little information on the risk of getting the infection in people who have a neurological

disorder. People with any of these conditions might be at an increased risk of severe illness from COVID-19:
- cerebrovascular disease
- stroke
- obesity
- dementia
- diabetes
- high blood pressure

There is evidence that COVID-19 seems to disproportionately affect some racial and ethnic populations, perhaps because of higher rates of preexisting conditions such as heart disease, diabetes, and lung disease. Social determinants of health (such as access to health care, poverty, education, ability to remain socially distant, and where people live and work) also contribute to increased health risks and outcomes.

CAN COVID-19 CAUSE OTHER NEUROLOGICAL DISORDERS?

In some people, response to the coronavirus has been shown to increase the risk of stroke, dementia, muscle and nerve damage, encephalitis, and vascular disorders. Some researchers think the unbalanced immune system caused by reacting to the coronavirus may lead to autoimmune diseases, but it is too early to tell.

Anecdotal reports of other diseases and conditions that may be triggered by the immune system response to COVID-19 include parainfectious conditions that occur within days to a few weeks after infection:
- multisystem inflammatory syndrome (MIS)—which causes inflammation in the body's blood vessels
- transverse myelitis—an inflammation of the spinal cord
- Guillain-Barré syndrome (sometimes known as "acute polyradiculoneuritis")—a rare neurological disorder that can range from brief weakness to nearly devastating paralysis, leaving the person unable to breathe independently
- dysautonomia—dysfunction of the autonomic nerve system, which is involved with functions such as breathing, heart rate, and temperature control

- acute disseminating encephalomyelitis (ADEM)—an attack on the protective myelin covering of nerve fibers in the brain and spinal cord
- acute necrotizing hemorrhagic encephalopathy—a rare type of brain disease that causes lesions in certain parts of the brain and bleeding (hemorrhage) that can cause tissue death (necrosis)
- facial nerve palsies—(lack of function of a facial nerve) such as Bell palsy
- symptoms similar to Parkinson disease (PD)—reported in a few individuals who had no family history or early signs of the disease

DOES THE COVID-19 VACCINE CAUSE NEUROLOGICAL PROBLEMS?

Almost everyone should get the COVID-19 vaccination. It will help protect you from getting COVID-19. The vaccines are safe and effective and cannot give you the disease. Most side effects of the vaccine may feel like flu and are temporary and go away within a day or two. The U.S. Food and Drug Administration (FDA) continues to investigate any report of adverse consequences of the vaccine. Consult your primary care doctor or specialist if you have concerns regarding any preexisting known allergic or other severe reactions and vaccine safety.

A recent study from the United Kingdom demonstrated an increase in Guillain-Barré syndrome related to the AstraZeneca COVID-19 vaccine (virally delivered) but not the Moderna (messenger RNA vaccine). Guillain-Barré syndrome (a rare neurological disorder in which the body's immune system damages nerve cells, causing muscle weakness and sometimes paralysis) has also occurred in some people who have received the Janssen COVID-19 Vaccine (also virally delivered). In most of these people, symptoms began within weeks following receipt of the vaccine. The chance of having this occur after these vaccines is very low, five per million vaccinated persons in the U.K. study. The chance of developing Guillain-Barré syndrome was much higher if one develops COVID-19 infection (i.e., has a positive COVID test) than after receiving the AstraZeneca vaccine. The general sense is that there are COVID-19 vaccines that are safe in individuals whose

Guillain-Barré syndrome was not associated with a previous vaccination and that actual infection is the greater risk for developing Guillain-Barré syndrome.

The U.S. Centers for Disease Control and Prevention (CDC) site offers (www.cdc.gov/coronavirus/2019-ncov/index.html) information on vaccine resources. The National Institutes of Health (NIH) has information on vaccines for the coronavirus. The CDC has made public its report on the association of Guillain-Barré syndrome with the Janssen COVID-19 Vaccine, and no increased incidence occurred after vaccination with the Moderna or Pfizer vaccines.[1]

---

[1] "Coronavirus and the Nervous System," National Institute of Neurological Disorders and Stroke (NINDS), July 25, 2022. Available online. URL: www.ninds.nih.gov/current-research/coronavirus-and-ninds/coronavirus-and-nervous-system#top. Accessed December 9, 2022.

Chapter 7 | Understanding Your Coronavirus Risk Factors

FACTORS THAT LOWER OR INCREASE THE RISK OF TRANSMISSION
Length of Time
How long were you with the infected person?
   Longer exposure time increases the risk of transmission (e.g., contact longer than 15 minutes is more likely to result in transmission than two minutes of contact).

Cough or Heavy Breathing
Was the infected person coughing, singing, shouting, or breathing heavily?
   Activities such as coughing, singing, shouting, or breathing heavily due to exertion increase the risk of transmission.

Symptoms
Did the infected person have symptoms at the time?
   Being around people who are symptomatic increases the risk of transmission.

Masks
Were you or the infected person or both wearing a respirator (e.g., N95) or high-quality mask?

If one person was wearing a mask, the risk of transmission is decreased, and if both people were wearing masks, the risk is substantially decreased. Risk is also lower if the mask or respirator is a type that offers greater protection.

Ventilation and Filtration
How well-ventilated was the space?

More outdoor air can decrease the risk of transmission. Being outside would be a lower exposure risk than being indoors, even with good ventilation and filtration; both of those options would be a lower risk than being indoors with poor ventilation or filtration.

Distance
How close was the infected person to you?

Being closer to someone who is infected with COVID-19 increases the risk of transmission. Crowded settings can raise your likelihood of being close to someone with COVID-19.[1]

FACTORS THAT RAISE YOUR RISK OF GETTING VERY SICK FROM COVID-19

Vaccination, past infection, or timely access to testing and treatment can help protect you from getting very sick if you get COVID-19. However, some people are more likely than others to get very sick if they get COVID-19. This includes people who are older, are immunocompromised, have certain disabilities, or have underlying health conditions. Understanding your COVID-19 risk and the risks that might affect others can help you make decisions to protect yourself and others.

Age
Older adults (especially those aged 50 years and older, with risk increasing with older age) are more likely than younger people

---

[1] "Understanding Exposure Risks," Centers for Disease Control and Prevention (CDC), August 11, 2022. Available online. URL: www.cdc.gov/coronavirus/2019-ncov/your-health/risks-exposure.html. Accessed December 9, 2022.

to get very sick if they get COVID-19. This means they are more likely to need hospitalization, intensive care, or a ventilator to help them breathe, or they could die. Most COVID-19 deaths occur in people older than 65.

Immunocompromised or Weakened Immune System

Having a weakened immune system, also known as "being immunocompromised," can make you likely to get very sick if you get COVID-19. People who are immunocompromised, or who are taking medicines that weaken their immune system, may not be protected as well as others, even if they are up-to-date on their vaccines. EVUSHELD™ is a medicine given by a health-care provider every six months to help prevent COVID-19 before you are exposed or test positive for COVID-19. EVUSHELD™ remains protective but may offer less protection against certain strains of the Omicron variant. It is important that even if EVUSHELD™ is provided, you take multiple prevention measures.

Talk to your health-care provider about whether EVUSHELD™ is the best option for you.

Underlying Health Conditions

Certain underlying health conditions you have (e.g., obesity or chronic obstructive pulmonary disorder) may affect your risk of becoming very sick if you get COVID-19.

Often, the more health conditions you have, the higher your risk. Certain conditions increase your risk more than others. For example, severe heart disease increases your risk more than high blood pressure.

FACTORS THAT CAN HELP PROTECT YOU FROM GETTING VERY SICK FROM COVID-19
Vaccination

COVID-19 vaccines are safe and effective. Staying up-to-date with your COVID-19 vaccines is the best way to protect yourself and others around you from getting very sick, being hospitalized, or dying from COVID-19. Booster doses can give you additional protection. They can help enhance or restore protection that might have decreased over time.

People who are vaccinated with all recommended vaccine doses, including boosters, are far less likely to be hospitalized or die from COVID-19 than people of the same age who have not been vaccinated or who are not up-to-date on their COVID-19 vaccines. However, even though vaccines reduce their risk, some people, particularly older adults with multiple underlying health conditions or people who are immunocompromised, can still get very sick from COVID-19.

Timely Testing and Treatment

If you are at an increased risk of getting very sick from COVID-19, free medications are available that can reduce your chances of severe illness and death. It is important to get tested quickly if you think you are sick with COVID-19 because most treatment needs to be started within a few days of infection. It can also help have a plan for what to do if you feel sick or are diagnosed with COVID-19, especially if you have barriers to testing or treatment, such as transportation challenges or lack of insurance.

Previous Infection

Having a previous infection with the virus that causes COVID-19 offers some protection from future illness. However, people who have had previous infections can still be reinfected and get severe COVID-19, especially if their previous infection was months ago or with a different variant (e.g., Delta variant). There are also risks to being repeatedly infected, including the potential of longer-term symptoms or development of post-COVID conditions.

Studies show that people with previous infections who are vaccinated are less likely to be hospitalized than those with previous infections who are not vaccinated. This means that people who have had previous infection should still get vaccinated and boosted to

Understanding Your Coronavirus Risk Factors

increase their protection against COVID-19. Getting a COVID-19 vaccination is a safer way to build protection than getting sick with COVID-19.[2]

---

[2] "Factors That Affect Your Risk of Getting Very Sick from COVID-19," Centers for Disease Control and Prevention (CDC), October 19, 2022. Available online. URL: www.cdc.gov/coronavirus/2019-ncov/your-health/risks-getting-very-sick.html#:~:text=Certain%20underlying%20health%20conditions%20you,your%20risk%20more%20than%20others. Accessed December 9, 2022.

Chapter 8 | Clinical Presentation in Specific Population

Chapter Contents
Section 8.1—COVID-19 in Pregnant and Recently
            Pregnant People..99
Section 8.2—COVID-19 in People with Preexisting
            Medical Conditions 103
Section 8.3—COVID-19 in People with Human
            Immunodeficiency Virus 111
Section 8.4—COVID-19 in People Who Are
            Immunocompromised.. 115
Section 8.5—COVID-19 in People with Asthma....................... 121
Section 8.6—COVID-19 Infections in Pets and Animals.......... 124

Section 8.1 | COVID-19 in Pregnant and Recently Pregnant People

INCREASED RISK OF SEVERE ILLNESS

If you are pregnant or were recently pregnant, you are more likely to get severely ill from COVID-19 than people who are not pregnant. Pregnancy causes changes in the body that could make it easier to get very sick from respiratory viruses such as the one that causes COVID-19. These changes in the body can continue after pregnancy.

Severe illness means that a person with COVID-19 may need the following:
- hospitalization
- admission into an intensive care unit (ICU)
- a ventilator or special equipment to help them breathe

People with COVID-19 who become severely ill can die.

Certain Factors Can Increase Risk

Other factors can further increase the risk of getting very sick from COVID-19 during or recently after pregnancy, such as the following:
- having certain underlying medical conditions
- being older than 25 years
- living or working in a community with high numbers of COVID-19 cases
- living or working in a community with low levels of COVID-19 vaccination
- working in places where it is difficult or not possible to avoid contact with people who might be sick with COVID-19
- being part of some racial and ethnic minority groups that experience social and health disparities

EFFECT ON PREGNANCY OUTCOMES

People with COVID-19 during pregnancy are more likely to experience complications that can affect their pregnancy and developing baby than people without COVID-19 during pregnancy. For example, COVID-19 during pregnancy increases the risk of delivering preterm (earlier than 37 weeks) or stillborn infants. People with COVID-19 during pregnancy may also be likely to have other pregnancy complications.

COVID-19 VACCINES AND PREGNANCY

COVID-19 vaccination is recommended for everyone aged six months and older, including people who are pregnant, breastfeeding, or trying to get pregnant now or might become pregnant in the future. This recommendation includes getting boosters when it is time to get one. If you have questions about getting vaccinated, talking with your health-care professional might help but is not required.

Getting vaccinated prevents severe illness, hospitalizations, and death. People who have not received a COVID-19 vaccine should get vaccinated as soon as possible and continue masking. To maximize protection from variants and prevent possibly spreading the virus to others, people who are up-to-date with their COVID-19 vaccines should wear a mask indoors in public in areas with a high COVID-19 community level. With the emergence of variants, this is more urgent than ever.

REDUCING YOUR RISK OF GETTING COVID-19

It is especially important for people who are or were recently pregnant, as well as those who visit or live with them, to take steps to protect themselves and others from getting COVID-19.

Limit in-person interactions with people who might have been exposed to COVID-19, including people within your household, as much as possible. If you or someone in your household is sick with COVID-19, follow guidance for isolation.

Clinical Presentation in Specific Population

STAYING HEALTHY DURING AND AFTER YOUR PREGNANCY

- Keep all of your health-care appointments during and after pregnancy. Visit your health-care provider for all recommended appointments. If you are concerned about going to your appointments in person because of COVID-19, ask your health-care professional what steps they are taking to protect patients from COVID-19 or ask about telemedicine options. If you need help finding a health-care professional, contact your nearest hospital, clinic, community health center, or health department.
- Talk to your health-care professional about how to stay healthy and take care of yourself and the baby.
- Ask any questions you have about the best place to deliver your baby. Delivering a baby is always safest under the care of trained health-care professionals.
- You should also talk to your health-care professional if you think you are experiencing depression during or after pregnancy.
- Get recommended vaccines during pregnancy. These vaccines can help protect you and your baby.
    - Get a flu vaccine every year. Others living in your household should also get vaccinated to protect themselves and you.
    - Get the Tdap vaccine to protect your baby against whooping cough, which can have similar symptoms to COVID-19. The Centers for Disease Control and Prevention (CDC) recommends all pregnant people receive a Tdap vaccine during each pregnancy. In addition, everyone who is around the baby should be up-to-date with their whooping cough vaccine.
- Call your health-care professional if you have any concerns about your pregnancy, if you get sick, or if you think that you may have COVID-19.
- Do not delay getting emergency care because of worries about getting COVID-19. Emergency departments have steps in place to protect you from getting COVID-19 if you need medical care.

- If you need emergency help, call 911 right away. If someone else is driving you to the emergency department, call the emergency facility while you are on the way.
- If you must drive yourself, call before you start driving.
- Tell them that you are pregnant or were recently pregnant and are having an emergency.
- Seek medical care immediately if you experience any urgent maternal warning signs and symptoms (e.g., a headache that would not go away, dizziness, fever, severe swelling of the hand, face, arm, or leg, trouble breathing, chest pain, fast-beating heart, severe nausea and throwing up, or vaginal bleeding or discharge during or after pregnancy). These symptoms could indicate a potentially life-threatening complication.

WHAT TO DO IF YOU ARE SICK OR THINK YOU WERE EXPOSED TO COVID-19

If you have any symptoms of COVID-19, contact your health-care professional within 24 hours and follow the steps for when you feel sick.

If you are diagnosed with COVID-19, learn about breastfeeding and caring for newborns when the mother has COVID-19. Current evidence suggests that breast milk is not likely to spread the virus to babies.[1]

---

[1] "Pregnant and Recently Pregnant People," Centers for Disease Control and Prevention (CDC), October 25, 2022. Available online. URL: www.cdc.gov/coronavirus/2019-ncov/need-extra-precautions/pregnant-people.html. Accessed December 12, 2022.

Clinical Presentation in Specific Population

Section 8.2 | **COVID-19 in People with Preexisting Medical Conditions**

Based on the current evidence, a person with any of the conditions listed later in this section is likely to get very sick from COVID-19. This means that a person with one or more of these conditions who get very sick from COVID-19 (has a severe illness from COVID-19) is likely to:
- be hospitalized
- need intensive care
- require a ventilator to help them breathe
- die

In addition, the following can be the reasons for people get very sick from COVID-19:
- Older adults are at the highest risk of getting very sick from COVID-19. More than 81 percent of COVID-19 deaths occur in people over age 65. The number of deaths among people over age 65 is 97 times higher than the number of deaths among people aged 18–29.
- A person's risk of severe illness from COVID-19 increases as the number of underlying medical conditions they have increased.
- Some people are at increased risk of getting very sick or dying from COVID-19 because of where they live or work or because they cannot get health care. This includes many people from racial and ethnic minority groups and people with disabilities.
  - Studies have shown people from racial and ethnic minority groups are also dying from COVID-19 at younger ages. People in racial and ethnic minority groups are often younger when they develop chronic medical conditions and may be more likely to have more than one medical condition.
  - People with disabilities are more likely than those without disabilities to have chronic health

conditions, live in shared group (also called "congregate") settings, and face more barriers in accessing health care. Studies have shown that some people with certain disabilities are likely to get COVID-19 and have worse outcomes.

Staying up-to-date with COVID-19 vaccines and taking COVID-19 prevention actions are important. This is especially important if you are older or have severe health conditions or more than one health condition, including those on this list.

MEDICAL CONDITIONS
Cancer
Having cancer can make you likely to get very sick from COVID-19. Treatments for many types of cancer can weaken your body's ability to fight off disease. At this time, based on available studies, having a history of cancer may increase your risk.

Chronic Kidney Disease
Having chronic kidney disease at any stage can make you likely to get very sick from COVID-19.

Chronic Liver Disease
Having a chronic liver disease can make you more likely to get very sick from COVID-19. Chronic liver disease can include alcohol-related liver disease, nonalcoholic fatty liver disease, autoimmune hepatitis, and cirrhosis (or scarring of the liver).

Chronic Lung Diseases
Having a chronic lung disease can make you more likely to get very sick from COVID-19. Chronic lung diseases can include:
- asthma, if it is moderate to severe
- bronchiectasis (thickening of the lungs' airways)
- bronchopulmonary dysplasia (chronic lung disease affecting newborns)

Clinical Presentation in Specific Population

- chronic obstructive pulmonary disease (COPD), including emphysema and chronic bronchitis
- having damaged or scarred lung tissue known as "interstitial lung disease" (including idiopathic pulmonary fibrosis)
- pulmonary embolism (blood clot in the lungs)
- pulmonary hypertension (high blood pressure in the lungs)

Cystic Fibrosis
Having cystic fibrosis (CF), with or without a lung transplant or other solid organ transplants (such as kidney, liver, intestines, heart, and pancreas), can make you likely to get very sick from COVID-19.

Dementia or Other Neurological Conditions
Having neurological conditions, such as dementia, can make you likely to get very sick from COVID-19.

Diabetes (Type 1 or 2)
Having either type 1 or type 2 diabetes can make you likely to get very sick from COVID-19.

Disabilities
People with some types of disabilities may be likely to get very sick from COVID-19 because of underlying medical conditions, living in congregate settings, or systemic health and social inequities, including people with:
- any type of disability that makes it more difficult to do certain activities or interact with the world around them, including people who need help with self-care or daily activities
- attention deficit hyperactivity disorder (ADHD)
- cerebral palsy
- birth defects

- intellectual and developmental disabilities
- learning disabilities
- spinal cord injuries
- Down syndrome

Heart Conditions

Having heart conditions such as heart failure, coronary artery disease, cardiomyopathies, and possibly high blood pressure (hypertension) can make you likely to get very sick from COVID-19.

HIV Infection

Having human immunodeficiency virus (HIV) can make you likely to get very sick from COVID-19.

Immunocompromised Condition or Weakened Immune System

Some people are immunocompromised or have a weakened immune system because of a medical condition or a treatment for a condition. This includes people who have cancer and are on chemotherapy or who have had a solid organ transplant, such as a kidney transplant or heart transplant, and are taking medication to keep their transplant. Other people have to use certain types of medicines for a long time, such as corticosteroids, that weaken their immune system. Such long-term uses can lead to secondary or acquired immunodeficiency. Other people have a weakened immune system because of lifelong conditions. For example, some people inherit problems with their immune systems. One example is called "primary immunodeficiency." Being immunocompromised can make you more likely to get very sick from COVID-19 or be sick for a longer period of time.

People who are immunocompromised or are taking medicines that weaken their immune system may not be protected even if they are up-to-date on their vaccines. Talk with your health-care provider about wearing a mask at a medium COVID-19 Community Level and what additional precautions may be necessary at medium or high COVID-19 Community Levels.

Clinical Presentation in Specific Population

Mental Health Conditions
Having mood disorders, including depression and schizophrenia spectrum disorders, can make you likely to get very sick from COVID-19.

Overweight and Obesity
Overweight (defined as a body mass index (BMI) is 25 kg/m² or higher but under 30 kg/m²), obesity (BMI is 30 kg/m² or higher but under 40 kg/m²), or severe obesity (BMI is 40 kg/m² or higher), can make you more likely to get very sick from COVID-19. The risk of severe illness from COVID-19 increases sharply with a higher BMI.

Physical Inactivity
People who do little or no physical activity are more likely to get very sick from COVID-19 than those who are physically active. Being physically active is important to being healthy.

Pregnancy
Pregnant and recently pregnant people (for at least 42 days following the end of pregnancy) are likely to get very sick from COVID-19 compared with nonpregnant people.

Sickle Cell Disease or Thalassemia
Having hemoglobin blood disorders such as sickle cell disease or thalassemia (inherited red blood cell disorders) can make you likely to get very sick from COVID-19.

Smoker, Current or Former
Being a current or former cigarette smoker can make you likely to get very sick from COVID-19. If you currently smoke, quit. If you used to smoke, do not start again. If you have never smoked, do not start.

Solid Organ or Blood Stem Cell Transplant
Having had a solid organ or blood stem cell transplant, which includes bone marrow transplants, can make you likely to get very sick from COVID-19.

Stroke or Cerebrovascular Disease
Having cerebrovascular disease, such as having a stroke that affects blood flow to the brain, can make you likely to get very sick from COVID-19.

Substance Use Disorders
Having a substance use disorder (such as alcohol, opioid, or cocaine use disorder) can make you likely to get very sick from COVID-19.

Tuberculosis
Having tuberculosis (TB) can make you likely to get very sick from COVID-19.

ADDITIONAL INFORMATION ABOUT CHILDREN AND TEENS
Current evidence suggests that children with medical complexity; genetic, neurologic, or metabolic conditions; or congenital heart disease can be at increased risk for getting very sick from COVID-19. Like adults, children with obesity, diabetes, asthma or chronic lung disease, or sickle cell disease or those who are immunocompromised can also be at increased risk for getting very sick from COVID-19.

ACTIONS YOU CAN TAKE
It is important to protect yourself and others by taking COVID-19 prevention actions:
- Stay up-to-date with your COVID-19 vaccines.
- Improve ventilation.
- Get tested if you have symptoms.
- Follow recommendations for what to do if you have been exposed.

Clinical Presentation in Specific Population

- Stay home if you have suspected or confirmed COVID-19.
- Seek treatment if you have COVID-19 and are at high risk of getting very sick.
- Avoid contact with people who have suspected or confirmed COVID-19.
- Wear a mask or respirator.
- Increase space and distance.

SEEK CARE WHEN NEEDED

- Call your health-care provider if you have any concerns about your medical conditions or if you get sick and think that you may have COVID-19. Discuss steps you can take to manage your health and risks. If you need emergency help, call 911 right away.
- Do not delay getting care for your medical condition because of COVID-19. Emergency departments, urgent care, clinics, and your health-care provider have infection prevention plans to help protect you from getting COVID-19 if you need care.

CONTINUE MEDICATIONS AND PREVENTIVE CARE

- Continue your medicines and do not change your treatment plan without talking to your health-care provider.
- Have at least a 30-day supply of prescription and nonprescription medicines. Talk to a health-care provider, insurer, or pharmacist about getting an extra supply (i.e., more than 30 days) of prescription medicines, if possible, to reduce your trips to the pharmacy.
- Follow your current treatment plan (e.g., Asthma Action Plan (www.cdc.gov/asthma/actionplan.html) Plan, dialysis schedule, blood sugar testing, nutrition, and exercise recommendations) to keep your medical condition(s) under control.
- When possible, keep your appointments (e.g., vaccinations and blood pressure checks) with your

health-care provider. Check with your health-care provider about safety precautions for office visits and ask about telemedicine or virtual health-care appointment options.
- Learn about stress and coping. You may feel increased stress during this pandemic. Fear and anxiety can be overwhelming and cause strong emotions. It can be helpful to talk with a professional such as a counselor, therapist, psychologist, or psychiatrist. Ask your primary care provider if you would like to speak with a professional. Getting regular exercise and being physically active is also a great way to reduce stress.

ACCOMMODATE DIETARY NEEDS AND AVOID TRIGGERS
- Have nonperishable food choices such as canned goods available that meet your needs based on your medical condition (e.g., kidney diet and KCER 3-Day Emergency Diet Plan, diabetic diet).
- Know the triggers for your condition and avoid them when possible (e.g., avoid asthma triggers by having another member of your household clean and disinfect your house for you or avoid possible sickle cell disease triggers to prevent pain crises).[2]

---

[2] "People with Certain Medical Conditions," Centers for Disease Control and Prevention (CDC), December 6, 2022. Available online. URL: www.cdc.gov/coronavirus/2019-ncov/need-extra-precautions/people-with-medical-conditions.html. Accessed December 12, 2022.

Clinical Presentation in Specific Population

Section 8.3 | COVID-19 in People with Human Immunodeficiency Virus

People with human immunodeficiency virus (HIV) may have concerns and questions about COVID-19, including the risk of serious illness and vaccine safety. The Centers for Disease Control and Prevention (CDC) will continue to provide updated information as it becomes available.

ARE PEOPLE WITH HUMAN IMMUNODEFICIENCY VIRUS AT A HIGHER RISK FOR SERIOUS ILLNESS FROM COVID-19 THAN OTHER PEOPLE?

We are still learning about COVID-19 and how it affects people with HIV. Nearly half of the people in the United States with diagnosed HIV are aged 50 and older. People with HIV also have higher rates of certain underlying health conditions. Older age and underlying health conditions can make people likely to become seriously ill if they get COVID-19. This is especially true for people with advanced HIV or people with HIV who are not on treatment.

People at an increased risk for severe illness, as well as those who live with or visit them, should take precautions (including getting vaccinated and wearing a well-fitting mask) to protect themselves and others from COVID-19.

DO COVID-19 TREATMENTS INTERACT WITH MEDICINE TO TREAT OR PREVENT HUMAN IMMUNODEFICIENCY VIRUS?

Some COVID-19 treatments can interact with antiretroviral therapy (ART) used to treat HIV. If you have HIV, let your health-care provider know before starting COVID-19 treatment. There are no known interactions between HIV treatment and the medicine used to prevent COVID-19 (Evusheld).

For people without HIV, there is no evidence that currently available medicine used to treat or prevent COVID-19 will interact with pre-exposure prophylaxis (PrEP) to prevent HIV.

If you have possible symptoms of COVID-19, have had a positive test, or have been exposed to the virus that causes COVID-19, talk to your health-care provider to see if you are eligible for COVID-19 treatment or preventive medicine.

DO COVID-19 VACCINES INCREASE THE RISK OF SOMEONE GETTING HUMAN IMMUNODEFICIENCY VIRUS?

No. There is no association between COVID-19 vaccines and the risk for HIV infection. COVID-19 vaccines improve the immune system's ability to prevent COVID-19 and protect vaccinated people from the more severe complications of COVID-19.

ARE COVID-19 VACCINES SAFE FOR PEOPLE WITH HUMAN IMMUNODEFICIENCY VIRUS?

Yes. COVID-19 vaccines are safe for people with HIV. COVID-19 vaccines meet the Food and Drug Administration's rigorous scientific standards for safety, effectiveness, and manufacturing quality, and people with HIV were included in vaccine clinical trials.

Authorized or approved COVID-19 vaccines will continue to undergo the most intensive safety monitoring. This includes using established and new safety monitoring systems to make sure that COVID-19 vaccines are safe.

HOW MANY DOSES OF THE COVID-19 VACCINE DO PEOPLE WITH HUMAN IMMUNODEFICIENCY VIRUS NEED TO GET?

COVID-19 Vaccine Primary Series

COVID-19 vaccines are recommended for everyone who is eligible. The number of vaccine doses you need depends on the type of vaccine you receive.

Additional Primary Shot

After completing the COVID-19 vaccine primary series, some people who have advanced HIV (including an acquired immune deficiency syndrome (AIDS) diagnosis) or who have HIV and are not taking HIV treatment should get an additional primary

Clinical Presentation in Specific Population

shot. The additional primary shot is intended to improve a person's immune response to their two-dose COVID-19 vaccine primary series. People who are eligible for an additional primary shot should receive this dose before they get a booster shot. Talk to your health-care provider to determine if getting an additional primary shot is right for you.

The CDC does not recommend an additional primary shot of the COVID-19 vaccine for people with HIV who are virally suppressed or who do not have advanced HIV.

Booster Shot
The CDC recommends that everyone, including people with HIV, get a booster shot when they are eligible.

WILL COVID-19 VACCINES INTERFERE WITH MEDICINE TO PREVENT OR TREAT HUMAN IMMUNODEFICIENCY VIRUS?
There is no evidence that COVID-19 vaccines interfere with PrEP to prevent HIV or with ART to treat HIV.

WHAT CAN PEOPLE WITH HUMAN IMMUNODEFICIENCY VIRUS DO TO PROTECT THEMSELVES FROM COVID-19?
People with HIV can protect themselves from COVID-19 by following the CDC's COVID-19 prevention recommendations.

If you have HIV and are taking your HIV medicine as prescribed, it is important to continue your treatment and follow your health-care provider's advice. This is the best way to keep your immune system healthy. People with HIV should also continue to maintain a healthy lifestyle.

Here are more steps that people with HIV can take:
- Make sure you have at least a 30-day (or longer) supply of your HIV medicine and any other medicines or medical supplies you need for managing HIV. Ask your health-care provider about getting your medicine by mail.
- Talk to your health-care provider and make sure all your vaccinations are up-to-date, including

vaccinations against seasonal influenza (flu) and bacterial pneumonia. These vaccine-preventable diseases affect people with HIV more than others.
- When possible, keep your medical appointments. Check with your health-care provider about safety precautions for office visits and ask about telemedicine or remote clinical care options.
- People with HIV can sometimes be more likely than others to need extra help from friends, family, neighbors, community health workers, and others. If you become sick, make sure you stay in touch by phone or email with people who can help you.

WHAT SHOULD YOU DO IF YOU THINK YOU MIGHT HAVE COVID-19?

Call your health-care provider if you develop symptoms that could be consistent with COVID-19.

It is important to continue taking your HIV medicine as prescribed. This will help keep your immune system healthy.

CAN HUMAN IMMUNODEFICIENCY VIRUS MEDICINE ANTIRETROVIRAL THERAPY BE USED TO TREAT COVID-19?

Currently, treatment for COVID-19 is limited. There are no HIV medicines approved to treat COVID-19. People with HIV should not switch their HIV medicine in an attempt to prevent or treat COVID-19.

Some clinical trials are looking at whether HIV medicines can treat COVID-19. Other trials are looking at the effectiveness of different drugs to treat COVID-19 in people with HIV. They are also looking to better understand how people with HIV manage COVID-19.

TRAVEL CONCERNS FOR PEOPLE WITH HUMAN IMMUNODEFICIENCY VIRUS

Everyone, including people with HIV, should follow the CDC's COVID-19 travel recommendations.

Clinical Presentation in Specific Population

WHAT CAN EVERYONE DO TO MINIMIZE STIGMA ABOUT COVID-19?

Minimizing stigma and misinformation about COVID-19 is very important. People with HIV have experience in dealing with stigma and can be allies in preventing COVID-19 stigma. Learn how you can reduce stigma and help prevent the spread of rumors about COVID-19.[3]

Section 8.4 | COVID-19 in People Who Are Immunocompromised

Some people who are immunocompromised (have a weakened immune system) are likely to get sick with COVID-19 or be sick for a longer period. People can be immunocompromised either due to a medical condition or from receipt of immunosuppressive medications or treatments.

Examples of medical conditions or treatments that may result in moderate-to-severe immunocompromise include but are not limited to the following:
- active treatment for solid tumor and hematologic malignancies
- hematologic malignancies associated with poor responses to COVID-19 vaccines regardless of current treatment status (e.g., chronic lymphocytic leukemia, non-Hodgkin lymphoma, multiple myeloma, acute leukemia)
- receipt of a solid-organ transplant or an islet transplant and taking immunosuppressive therapy
- receipt of chimeric antigen receptor (CAR) T-cell therapy or hematopoietic stem cell transplant (within two years of transplantation or taking immunosuppressive therapy)
- moderate or severe primary immunodeficiency (e.g., common variable immunodeficiency disease, severe

---

[3] "HIV and COVID-19 Basics," Centers for Disease Control and Prevention (CDC), July 12, 2022. Available online. URL: www.cdc.gov/hiv/basics/covid-19.html. Accessed December 12, 2022.

combined immunodeficiency, DiGeorge syndrome, Wiskott-Aldrich syndrome)
- advanced or untreated human immunodeficiency virus (HIV) infection (people with HIV and clusters of differentiation 4 (CD4) cell counts less than 200/mm^3, history of an acquired immune deficiency syndrome (AIDS) defining illness without immune reconstitution, or clinical manifestations of symptomatic HIV)
- active treatment with high-dose corticosteroids (i.e., 20 mg or more of prednisone or equivalent per day when administered for two or more weeks), alkylating agents, antimetabolites, transplant-related immunosuppressive drugs, cancer chemotherapeutic agents classified as severely immunosuppressive, tumor necrosis factor (TNF) blockers, and other biologic agents that are immunosuppressive or immunomodulatory

Talk to your health-care provider if you have another medical condition or are on medication that may not be reflected above.

If you or someone you live or spend time with is immunocompromised, it is important to have a COVID-19 plan to protect yourself from infection and prepare for what to do if you get sick. Information on this page can help you build a COVID-19 plan for preventing, diagnosing, and treating COVID, so you know what to do and can act quickly if you are exposed, develop symptoms, or test positive and when COVID-19 levels are increasing in your community.

HOW TO PROTECT YOURSELF
Stay Up-to-Date on COVID-19 Vaccinations
COVID-19 vaccines are effective at protecting people—especially those who are up-to-date—from getting seriously ill, being hospitalized, and even dying. As with vaccines for other diseases, you are protected best when you stay up-to-date with your COVID-19 vaccines. The people you live or spend time with can help protect you and themselves by staying up-to-date on their COVID-19 vaccines too.

Clinical Presentation in Specific Population

You are up-to-date with your COVID-19 vaccines when you have received all doses in the primary series and all boosters recommended for you, when eligible. Since your immune response to COVID-19 vaccination may not be as strong as in people who are not immunocompromised, you have different recommendations for COVID-19 vaccines, including boosters.

Take Extra Precautions

Even if you stay up-to-date on COVID-19 vaccines and receive Evusheld™, taking multiple prevention steps can provide additional layers of protection from COVID-19:
- Wear a well-fitting, high-quality mask or respirator. Properly fitting respirators provide the highest level of protection.
- Avoid poorly ventilated or crowded indoor settings.
- When indoors with others, try to improve ventilation as much as possible.
- Wash your hands often with soap and water or use a hand sanitizer that contains at least 60 percent alcohol.

KNOW WHAT TO DO IF YOU GET SICK

It is important to be prepared and know what to do if you get sick with COVID-19. Do not delay seeking medical care.

What You Can Do Now
- Know the symptoms of COVID-19.
- Learn how to check your COVID-19 Community Level. Knowing your COVID-19 Community Levels will help you decide when to add layers of protection, such as wearing a mask.
- Know how to get tested as soon as possible if you develop symptoms.
  - Order free at-home tests to have when you need them. If you need more tests, check with your health insurance, Medicaid, or Medicare plan to learn what tests are available.

- Know where free or low-cost testing locations are near you, so you know where to go.
- Know how to reach a health-care provider right away, including after-hours or on weekends. Ask them about telehealth appointment options.
- Have an updated list of all your current medications in case you need to see a different provider.

What to Do If You Were Exposed to COVID-19
- Determine if you should stay home.
- Monitor your health for COVID-19 symptoms and get tested at least five days after you had close contact with someone with COVID-19, even if you do not develop symptoms.
- Wear a high-quality mask for 10 full days any time you are around others inside your home or in public. Do not go to places where you are unable to wear a mask.

What to Do If You Have COVID-19 Symptoms
- Stay home.
- Get tested right away. Use a self-test at home or find a testing location near you.

What to Do If You Test Positive for COVID-19
Effective treatments are now widely available and free, and you may be eligible.
- Contact your health-care provider, health department, or community health center to learn about treatment options. Do not delay! Treatment must be started soon after you first develop symptoms to be effective.
- If you do not have timely access to a health-care provider, check if a test-to-treat location is in your community. You can get tested, receive a prescription

from a health-care provider (either on-site or by telehealth), and have it filled all at one location.
- Isolate until it is safe to be around others. The Centers for Disease Control and Prevention (CDC) recommends that you isolate for at least 10 and up to 20 days. Check with your health-care provider to learn when you can be around others.
- Monitor your symptoms. Call your health-care provider if you develop symptoms that are severe or concerning to you. If you notice emergency warning signs, call 911 or call ahead to your local emergency facility.

GET TREATMENT QUICKLY

If you test positive for COVID-19, oral antiviral treatments are available for people who are likely to get very sick.

Do not delay. Treatment must be started right away to be effective. Talk to your health-care provider about what treatment options are best for you.

Antiviral Treatments

Antiviral treatments may help your body fight COVID-19 by stopping the severe acute respiratory syndrome coronavirus 2 (SARS-CoV-2, the virus that causes COVID-19) from multiplying in your body or by lowering the amount of the virus within your body. You can get a prescription from your health-care provider or a test-to-treat location. Oral antivirals can be taken at home and must be given within five days after the first symptoms of COVID-19 appear.

Convalescent Plasma

Some people with COVID-19 who are immunocompromised or are receiving immunosuppressive treatment may benefit from a treatment called "convalescent plasma." Your health-care provider can help decide whether this treatment is right for you.

BUILD YOUR PERSONAL COVID-19 PLAN

Make a COVID-19 plan now, so you are prepared. Consider the ways you will protect yourself and how to be prepared if you get sick with COVID-19. Include how you will adjust your plan if the COVID-19 situation changes in your community.

Your plan should include the following:
- What are you doing to protect yourself and prepare (in case you get COVID-19)?
- What will you do if you are exposed or develop symptoms?
- What will you do if you test positive?

Talk with your family, friends, and health-care provider about your plan.

Share your COVID-19 plan with your family, friends, and health-care providers, so they can support your prevention and preparation steps. Consider how others may help you if you get sick and identify the supplies you may need. Be sure to stick to your treatment plans, to stick to your routine health-care appointments, and to have all your prescriptions filled. Plan for options for work, childcare, and other responsibilities that may cause stress if you were to become sick.

COVID-19 remains a major health concern, and this can be stressful to manage. Understanding what you can do to protect yourself and what to do if you get sick can help minimize that stress. Take as many steps as you can to prevent COVID-19 and get treated quickly if you test positive for COVID-19.[4]

---

[4] "People Who Are Immunocompromised," Centers for Disease Control and Prevention (CDC), December 5, 2022. Available online. URL: www.cdc.gov/coronavirus/2019-ncov/need-extra-precautions/people-who-are-immuno-compromised.html#:~:text=Some%20people%20who%20are%20immunocompromised,of%20immunosuppressive%20medications%20or%20treatments. Accessed December 13, 2022.

Clinical Presentation in Specific Population

Section 8.5 | COVID-19 in People with Asthma

People with moderate-to-severe or uncontrolled asthma are likely to be hospitalized from COVID-19. Take steps to protect yourself.

FOLLOW YOUR ASTHMA ACTION PLAN
- Keep your asthma under control by following your asthma action plan.
- Avoid your asthma triggers.
- Continue current medications, including any inhalers with steroids in them ("steroids" is another word for corticosteroids). Know how to use your inhaler.
- Do not stop any medications or change your asthma treatment plan without talking to your health-care provider.
- Talk to your health-care provider, insurer, and pharmacist about creating an emergency supply of prescription medications, such as asthma inhalers. Make sure that you have 30 days of nonprescription medications and supplies on hand in case you need to stay home for a long time.
- Be careful around cleaning agents and disinfectants.

Follow the recommendations below to reduce your chance of an asthma attack while cleaning. Follow recommendations for cleaning your home and your facility.

CLEANING AND DISINFECTING YOUR HOME
- If you have asthma, do the following:
  - Ask an adult without asthma to clean and disinfect surfaces and objects for you.
  - Stay in another room when cleaners or disinfectants are being used and right after their use.
  - Use cleaning agents and disinfectants only when necessary. In routine situations, high-touch surfaces

and objects might be cleaned effectively with soap and water.
- Make a list of the urgent care or health facilities near you that provide nebulizer/asthma treatments and keep it close to your phone.
- If you have an asthma attack, move away from the trigger, such as the cleaning agent or disinfectant or the area that was disinfected. Follow your asthma action plan. Call 911 for medical emergencies.
- The person cleaning and disinfecting should do the following:
  - Choose disinfectants that are less likely to cause an asthma attack, using the list of products approved by the U.S. Environmental Protection Agency (EPA), such as the following:
    - Products with hydrogen peroxide (no stronger than 3%) or ethanol (ethyl alcohol). Ensure that products with hydrogen peroxide do not contain other chemicals that can trigger asthma attacks, such as peroxyacetic acid or peracetic acid.
  - Limit the use of chemicals that can trigger asthma attacks, such as bleach (sodium hypochlorite) or quaternary ammonium compounds (e.g., benzalkonium chloride), and do not use them in enclosed spaces.
  - Follow additional precautions for cleaning and disinfecting places where people with asthma might be, to reduce exposure to asthma triggers.
- Use products safely and correctly:
  - Always read and follow the directions on the product label to ensure you are using it safely and effectively.
  - Wear skin protection such as gloves and consider eye protection to protect yourself against splashes.
  - Make sure there is enough airflow (ventilation).
  - Use only the amount recommended on the label.
  - Use water at room temperature for dilution (unless stated otherwise on the label).

Clinical Presentation in Specific Population

- Do not mix chemical products. Label diluted cleaning solutions.
- Spray or pour spray products onto a cleaning cloth or paper towel instead of spraying the product directly onto the cleaning surface (if the product label allows).
- Store products safely and correctly:
  - Store and use chemicals out of the reach of children and pets.
  - Label diluted cleaning solutions.
  - Follow the EPA's six steps (www.epa.gov/coronavirus/six-steps-safe-effective-disinfectant-use) for safe and effective disinfectant use.

IF YOU FEEL ILL

Call your health-care provider to ask about your symptoms. If you do not have a health-care provider, contact your nearest community health center or health department. Remember to call 911 for medical emergencies.

TAKE STEPS TO HELP YOURSELF COPE WITH STRESS AND ANXIETY

It is natural for some people to feel concerned or stressed as more cases of COVID-19 are discovered, and our communities act to combat the spread of disease. Strong emotions can trigger an asthma attack.[5]

---

[5] "People with Moderate to Severe Asthma," Centers for Disease Control and Prevention (CDC), April 7, 2022. Available online. URL: www.cdc.gov/coronavirus/2019-ncov/need-extra-precautions/asthma.html. Accessed December 13, 2022.

Section 8.6 | COVID-19 Infections in Pets and Animals

CAN PEOPLE GET COVID-19 FROM PETS OR OTHER ANIMALS?
Based on the information available to date, the risk of pets or other animals spreading COVID-19 to people is considered to be low.

CAN PETS OR OTHER ANIMALS GET COVID-19 FROM PEOPLE?
The virus that causes COVID-19 can spread from people to animals, including pets, zoo animals, and wildlife, and may spread to other animals, especially during close contact. If a person inside the household becomes sick, isolate that person from everyone else, including pets and other animals.

If you are sick with COVID-19 (either suspected or confirmed by a test), you should avoid contact with your pets and other animals, just like you would with people. Contact includes petting, snuggling, kissing, licking, sharing food, and sleeping in the same bed.

We know that most pets that get infected do so after close contact with their owner or other household members with COVID-19. Talk to your veterinarian if your pet gets sick or if you have any concerns about your pet's health.

SHOULD YOU GET YOUR PET TESTED FOR COVID-19?
Routine testing of pets for COVID-19 is not recommended at this time. There is currently no evidence that pets are a source of COVID-19 infection in people in the United States. Based on the limited information available to date, the risk of pets spreading the virus to people is considered to be low. If your pet is sick, consult your veterinarian.

Animal testing is reserved for situations when the results may affect the treatment or management of people and animals. If your veterinarian thinks your pet is a candidate for testing, they will consult the state veterinarian and public health officials. Do not contact your state veterinarians directly: They do not have the client/patient–veterinarian relationship that would allow them to fully understand the situation, and they are also actively involved

Clinical Presentation in Specific Population

in other animal disease-related emergencies as well as response to COVID-19.

WHAT ANIMAL SPECIES CAN GET COVID-19?

The National Veterinary Services Laboratories of the U.S. Department of Agriculture (USDA) maintains an overview and list of confirmed cases of severe acute respiratory syndrome coronavirus 2 (SARS-CoV-2) on its website (www.aphis.usda.gov/aphis/dashboards/tableau/sars-dashboard).

More studies are needed to understand if and how different animals could be affected by COVID-19. The Centers for Disease Control and Prevention (CDC) updates its site with research and findings from experimental studies (www.cdc.gov/coronavirus/2019-ncov/daily-life-coping/animals.html).

CAN PETS CARRY THE VIRUS THAT CAUSES COVID-19 ON THEIR SKIN OR FUR?

Although you know certain bacteria and fungi can be carried on fur and hair, there is no evidence that viruses, including the virus that causes COVID-19, can spread to people from the skin, fur, or hair of pets.

However, because animals can sometimes carry other germs that can make people sick, it is always a good idea to practice healthy habits around pets and other animals, including washing hands before and after interacting with them and especially after cleaning up their waste.

Do not put masks on pets. A mask can cause harm to a pet. Do not wipe or bathe your pet with chemical disinfectants, alcohol, hydrogen peroxide, or other products, such as hand sanitizer, counter-cleaning wipes, or other industrial or surface cleaners. If you have questions about appropriate products for bathing or cleaning your pet, talk to your veterinarian. If your pet gets hand sanitizer on their skin or fur, rinse or wipe down your pet with water immediately. If your pet ingests hand sanitizer (such as by chewing the bottle) or is showing signs of illness after use, contact your veterinarian or pet poison control immediately.

ARE THERE ANY APPROVED PRODUCTS THAT CAN PREVENT OR TREAT COVID-19 IN ANIMALS?

No. The Federal Food, Drug, and Cosmetic (FD&C) Act defines drugs as "articles intended for use in the diagnosis, cure, mitigation, treatment, or prevention of disease in man or other animals." The U.S. Food and Drug Administration (FDA) has not approved any drugs for the diagnosis, cure, mitigation, treatment, or prevention of COVID-19 in animals. The USDA Animal and Plant Health Inspection Service (APHIS) Center for Veterinary Biologics (CVB) regulates veterinary biologics, including vaccines, diagnostic kits, and other products of biological origin.

The FDA has taken action against unapproved products claiming to prevent or cure COVID-19. The public can help safeguard human and animal health by reporting any products claiming to do so to FDA-COVID-19-Fraudulent-Products@fda.hhs.gov or 888-INFO-FDA (888-463-6332).

ARE THERE SHORTAGES OR DISRUPTIONS TO THE U.S. PET FOOD SUPPLY?

In general, pet food is available. There may be intermittent decreased availability of certain brands/flavors, but the products have been and continue to be available to meet pets' nutritional needs.

If a specific preferred flavor or brand is temporarily unavailable, pet owners may need to opt for a short-term alternative.

There have been some reports of decreased availability of some specially formulated veterinary diets that are used to both provide nutrition and address a diagnosed medical condition, which may make it more difficult to find an alternative diet. If a pet needs a specialty diet, it may be helpful for pet owners to consult a veterinarian to find a recommended alternative diet.

ARE THERE ANY ANIMAL DRUG SHORTAGES DUE TO THE COVID-19 OUTBREAK?

The FDA has been and is continuing to closely monitor how the COVID-19 outbreak may impact the animal medical product supply chain.

Clinical Presentation in Specific Population

While the FDA does not have regulatory authority requiring the animal drug industry to report shortages, you have been reaching out to manufacturers as part of your approach to identifying potential disruptions or shortages. We will use all available tools to react swiftly to help mitigate the impact if a potential disruption or shortage is identified.[6]

---

[6] "COVID-19 Frequently Asked Questions," U.S. Food and Drug Administration (FDA), December 8, 2022. Available Online. URL: www.fda.gov/emergency-preparedness-and-response/coronavirus-disease-2019-covid-19/covid-19-frequently-asked-questions#animals. Accessed December 13, 2022.

Chapter 9 | Disparities in COVID-19

Though everybody is at risk of COVID-19 and its effects, research shows that some racial and ethnic minority groups, older adults, people with disabilities, and people with lower incomes are disproportionately affected by COVID-19 and its impacts. COVID-19 data show that Black, African American, Hispanic, Latino, American Indian, and Alaska Native persons in the United States experience higher rates of COVID-19-related hospitalization and death than non-Hispanic White populations and that these disparities persist even when accounting for other demographic and socioeconomic factors. Age-adjusted case, hospitalization, and death rates were highest in American Indian and Alaska Native individuals. Non-Hispanic Black or African American people and Hispanic people are both more than twice as likely to be hospitalized due to COVID-19 than non-Hispanic White people.

In 2020, residents of long-term care facilities made up less than one percent of the U.S. population but accounted for more than 35 percent of all COVID-19 deaths, with even more disproportionate impacts in nursing homes with higher percentages of residents from racial and ethnic minority groups. Compared with ages 18–29, the rate of death is 330 times higher in those who are aged 85 and older. In addition, people aged 18 and older with certain underlying medical conditions and certain disabilities are at an increased risk for severe illness from COVID-19. In addition, immunocompromised individuals may experience weaker immune responses to COVID-19 vaccines.

Social determinants of health (SDOH) are conditions in the environment that affect a wide range of health outcomes and risks. These SDOH include neighborhood and the physical environment, health and health care, occupation and job conditions, income and wealth, and education. Discrimination, including racism, ableism, and associated chronic stress, influences each of these important topic areas. Together, disparities in each of these areas have contributed to disproportionately worse COVID-19-related outcomes for people from racial and ethnic minority groups, people with disabilities, and older people.

RACIAL AND ETHNIC MINORITY POPULATIONS
- They had higher rates of positive test results, hospitalizations, severe illness, and death from COVID-19, even after adjusting for age.
- They experienced greater unemployment and were likely to be behind on rent.
- They had higher rates of anxiety symptoms, depressive symptoms, and suicidal ideation.
- They were twice as likely to report having lost a relative or close friend to COVID-19.

OLDER ADULTS
- Age is the strongest risk factor for severe COVID-19 outcomes.
- U.S. adults aged 65 years and older accounted for 81 percent of COVID-19-related deaths in 2020.

PEOPLE WITH DISABILITIES
People with disabilities, including attention deficit hyperactivity disorder (ADHD), cerebral palsy (CP), intellectual and developmental disabilities, spinal cord injuries, Down syndrome (DS), and other chronic health conditions such as human immunodeficiency virus/acquired immune deficiency syndrome (HIV/AIDS), may

Disparities in COVID-19

be likely to get very sick from COVID-19 because of underlying medical conditions, living in congregate settings, or systemic health and social inequities.[1]

---

[1] "Services and Supports for Longer-Term Impacts of COVID-19," U.S. Department of Health and Human Services (HHS), August 1, 2022. Available online. URL: www.covid.gov/assets/files/Services-and-Supports-for-Longer-Term-Impacts-of-COVID-19-08012022.pdf. Accessed December 9, 2022.

Chapter 10 | COVID-19 Statistics in United States

Chapter Contents
Section 10.1—U.S. COVID-19 Cases and Deaths...................... 135
Section 10.2—Excess Deaths Associated with
          COVID-19 138

Section 10.1 | U.S. COVID-19 Cases and Deaths

AGGREGATE DATA COLLECTION PROCESS
Since the start of the COVID-19 pandemic, data have been gathered through a robust process with the following steps:
- A Centers for Disease Control and Prevention (CDC) data team reviews and validates the information obtained from jurisdictions' state and local websites via an overnight data review process.
- If more than one official county data source exists, the CDC uses a comprehensive data selection process comparing each official county data source and takes the highest case and death counts, unless otherwise specified by the state.
- The CDC compiles these data and posts the finalized information on COVID Data Tracker (https://covid.cdc.gov/covid-data-tracker/#datatracker-home).
- County-level data are aggregated to obtain state- and territory-specific totals.

This process is collaborative, with the CDC and jurisdictions working together to ensure the accuracy of COVID-19 case and death numbers. County counts provide the most up-to-date numbers on cases and deaths by report date. The CDC may retrospectively update counts to correct data quality issues.

Relation to the Archived Data Set
Prior to October 20, 2022, the CDC collected aggregate case and death data at the state level. These data were compiled and published daily on data.cdc.gov in a data set called "United States COVID-19 Cases and Deaths by State over Time" (https://data.cdc.gov/Case-Surveillance/United-States-COVID-19-Cases-and-Deaths-by-State-o/9mfq-cb36) As of October 20, 2022, this data set has been archived and will no longer update.

Methodology Changes
Several differences exist between the current, weekly updated data set and the archived version of the United States COVID-19 Cases and Deaths by State over Time (https://data.cdc.gov/Case-Surveillance/United-States-COVID-19-Cases-and-Deaths-by-State-o/9mfq-cb36) data set:
- **Source**. The current, weekly updated version is based on county-level aggregate count data, while the archived version is based on state-level aggregate count data.
- **Confirmed/probable cases/death breakdown**. While the probable cases and deaths are included in the total case and total death counts in both versions (if applicable), they were reported separately from the confirmed cases and deaths by the jurisdiction in the archived version. In the current weekly updated version, the counts by jurisdiction are not reported by confirmed or probable status.
- **Time series frequency**. The current weekly updated version contains weekly time series data (i.e., one record per week per jurisdiction), while the archived version contains daily time series data (i.e., one record per day per jurisdiction).
- **Update frequency**. The current weekly updated version is updated weekly, while the archived version was updated twice daily up to October 20, 2022.

Note. The counts reflected during a given time period in this data set may not match the counts reflected for the same time period in the archived data set noted above. Discrepancies may exist due to differences between county and state COVID-19 case surveillance and reconciliation efforts.

Confirmed and Probable Counts
In this data set, counts by jurisdiction are not displayed by confirmed or probable status. Instead, confirmed and probable cases and deaths are included in the "total cases" and "total deaths" columns, when available. Not all jurisdictions report probable cases and deaths to the CDC.

COVID-19 Statistics in United States

Deaths

The CDC reports death data on other sections of the website: CDC COVID Data Tracker: Home (https://covid.cdc.gov/covid-data-tracker/#datatracker-home), CDC COVID Data Tracker: Cases, Deaths, and Testing (https://covid.cdc.gov/covid-data-tracker/?CDC_AA_refVal=https%3A%2F%2Fwww.cdc.gov%2Fcoronavirus%2F2019-ncov%2Fcases-updates%2Fcases-in-us.html#cases_newcaserateper100k), and National Center for Health Statistics (NCHS) Provisional Death Counts (https://www.cdc.gov/nchs/nvss/covid-19.htm). Information presented on the COVID Data Tracker pages is based on the same source (total case counts) as the present data set; however, NCHS death counts are based on death certificates that use information reported by physicians, medical examiners, or coroners in the cause-of-death section of each certificate. Data from each of these pages are considered provisional (not complete and pending verification) and are, therefore, subject to change. Counts from previous weeks are continually revised as more records are received and processed.

Number of Jurisdictions Reporting

There are currently 60 public health jurisdictions reporting cases of COVID-19. This includes the 50 states, the District of Columbia (DC), New York City, the U.S. territories of American Samoa, Guam, the Commonwealth of the Northern Mariana Islands, Puerto Rico, and the U.S Virgin Islands, as well as three independent countries in compacts of free association with the United States, the Federated States of Micronesia, the Republic of the Marshall Islands, and the Republic of Palau. New York state's reported case and death counts do not include New York City's counts as they separately report nationally notifiable conditions to the CDC.

CDC COVID-19 data are available to the public as summary or aggregate count files, including total counts of cases and deaths, available by state and by county.[1]

---

[1] "Weekly United States COVID-19 Cases and Deaths by State," Centers for Disease Control and Prevention (CDC), December 16, 2022. Available online. URL: https://data.cdc.gov/Case-Surveillance/Weekly-United-States-COVID-19-Cases-and-Deaths-by-/pwn4-m3yp. Accessed December 20, 2022.

Section 10.2 | Excess Deaths Associated with COVID-19

Estimates of excess deaths can provide information about the burden of mortality potentially related to the COVID-19 pandemic, including deaths that are directly or indirectly attributed to COVID-19. Excess deaths are typically defined as the difference between the observed numbers of deaths in specific time periods and the expected numbers of deaths in the same time periods. This visualization provides weekly estimates of excess deaths by the jurisdiction in which the death occurred. Weekly counts of deaths are compared with historical trends to determine whether the number of deaths is significantly higher than expected.

Counts of deaths from all causes of death, including COVID-19, are presented. As some deaths due to COVID-19 may be assigned to other causes of deaths (e.g., if COVID-19 was not diagnosed or not mentioned on the death certificate), tracking all-cause mortality can provide information about whether an excess number of deaths is observed, even when COVID-19 mortality may be undercounted. Additionally, deaths from all causes, excluding COVID-19, were also estimated. Comparing these two sets of estimates—excess deaths with and without COVID-19—can provide insight about how many excess deaths are identified as due to COVID-19 and how many excess deaths are reported as due to other causes of death. These deaths could represent misclassified COVID-19 deaths or potentially could be indirectly related to the COVID-19 pandemic (e.g., deaths from other causes occurring in the context of health-care shortages or overburdened health-care systems).

As of June 3, 2020, additional information on weekly counts of deaths by cause of death has been added to this release. Similar to all causes of death, these weekly counts can be compared to values from the same weeks in prior years to determine whether recent increases have occurred for specific causes of death. The causes shown here were chosen based on analyses of the most prevalent comorbid conditions reported on death certificates where COVID-19 was listed as a cause of death. Cause-of-death counts are based on the underlying cause of death and presented for respiratory diseases, circulatory diseases, malignant neoplasms, and Alzheimer

COVID-19 Statistics in United States

disease (AD) and dementia. Deaths due to external causes (i.e., injuries) or unknown causes are excluded.

Estimates of excess deaths can be calculated in a variety of ways and will vary depending on the methodology and assumptions about how many deaths are expected to occur. Estimates of excess deaths presented in this web page were calculated using Farrington surveillance algorithms. A range of values for the number of excess deaths was calculated as the difference between the observed count and one of two thresholds (either the average expected count or the upper bound of the 95% prediction interval), by week and jurisdiction.

Provisional death counts are weighted to account for incomplete data. However, data for the most recent week(s) are still likely to be incomplete. Weights are based on the completeness of provisional data in prior years, but the timeliness of data may have changed in 2020 relative to prior years, so the resulting weighted estimates may be too high in some jurisdictions and too low in others. As more information about the accuracy of the weighted estimates is obtained, further refinements to the weights may be made, which will impact the estimates. Any changes to the methods or weighting algorithm will be noted in the Technical Notes (www.cdc.gov/nchs/nvss/vsrr/covid19/excess_deaths.htm#techNotes) when they occur. More detail about the methods, weighting, data, and limitations can be found in the Technical Notes.

This visualization includes several different estimates:
- **The number of excess deaths**. A range of estimates for the number of excess deaths was calculated as the difference between the observed count and one of two thresholds (either the average expected count or the upper bound threshold), by week and jurisdiction. Negative values, where the observed count fell below the threshold, were set to zero.
- **Percent excess**. The percent excess was defined as the number of excess deaths divided by the threshold.
- **The total number of excess deaths**. The total number of excess deaths in each jurisdiction was calculated by summing the excess deaths in each week, from February 1, 2020, to the present. Similarly, the total

number of excess deaths for the United States overall was computed as a sum of jurisdiction-specific numbers of excess deaths (with negative values set to zero) and not directly estimated using the Farrington surveillance algorithms.

TECHNICAL NOTES
Methods

Counts of deaths in the most recent weeks were compared with historical trends (from 2013 to the present) to determine whether the number of deaths in recent weeks was significantly higher than expected, using Farrington surveillance algorithms. The "surveillance" package in R was used to implement the Farrington algorithms, which use overdispersed Poisson generalized linear models with spline terms to model trends in counts, accounting for seasonality. For each jurisdiction, a model is used to generate a set of expected counts, and an upper bound threshold based on a one-sided 95 percent prediction interval of these expected counts is used to determine whether a significant increase in deaths has occurred. Estimates of excess deaths are provided based on the observed number of deaths relative to two different thresholds. The lower end of the excess death estimate range is generated by comparing the observed counts to the upper bound threshold, and a higher end of the excess death estimate range is generated by comparing the observed count to the average expected number of deaths. Reported counts were weighted to account for potential underreporting in the most recent weeks.

This method is useful in detecting when jurisdictions may have higher than expected numbers of deaths but cannot be used to determine whether a given jurisdiction has fewer deaths than expected given that the data are provisional. Provisional counts of deaths are known to be incomplete, and the degree of completeness varies considerably by jurisdiction and time. Incomplete data in recent weeks can contribute to observed counts below the threshold. Thus, the estimates of excess deaths—the numbers of deaths falling above the threshold—may be underestimated. While reported counts are weighted to account for potential underreporting in

COVID-19 Statistics in United States

the most recent weeks, the true magnitude of underreporting is unknown. Therefore, weighted counts of deaths may overestimate or underestimate the true number of deaths in a given jurisdiction.

A range of estimates of excess deaths is provided based on comparing the observed numbers of deaths to two different thresholds, by week and jurisdiction: the average expected number of deaths and the upper bound of the 95 percent prediction interval of the expected number of deaths. Negative values, where the observed count fell below the thresholds, were set to zero. The percent excess was defined as the number of excess deaths divided by the threshold. The total number of excess deaths in each state was calculated by summing the excess deaths in each week, from February 1, 2020, to the present. Similarly, the total number of excess deaths in the United States was calculated by summing the total numbers of excess deaths across the jurisdictions.

Estimates of excess deaths for the United States overall were computed as a sum of jurisdiction-specific numbers of excess deaths (with negative values set to zero) and not directly estimated using the Farrington surveillance algorithms. Summation (rather than estimation) was chosen to account for the possibility that some jurisdictions may have substantially incomplete data while other jurisdictions report many more deaths than expected; these negative and positive values will cancel each other out when estimating excess deaths for the United States directly using the Farrington surveillance algorithms. Until data are finalized (typically 12 months after the close of the data year), it is not possible to determine whether observed decreases in mortality using provisional data are due to true declines or to incomplete reporting. Thus, when computing excess deaths directly for the United States, negative values due to incomplete reporting in some jurisdictions will offset excess deaths observed in other jurisdictions. For example, the total number of excess deaths in the United States computed directly for the United States using the Farrington algorithms was approximately 25 percent lower than the number calculated by summing across the jurisdictions with excess deaths. This difference is likely due to several jurisdictions reporting lower-than-expected numbers of deaths—which could be a function of underreporting, true declines in mortality in certain areas, or a combination of these factors. In addition, potential discrepancies between the number of excess deaths in the United States when estimated directly and the sum of jurisdiction-specific estimates could be related to different estimated thresholds for the expected number of deaths in the United States and across the jurisdictions.

Different definitions of excess deaths result in different estimates, for example, defining excess deaths as the difference between the observed counts and the expected (not the upper bound estimate) results in larger estimates of excess deaths. The upper bound more readily identifies areas experiencing statistically significantly higher than normal mortality. Using the expected count, by contrast, would indicate which areas are experiencing higher-than-average mortality. Expected counts are now provided so that users can evaluate excess deaths relative to different thresholds.

Finally, the estimates of excess deaths reported here may not be due to COVID-19, either directly or indirectly. The pandemic may have changed mortality patterns for other causes of death. Upward trends in other causes of death (e.g., suicide, drug overdose, heart disease) may contribute to excess deaths in some jurisdictions. Future analyses of cause-specific excess mortality may provide additional information about these patterns.

As more information about the accuracy of the weighted estimates is obtained, further refinements may be made, and changes to the weighting methods will impact the estimates. Any changes to the methods or weighting algorithm will be noted in the Technical Notes when they occur.

Completeness

Methods to address reporting lags (i.e., underreporting) were updated as of September 9, 2020. Generally, these updates resulted in estimates of the total number of excess deaths that were approximately five percent smaller than the previous method, as weights in some jurisdictions with improved timeliness were reduced. While these adjustments likely reduce potential overestimation for those jurisdictions with improved timeliness, estimates for the most recent weeks for the United States overall are likely underestimated to a larger extent than in previous releases. Some jurisdictions have few to no provisional data available in the most recent week(s) (CT, NC, WV); together, these jurisdictions represent approximately five percent of U.S. deaths. In previous releases, some of the underestimation or lack of provisional data from certain jurisdictions was offset by the overestimation in other jurisdictions with improved timeliness when considering trends for the United States overall. Because the updated weighting methods mitigate the impact of the previous overestimation for some jurisdictions with improved timeliness but provide no additional adjustments for underestimation or a lack of recent provisional data in other jurisdictions, the excess death estimates for the United States overall are expected to result in a larger degree of underestimation than in previous releases.

To account for potential underreporting in the most recent weeks, counts were weighted by the inverse of completeness. Completeness was estimated as follows. Using provisional data from 2018 to 2019, weekly provisional counts were compared to final data (with final data for 2019 approximated by the data available as of April 9, 2020), at various lag times (e.g., one week following the death, two weeks, three weeks, up to 26 weeks) by reporting jurisdiction. Completeness by week, lag, and jurisdiction was modeled using zero-inflated binomial hierarchical Bayesian models with state-level and temporal random effects. Temporal random effects were included for both the time trend in the provisional counts and the lag or reporting delay. These random effects were specified using a type-I random walk distribution, where counts in a given time period depend on the value for the prior time period, plus an error term. These models were implemented using R-INLA. Posterior predicted median values of completeness by jurisdiction and lag time were obtained from the models, and the weekly estimates for 2019 were averaged to provide the most recent possible estimates of completeness by jurisdiction, at given lag times. The inverse of these completeness values was applied as weights to adjust for incomplete reporting of provisional mortality data. For example, if provisional mortality data in 2019 for a given jurisdiction were 50 percent complete within one week of death and 75 percent complete within two weeks of death, then the weights for that jurisdiction would be two for data presented with a one-week lag and 1.3 for data presented with a two-week lag. Of note, these estimates of completeness differ from the estimates provided elsewhere (www.cdc.gov/nchs/nvss/vsrr/covid19/), which rely on the current counts of deaths relative to the expected number (i.e., percent over expected).

Weights in the first few weeks following the date of death were highly inflated and variable for some jurisdictions with relatively small numbers of deaths and where completeness of provisional data is typically very low (0–2%) in the first few weeks following the date of death. These jurisdictions include Alaska, Connecticut, Louisiana, North Carolina, Ohio, Puerto Rico, Rhode Island, and West Virginia. To avoid highly inflated estimates in these jurisdictions, weights were trimmed at the 90th percentile for weeks reported with shorter lag times (e.g., 1–6 weeks). Additionally, as of September 9, weights for several jurisdictions were adjusted downward based on preliminary analyses of the timeliness of provisional data for deaths occurring from April to May 2020. These analyses have suggested that timeliness has improved at shorter lags in Alaska, Mississippi, New York (excluding New York City), Ohio, Pennsylvania, South Carolina, Texas, Vermont, Virginia, West Virginia, and Puerto Rico. Weights for these jurisdictions were adjusted downward accordingly to improve the accuracy of the predicted counts.

Unweighted estimates are shown in one of the dashboards so that readers can examine the impact of weighting on estimates of excess deaths. For some jurisdictions, improvements in timeliness in 2020 relative to prior years will lead to weighted estimates that are too large. For other jurisdictions, the weighting may be insufficient to address reporting lags, particularly for data reported with shorter lag times (e.g., within 4–6 weeks). As an additional step to guard against underreporting, the weighted counts of deaths by week and jurisdiction were compared with control counts of deaths based on available demographic information from the death certificate. Demographic data are typically available prior to the cause of death data, which can take 1–8 weeks or more, depending on the jurisdiction and cause of death. For weeks and jurisdictions where the weighted count of deaths was less than the control count based on the demographic data, the

COVID-19 Statistics in United States

weighted values were replaced with the control count. For example, if the weighted count for a given jurisdiction and week was 400, while the control count for that same jurisdiction and week was 800, this indicates that the weights are not fully accounting for incomplete data. In this case, the value of 800 would be used, as it represents a more complete estimate of the total number of deaths occurring in that jurisdiction and week.

Data for jurisdictions where counts are between one and nine are suppressed. Additionally, data for weeks where the counts are less than 50 percent of the expected number are also suppressed, as these provisional counts are highly incomplete and potentially misleading. This change resulted in showing estimates with a lag of one week for most jurisdictions and the United States. For some jurisdictions (Connecticut, North Carolina, Puerto Rico), lags may be greater. Declines in the observed numbers of deaths in recent weeks should not be interpreted to mean that the numbers of deaths are decreasing, as these declines are expected when relying on provisional data that are generally less complete in recent weeks. While the weighting method is intended to mitigate the impact of underreporting, it may not be sufficient to eliminate the problem of underreporting entirely. Therefore, it is not yet possible to determine whether decreases in the number of deaths are due to underreporting or to true declines until more complete data are obtained.

Mortality Outcomes

Weekly counts of deaths from all causes were examined, including deaths due to COVID-19. As many deaths due to COVID-19 may be assigned to other causes of deaths (e.g., if COVID-19 was not mentioned on the death certificate as a suspected cause of death), tracking all-cause mortality can provide information about whether the excess number of deaths is observed, even when COVID-19 mortality may be undercounted. These estimates can also provide information about deaths that may be indirectly related to COVID-19. For example, deaths due to other causes may increase as a result of health-care shortages due to COVID-19. Additionally, deaths from all causes excluding COVID-19 were also estimated.

These counts excluded deaths with U07.1 as an underlying cause or multiple causes of death.

Comparing these two sets of estimates—excess deaths with and without COVID-19—can provide insight about how many excess deaths are identified as due to COVID-19 and how many excess deaths are due to other causes of death. These deaths could represent misclassified COVID-19 deaths or potentially could be indirectly related to COVID-19. Additionally, death certificates are often initially submitted without a cause of death and then updated when the cause of death information becomes available. It may be the case that some excess deaths that are not attributed directly to COVID-19 will be updated in coming weeks with cause-of-death information that includes COVID-19. These analyses will be updated periodically, and the numbers presented will change as more data are received.

Cause of Death

As of June 3, 2020, weekly counts of deaths due to select causes of death are presented. These causes were selected based on analyses of comorbid conditions reported on death certificates where COVID-19 was listed as a cause of death (see www.cdc.gov/nchs/nvss/vsrr/covid_weekly/index.htm#Comorbidities). Some causes with insufficient numbers of deaths by week and jurisdiction were combined with other categories, and one cause was added to the AD and dementia category (ICD–10 code G31). These estimates are based on the underlying cause of death and include respiratory diseases, circulatory diseases, malignant neoplasms, and AD and dementia. ICD–10 codes were used to classify deaths according to the following causes:
- respiratory diseases
  - influenza and pneumonia (J09–J18)
  - chronic lower respiratory diseases (J40–J47)
  - other diseases of the respiratory system (J00–J06, J20–J39, J60–J70, J80–J86, J90–J96, J97–J99, R09.2, U04)
- circulatory diseases
  - hypertensive diseases (I10–I15)

COVID-19 Statistics in United States

- ischemic heart disease (I20–I25)
- heart failure (I50)
- cerebrovascular diseases (I60–I69)
- other disease of the circulatory system (I00–I09, I26–I49, I51, I52, I70–I99)
- malignant neoplasms (C00–C97)
- AD and dementia (G30, G31, F01, F03)
- other select causes of death
  - diabetes (E10–E14)
  - renal failure (N17–N19)
  - sepsis (A40–A41)

Estimated numbers of deaths due to these other causes of death could represent misclassified COVID-19 deaths or potentially could be indirectly related to COVID-19 (e.g., deaths from other causes occurring in the context of health-care shortages or overburdened health-care systems). Deaths with an underlying cause of death of COVID-19 are not included in these estimates of deaths due to other causes, but deaths where COVID-19 appeared on the death certificate as multiple causes of death may be included in the cause-specific estimates. For example, in some cases, COVID-19 may have contributed to the death, but the underlying cause of death was another cause, such as terminal cancer. For the majority of deaths where COVID-19 is reported on the death certificate (approximately 95%), COVID-19 is selected as the underlying cause of death.

Deaths due to all other natural causes were excluded (ICD-10 codes: A00–A39, A42–B99, D00–E07, E15–E68, E70–E90, F00, F02, F04–G26, G31–H95, K00–K93, L00–M99, N00–N16, N20–N98, O00–O99, P00–P96, Q00–Q99). External causes of death (i.e., injuries) were excluded, as the reporting lag is substantially longer for external causes of death. Additionally, causes of death where the underlying cause was unknown or ill-specified (i.e., R-codes) were excluded (except for R09.2, which is included under the "respiratory diseases" category). Counts of deaths with an unknown cause are typically substantially higher in provisional data, as many records are initially submitted without a specific cause of death and are then updated when more information becomes available. For deaths due to external causes of death or unknown cause, provisional data are highly unreliable and inaccurate in recent weeks, and it can take 6–9 months to ensure sufficiently accurate estimates. Counts by cause provided here will not sum to the total number of deaths, given that some causes are excluded.

Estimates by cause of death and age at death are weighted, using the methods described above. The total count of deaths above average levels is shown for select causes of death. These totals are calculated by summing the number of deaths above average levels (based on weekly counts from 2015 to 2019) since February 1, 2020. Negative values were set to zero and therefore excluded from these sums. Because not all causes of death are shown and due to differences in how the average expected numbers of deaths are estimated, the total numbers of deaths across all the selected causes will not match the numbers of excess deaths from all causes excluding COVID-19.

Estimates by race and Hispanic origin are weighted using the methods described above. Weekly counts are shown for deaths due to all causes, all causes excluding COVID-19, and COVID-19. Because estimates are weighted to account for incomplete reporting in recent weeks, counts of death due to COVID-19 will not match other data sources. For data years 2018–2020, race and Hispanic-origin categories are based on the 1997 Office of Management and Budget (OMB) standards, allowing for the presentation of data by single race and Hispanic origin. These race and Hispanic-origin groups—non-Hispanic single-race White, non-Hispanic single-race Black or African American, non-Hispanic single-race American Indian or Alaska Native (AIAN), and non-Hispanic single-race Asian—differ from the bridged-race categories used in previous data years when not all jurisdictions reported race and Hispanic origin using the 1997 OMB standards. Numbers may therefore differ from previous reports and other sources of data on mortality by race and Hispanic origin.

Limitations

These estimates are based on provisional data, which are incomplete. The weighting method applied may not fully account for reporting lags if there are longer delays at present than in past

COVID-19 Statistics in United States

years. For example, in Pennsylvania, reporting lags are currently much longer than they have been in past years, and death counts for 2020 are therefore underestimated. Conversely, the weighting method may overadjust for underreporting, given improvements in data timeliness in certain jurisdictions. Unweighted estimates are provided so that users can see the impact of weighting the provisional counts. However, these unweighted provisional counts are incomplete, and the extent to which they may underestimate the true count of deaths is unknown. Some jurisdictions exhibit recent increases in deaths when using weighted estimates but not the unweighted. The estimates presented may be an early indication of excess mortality related to COVID-19 but should be interpreted with caution, until confirmed by other data sources such as state or local health departments. It is possible that recent improvements in the timeliness of data could also contribute to the pattern where a jurisdiction exhibits recent increases with the weighted data but not the unweighted. Conversely, recent increases may be missed in jurisdictions with historically low levels of completeness (e.g., Connecticut, North Carolina) either due to the lack of provisional data or insufficient weighting to address incomplete data.

The completeness of provisional data varies by cause of death and by age group. However, the weights applied do not account for this variability. It is unknown whether completeness varies by race and Hispanic origin. Therefore, the predicted numbers of deaths may be too low for some age groups, race/ethnicity groups, and causes of death. For example, provisional data on deaths among younger age groups are typically less complete than those among older age groups. Predicted counts may therefore be too low among the younger age groups. Since the weights were based on the completeness of all-cause mortality data in past years, the weighted estimates for specific causes of death are likely too low, as reporting lags are typically larger for specific causes of death than for all-cause mortality. To minimize the degree of underreporting, cause-specific estimates are presented with a two-week lag.[2]

---

[2] "Excess Deaths Associated with COVID-19," Centers for Disease Control and Prevention (CDC), December 14, 2022. Available online. URL: www.cdc.gov/nchs/nvss/vsrr/covid19/excess_deaths.htm. Accessed December 20, 2022.

Chapter 11 | Worldwide COVID-19 Cases and Deaths

Since the COVID-19 pandemic began in late 2019, the virus has spread worldwide, resulting in a significant number of infections and deaths. The World Health Organization (WHO) has reported more than 750 million confirmed cases of COVID-19 as of February 2023. The pandemic has negatively affected the international economy, health systems, travel, and societies, posing a major public health challenge and a global concern.

The top 10 countries with the highest number of confirmed cases are provided in Table 11.1. In some countries, low vaccination rates, inconsistent public health measures, and other factors contributed to the number of confirmed cases. Additionally, virus variants such as the omicron and Delta have led to increased transmission in some areas.

Table 11.1. COVID-19: Total Number of Confirmed Cases in Top 10 Countries as of February 24, 2023

Rank	Country	Total Number of Cases
1	USA	101,752,396
2	China	98,932,687
3	India	44,685,132
4	France	38,487,043

Table 11.1. Continued

Rank	Country	Total Number of Cases
5	Germany	38,018,111
6	Brazil	36,989,373
7	Japan	33,097,952
8	Republic of Korea	30,445,775
9	Italy	25,547,414
10	United Kingdom	24,341,615

(Source: "WHO Coronavirus (COVID-19) Dashboard," World Health Organization (WHO).)

These numbers change daily and are likely to rise with time. Furthermore, these figures only represent confirmed, reported cases. The actual number of people infected with the virus is estimated to be higher with many cases left unreported.

According to the WHO, the highest number of confirmed deaths from COVID-19-related causes crossed more than 6.85 million worldwide as of February 24, 2023, mainly affecting the elderly and individuals with underlying health conditions such as cardiovascular disease, diabetes, chronic respiratory disease, and the elderly. The top 10 countries with the highest death rates are listed in Table 11.2.

Table 11.2. COVID-19: Total Number of Deaths in Top 10 Countries as of February 24, 2023

Rank	Country	Total Number of Deaths
1	USA	1,106,783
2	Brazil	698,056
3	India	530,761
4	Russia	395,867
5	Mexico	332,839
6	Peru	219,344

Worldwide COVID-19 Cases and Deaths

Table 11.2. Continued

Rank	Country	Total Number of Deaths
7	United Kingdom	206,246
8	Italy	187,850
9	Germany	167,387
10	France	161,083

(Source: "WHO Coronavirus (COVID-19) Dashboard," World Health Organization (WHO).)

Factors such as underreporting, misclassification, and variations in testing and reporting practices mean that the reported deaths from COVID-19 may not represent exactly the actual number. This is mainly an issue in developing and underdeveloped countries with poor economic status, which can lead to discrepancies in the data they collect.

To combat, control, and contain the spread of the coronavirus and reduce the number of severe cases, hospitalizations, and deaths, the most effective weapon is the COVID-19 vaccination. Vaccination helps protect individuals at higher risk of severe illness or death, such as the elderly, those with underlying medical conditions, and frontline workers. Furthermore, widespread vaccination also reduces the spread of the virus in the community, thereby providing herd immunity when a significant portion of the population is immune to the virus, making it difficult for the virus to spread. Refer to Table 11.3 for the total number of vaccine doses administered in the top 10 countries.

Table 11.3. COVID-19: Total Number of Vaccine Doses Administered in Top 10 Countries as of March 7, 2023

Rank	Country	Total Number of Vaccine Doses Administered
1	China	3,465,113,661
2	India	2,205,113,973
3	USA	662,514,513

Table 11.3. Continued

Rank	Country	Total Number of Vaccine Doses Administered
4	Brazil	502,262,440
5	Indonesia	444,303,130
6	Japan	381,845,653
7	Bangladesh	354,990,838
8	Pakistan	333,759,565
9	Vietnam	266,252,632
10	Mexico	225,063,079

(Source: "WHO Coronavirus (COVID-19) Dashboard," World Health Organization (WHO).)

The effectiveness of COVID-19 vaccinations has been proven in numerous studies. A study conducted in Israel in the first quarter of 2021 found that the Pfizer-BioNTech vaccine was 94 percent effective in preventing symptomatic COVID-19 infection and 92 percent effective in preventing severe illness and hospitalization. Another study conducted at the end of 2020 in the United States found that the Moderna vaccine was 94.1 percent effective in preventing COVID-19 infection.

However, the effectiveness of the vaccines can vary depending on various factors, such as the type of vaccine, the age of the person being vaccinated, and the prevalence of variants in the region. Nevertheless, since the start of vaccination campaigns, millions of people have been vaccinated globally, and the vaccines have proven to be highly effective in preventing COVID-19 infections. Studies have shown that vaccines significantly reduce the risk of severe disease and death, even against emerging virus variants.

Countries that have achieved high vaccination rates through successful vaccination campaigning have decreased COVID-19 cases, hospitalizations, and deaths and has helped ease the burden on health-care systems, allowing hospitals to manage the demand for medical services better, and has propelled the COVID-19 pandemic status toward an endemic one.

Worldwide COVID-19 Cases and Deaths

The COVID-19 pandemic has significantly impacted the world, with the United States, China, India, France, Germany, and Brazil having the highest number of confirmed cases and the United States, Brazil, India, and Russia having the highest number of deaths. It is imperative that adequate measures are taken to boost the number of recoveries and reduce the overall infection rate to effectively control the spread of the virus and minimize its toll.

References

Baden, Lindsey R; El Sahly, Hana M; Essink, Brandon, et al. "Efficacy and Safety of the mRNA-1273 SARS-CoV-2 Vaccine," The New England Journal of Medicine (NEJM), February 4, 2021. Available online. URL: www.nejm.org/doi/full/10.1056/NEJMoa2035389. Accessed March 7, 2023.

"Characteristics of COVID-19 Recurrence: A Systematic Review and Meta-Analysis," National Center for Biotechnology Information (NCBI), March 24, 2021. Available online. URL: www.ncbi.nlm.nih.gov/pmc/articles/PMC7996451. Accessed January 17, 2023.

"COVID-19 Projections," University of Washington, December 16, 2022. Available online. URL: https://covid19.healthdata.org/global?view=cumulative-deaths&tab=trend. Accessed March 7, 2023.

"COVID-19 Coronavirus Pandemic," Worldometer, January 12, 2023. Available online. URL: www.worldometers.info/coronavirus/#countries. Accessed January 12, 2023.

"Coronavirus Pandemic (COVID-19)," Our World In Data, March 5, 2020. Available online. URL: https://ourworldindata.org/coronavirus#coronavirus-country-profiles. Accessed January 17, 2023.

Dagan, Noa; Barda, Noam, Kepten, Eldad, et al. "BNT162b2 mRNA COVID-19 Vaccine in a Nationwide Mass Vaccination Setting," The New England Journal of Medicine (NEJM), April 15, 2021. Available online.

URL: www.nejm.org/doi/full/10.1056/NEJMoa2101765. Accessed March 7, 2023.

"Number of Coronavirus (COVID-19) Cases, Recoveries, and Deaths Worldwide as of January 9, 2023," Statista, January 9, 2023. Available online. URL: www.statista.com/statistics/1087466/covid19-cases-recoveries-deaths-worldwide. Accessed January 17, 2023.

"WHO Coronavirus (COVID-19) Dashboard," World Health Organization (WHO), January 3, 2023. Available online. URL: https://covid19.who.int/table. Accessed January 13, 2023.

Part 2 | Prevention and Control Measures of COVID-19

Chapter 12 | How to Protect Yourself and Others from the COVID-19 Infection

Chapter Contents
Section 12.1—Face Masks and Social Distancing 161
Section 12.2—Cleaning and Disinfecting at Home 169

Section 12.1 | Face Masks and Social Distancing

The Centers for Disease Control and Prevention (CDC) advises the use of simple cloth face coverings to slow the spread of the virus and to prevent people who are unaware they have the virus from spreading it to others. Respirators, disposable face masks, or cloth face coverings are designed and worn for different purposes.

If, prior to the COVID-19 pandemic, you were required to wear a respirator or disposable face mask on the job, based on a workplace hazard assessment, you should continue to do so.

RESPIRATORS, DISPOSABLE FACE MASKS, AND CLOTH FACE COVERINGS
Respirators
- Respirators protect wearers from breathing in hazardous contaminants in the air.
- Respirators are required equipment for workers performing some jobs in the food and agriculture sector.
- If you are required to use a respirator for your job, you should continue to do so.

Disposable Face Masks
- Disposable face masks, such as surgical or medical masks, are not respirators and do not protect the wearer from breathing in small particles, gases, or chemicals in the air.
- They act as a protective barrier to prevent splashes, sprays, large droplets, or splatter from entering the wearer's mouth and nose. The protective quality of disposable face masks varies depending on the type of material used to make the face mask.
- They also help prevent the wearer from spreading respiratory droplets.
- Because disposable face masks help prevent the wearer from spreading respiratory droplets, they may slow the spread of the virus that causes COVID-19. Wearing them

may help people who unknowingly have the virus from spreading it to others.

Cloth Face Coverings
- Cloth face coverings, whether provided by the employer or brought from home by the worker, are not respirators or disposable face masks and do not protect the worker wearing them from exposure.
- They are only intended to help contain the wearer's respiratory droplets from being spread.
- Used in this way, the CDC has recommended cloth face coverings to slow the spread of the virus that causes COVID-19. Wearing them may prevent people who unknowingly have the virus from spreading it to others.
- Workers can wear a cloth face covering if the employer has determined that a respirator or a disposable face mask is not required based on the workplace hazard assessment.
- When it is not practicable for workers to wear a single cloth face covering for the full duration of a work shift, particularly if they become wet, soiled, or otherwise visibly contaminated, a clean cloth face covering (or disposable face mask option) should be used and changed out as needed.
- Review information provided on how to wear and care for cloth face coverings.

CONSIDERATIONS FOR USE OF CLOTH FACE COVERINGS
Consider the following if you choose to wear a cloth face covering to slow the spread of COVID-19:
- Maintain face coverings in accordance with parameters in the Model Food Code Section 4-801.11 Clean Linens and Section 4.802.11 Specifications of the U.S. Food and Drug Administration (FDA; www.fda.gov/food/retail-food-protection/fda-food-code), as applicable.
- Launder reusable face coverings before each daily use.

How to Protect Yourself and Others from the COVID-19 Infection

Cloth face coverings should:
- cover the nose and below the chin
- fit snuggly but comfortably against the side of the face
- be secured with ties or ear loops
- include multiple layers of fabric
- allow for breathing without restriction
- be able to be laundered and machine dried without damage or change in shape[1]

OCCUPATIONAL SAFETY AND HEALTH ADMINISTRATION'S RESPIRATORY PROTECTION GUIDANCE

The Occupational Safety and Health Administration (OSHA) is committed to protecting the health and safety of America's workers. This guidance is designed specifically for nursing homes, assisted living, and other long-term care facilities (LTCFs; e.g., skilled nursing facilities, inpatient hospices, convalescent homes, and group homes with nursing care). LTCFs are different from other healthcare settings because they assist residents and clients with tasks of daily living in addition to providing skilled nursing care.

While this guidance focuses on protecting workers from occupational exposure to severe acute respiratory syndrome coronavirus 2 (SARS-CoV-2; the virus that causes COVID-19 disease) by the use of respirators, primary reliance on engineering and administrative controls for controlling exposure is consistent with good industrial hygiene practice and with the OSHA's traditional adherence to a "hierarchy of controls." Under this hierarchy, engineering and administrative controls are preferred to personal protective equipment (PPE). Therefore, employers should always reassess their engineering controls (e.g., ventilation) and administrative controls (e.g., hand hygiene, physical distancing, cleaning/disinfection of surfaces) to identify any changes they can make to avoid overreliance on respirators and other PPE. This is especially vital

---

[1] "Use of Respirators, Facemasks, and Cloth Face Coverings in the Food and Agriculture Sector during Coronavirus Disease (COVID-19) Pandemic," U.S. Food and Drug Administration (FDA), April 24, 2020. Available online. URL: www.fda.gov/food/food-safety-during-emergencies/use-respirators-facemasks-and-cloth-face-coverings-food-and-agriculture-sector-during-coronavirus. Accessed December 12, 2022.

considering the current supply chain demand for N95 filtering facepiece respirators (FFRs).

Even when control strategies are in place, PPE, including respirators, will be needed for workers when close contact with someone who is known or suspected of having COVID-19 cannot be avoided. Whenever respirators are required, employers must implement a written, worksite-specific respiratory protection program (RPP), including medical evaluation, fit testing, training, and other elements, as specified in the OSHA's Respiratory Protection standard (29 CFR 1910.134). OSHA requirements for other PPE (e.g., eye protection, protective clothing) can be found in the OSHA's General PPE standard (29 CFR 1910.132) and Eye and Face Protection standard (29 CFR 1910.133).

FDA-AUTHORIZED MASKS AND OTHER FACE COVERINGS

There are multiple products/devices that can be used during the COVID-19 pandemic to cover a wearer's mouth and nose, and it is important to select the right one for the situation. These products/devices can provide source control, and some of them are also considered PPE that will protect the wearer. Source control refers to the use of a product/device to cover a person's mouth and nose to reduce the spread of respiratory secretions and aerosols when that person is breathing, talking, sneezing, or coughing. Because of the potential for asymptomatic and presymptomatic transmission, source control measures are currently recommended for everyone in health-care facilities, including in LTCFs, even if they do not have symptoms of COVID-19. Health-care providers should wear source control products/devices at all times while they are in an LTCF, including in break rooms or other spaces where they might encounter other people, including coworkers. The source control product/device should be appropriate for the anticipated exposure(s). These products/devices include the following:

- **Cloth face coverings.** These are homemade or commercially available products made of cloth that cover the nose and mouth. Cloth face coverings should not be worn instead of the FDA-cleared or FDA-authorized surgical mask if protection against exposure to splashes and sprays of infectious material from others is needed. Cloth face coverings do not provide effective respiratory protection for workers when protection against airborne hazards is needed and do not fall under the OSHA's Respiratory Protection standard (www.osha.gov/laws-regs/regulations/standardnumber/1910/1910.134). They are not considered PPE for the wearer but can assist in source control. LTCF patients and visitors should wear their own cloth face covering upon arrival at and throughout their stay in an LTCF for source control. If they do not have a cloth face covering, they should be offered a face mask, surgical mask, or cloth face covering by the LTCF, as supplies allow.

- **Face masks**. These products look similar to, and are often mistaken for, surgical masks but do not provide fluid resistance. They do not provide effective respiratory protection for workers when protection against airborne hazards is needed and do not fall under the OSHA's Respiratory Protection standard (www.osha.gov/laws-regs/regulations/standardnumber/1910/1910.134). They are not considered PPE for the wearer but can assist in source control. The FDA has authorized the emergency use of face masks, including cloth face coverings, that meet certain criteria for use as source control by the general public and health-care personnel in accordance with the CDC recommendations during the COVID-19 public health emergency. An example of this type of product would be a KN95 respirator with ear loops instead of head straps and that has not undergone rigorous fit testing to demonstrate a proper fit/effective seal to the wearer's face.
- **FDA-cleared or FDA-authorized surgical masks**. Surgical masks are cleared, or are authorized for emergency use, by the FDA and are jointly regulated by the OSHA under the PPE standard (29 CFR 1910.132) and the Bloodborne Pathogens standard

(29 CFR 1910.1030). When available, FDA-cleared or FDA-authorized surgical masks are preferred over cloth face coverings for health-care workers, as they offer both source control and protection for the wearer against exposure to splashes and sprays of infectious material from others. They are loose-fitting devices that do not provide effective respiratory protection for workers when the wearer might be exposed to airborne hazards and do not fall under the OSHA's Respiratory Protection standard.

- **Respirators (including FDA-cleared or FDA-authorized surgical N95 FFRs).** Health-care providers who are in close contact with an LTCF resident with suspected or confirmed SARS-CoV-2 infection must use an N95 FFR approved by the National Institute for Occupational Safety and Health (NIOSH) or equivalent or higher-level respirator (29 CFR 1910.134). When protection against exposure to splashes and sprays of infectious material from others is also needed, an FDA-cleared or FDA-authorized surgical N95 FFR must be worn by health-care workers (29 CFR 1910.134 and 29 CFR 1910.1030). Surgical N95 respirators provide the same level of respiratory protection as an N95 respirator; however, a surgical N95 respirator meets the FDA requirements for fluid penetration, flammability, and biocompatibility. The OSHA regulates respirators under the Respiratory Protection standard (29 CFR 1910.134). In order for a respirator to provide the expected level of protection, it must be used in the context of an RPP (29 CFR 1910.134).[2]

---

[2] "Respiratory Protection Guidance for the Employers of Those Working in Nursing Homes, Assisted Living, and Other Long-Term Care Facilities during the COVID-19 Pandemic," Occupational Safety and Health Administration (OSHA), March 14, 2020. Available online. URL: www.osha.gov/sites/default/files/respiratory-protection-covid19-long-term-care.pdf. Accessed December 12, 2022.

How to Protect Yourself and Others from the COVID-19 Infection

SOCIAL DISTANCING

The OSHA is committed to protecting the health and safety of America's workers and workplaces during these unprecedented times. The agency will be issuing a series of alerts designed to keep workers safe.

Social (physical) distancing involves maintaining at least six feet of distance between people and is an effective way to help reduce the risk of exposure to the coronavirus. The following steps can help employers implement social distancing in the workplace:

- Encourage workers to stay home if they are sick.
- Isolate any worker who begins to exhibit symptoms until they can either go home or leave to seek medical care.
- Establish flexible worksites (e.g., telecommuting) and flexible work hours (e.g., staggered shifts), if feasible.
- In workplaces where customers are present, mark six-foot distances with a floor tape in areas where lines form, use drive-through windows or curbside pickup, and limit the number of customers allowed at one time.
- Stagger breaks and rearrange seating in common break areas to maintain physical distance between workers.
- Move or reposition workstations to create more distance and install plexiglass partitions.
- Encourage workers to bring any safety and health concerns to the employers' attention.[3]

STAYING AWAY FROM PEOPLE WHEN YOU HAVE COVID-19
Steps to Follow If You Have COVID-19 and Feel Sick

- Stay at home when you have COVID-19.
- Stay away from other people.
- Stay in your own room.
- Clean your room by yourself.

---

[3] "COVID-19 Guidance on Social Distancing at Work," Occupational Safety and Health Administration (OSHA), February 13, 2021. Available online. URL: www.osha.gov/sites/default/files/publications/OSHA4027.pdf. Accessed December 12, 2022.

- Use your own bathroom.
- Clean your bathroom by yourself.
- Stay home until you feel better.
- Stay away from pets and service animals.
- Stay home for at least five days.
- Tell someone if you are worried about how you feel.
- Take a COVID-19 test to know if you are better or if a doctor/the health department advised you to take one.

Steps to Follow If You Have COVID-19 and Feel Well
- Stay at home when you have COVID-19.
- Stay away from other people.
- Stay in your own room.
- Clean your room by yourself.
- Use your own bathroom.
- Clean your bathroom by yourself.
- Stay away from pets and service animals.
- Stay home for at least five days.
- Take a COVID-19 test to know if you are better or if a doctor/the health department advised you to take one.

Be Safer after Being with a Person with COVID-19
- Stay home after being near a person with COVID-19.
- Stay home for at least five days.
- Watch for ways COVID-19 can make you feel sick.
- See a doctor if you feel sick.
- Take a COVID-19 test to know if you are better or if a doctor/the health department advised you to take one.[4]

---

[4] "Staying Away from People When You Have COVID-19," Centers for Disease Control and Prevention (CDC), February 10, 2022. Available online. URL: www.cdc.gov/coronavirus/2019-ncov/easy-to-read/end-home-isolation.html. Accessed December 12, 2022.

How to Protect Yourself and Others from the COVID-19 Infection

Section 12.2 | Cleaning and Disinfecting at Home

CLEANING

- Cleaning with commercial cleaners that contain soap or detergent decreases the number of germs on surfaces and reduces the risk of infection from surfaces in your facility. Cleaning alone removes most types of harmful germs (such as viruses, bacteria, parasites, or fungi) from surfaces.
- Sanitizing reduces the remaining germs on surfaces after cleaning.
- Disinfecting can kill harmful germs that remain on surfaces after cleaning. By killing germs on a surface after cleaning, disinfecting can further lower the risk of spreading disease.

If you sanitize or disinfect, clean surfaces first because impurities such as dirt may make it harder for sanitizing or disinfecting chemicals to get to and kill germs.

Consider the type of surface and how often the surface is touched. Generally, high-touch surfaces are likely to spread germs. If the space is a high-traffic area, you may choose to clean more frequently or disinfect it in addition to cleaning.

When to Clean Surfaces
- Clean high-touch surfaces regularly (e.g., pens, counters, shopping carts, door handles, stair rails, elevator buttons, touch pads, restroom fixtures, and desks).
- Clean other surfaces when they are visibly dirty.

How to Safely Clean Various Surfaces
In most situations, cleaning regularly is enough to prevent the spread of germs. Always wash your hands with soap and water

for 20 seconds after cleaning. Follow the tips given below to safely clean different surfaces in your facility:
- hard surfaces, such as counters, light switches, desks, and floors:
  - Clean surfaces with soap and water or with cleaning products appropriate for use on the surface.
- soft surfaces, such as carpets, rugs, and drapes:
  - Clean the surface using a product containing soap, detergent, or other types of cleaner appropriate for use on these surfaces.
  - Launder items if possible, according to the label instructions. Use the warmest appropriate water setting and dry items completely.
  - Vacuum surfaces such as carpets and rugs and dispose of the dirt safely.
- laundry items, such as clothing, towels, and linens:
  - Use the warmest appropriate water setting and dry items completely.
  - It is safe to wash dirty laundry from a person who is sick with other people's items.
  - Clean clothes hampers or laundry baskets according to guidance for surfaces.
- electronics, such as tablets, touch screens, keyboards, remote controls, and automated teller machines (ATMs):
  - Consider putting a wipeable cover on electronics, which makes cleaning and disinfecting easier.
  - Follow the manufacturer's instructions and recommendations for cleaning the electronic device.
- outdoor areas, such as patios and sidewalks:
  - Do not spray cleaning or disinfection products on low-touch surfaces in outdoor areas—such as on sidewalks, roads, or ground cover—which is not necessary, effective, or recommended.
  - Clean high-touch surfaces made of plastic or metal, such as grab bars, play structures, and railings when visibly dirty.
  - Do not clean and disinfect wooden surfaces (such as wood play structures, benches, and tables).

DISINFECTING SAFELY
When to Disinfect
In addition to cleaning, disinfect areas of your facility where people have obviously been ill (e.g., vomiting on facility surfaces). If the space is a high-traffic area, you may choose to clean more frequently or disinfect it in addition to cleaning. During certain disease outbreaks, local health authorities might recommend specific disinfection procedures to reduce the risk of spreading disease within the facility.

How to Disinfect Safely
To disinfect, use a disinfecting product registered with the U.S. Environmental Protection Agency (EPA) for the specific harmful germ (such as viruses or bacteria) if known. Not all disinfectants are effective for all harmful germs.

Clean the surface with soap and water first. Always read the label on disinfecting products to make sure the products can be used on the type of surface you are disinfecting (such as a hard or soft surface, food contact surface, or residual surface).

Follow the important safety guidelines given below when using chemical disinfectants:
- Open doors and windows and use fans or heating, ventilation, and air conditioning (HVAC) settings to increase air circulation in the area.
- Wear the recommended protective equipment (e.g., gloves or goggles) to protect your skin and eyes from potential splashes, as recommended by Section 8 of the product's Safety Data Sheet (www.osha.gov/sites/default/files/publications/OsHA3514.pdf).
- After you apply the disinfectant to the surface, leave the disinfectant on the surface long enough to kill the germs. This is called the "contact/wet time." You can find the contact time listed in the Safety Data Sheet and in the directions. The surface should stay wet during the entire contact time to make sure germs are killed.
- Ensure safe use and proper storage of cleaning and disinfection products, including storing them securely

and using personal protective equipment (PPE) needed for the products.
- If the product instructions tell you to dilute the product with water, use water at room temperature (unless the label says otherwise). Note: Disinfectants activated or diluted with water may have a shorter shelf life.
- Clearly label all cleaning or disinfection solutions.
- Store and use chemicals out of the reach of children and animals.
- Do not mix products or chemicals with each other as this could be hazardous and change the chemical properties.
- Do not eat, drink, or breathe cleaning or disinfection products into your body or apply them directly to your skin. These products can cause serious harm.
- Do not wipe or bathe pets with any disinfection products.
- Immediately after disinfecting, wash your hands with soap and water for 20 seconds.

In most cases, fogging, fumigation, and wide-area or electrostatic spraying are not recommended as primary methods of surface disinfection and have several safety risks unless the product label says these methods can be used.[5]

WASH YOUR HANDS

The best way to prevent illness is to avoid being exposed (or exposing others) to this virus. First, practice simple hygiene. Wash your hands regularly with soap and water for 20 seconds—especially after going to the bathroom, before eating, and after coughing, sneezing, or blowing your nose.

If soap and water are not available, the Centers for Disease Control and Prevention (CDC) recommends that consumers use

---

[5] "When and How to Clean and Disinfect a Facility," Centers for Disease Control and Prevention (CDC), November 2, 2022. Available online. URL: www.cdc.gov/coronavirus/2019-ncov/community/disinfecting-building-facility.html. Accessed December 12, 2022.

How to Protect Yourself and Others from the COVID-19 Infection

alcohol-based hand sanitizers containing at least 60 percent ethanol (also known as "ethyl alcohol").

The U.S. Food and Drug Administration (FDA) continues to warn consumers about hand sanitizers that contain methanol, also called "wood alcohol." Methanol is very toxic and should never be used in the hand sanitizer. If absorbed through the skin or swallowed, methanol can cause serious health problems, such as seizures and blindness, or even death.

Before you buy a hand sanitizer or use some you already have at home, check the FDA's list (www.fda.gov/drugs/drug-safety-and-availability/fda-updates-hand-sanitizers-consumers-should-not-use#products) to see if the hand sanitizer may have methanol. Most hand sanitizers found to contain methanol do not list it as an ingredient on the label (because it is not an acceptable ingredient in the product), so it is important to check the FDA's list to see if the company or product is included. Continue checking this list often, as it is being updated routinely.

The FDA has also expanded the list (www.fda.gov/drugs/drug-safety-and-availability/fda-updates-hand-sanitizers-consumers-should-not-use) to include hand sanitizers that contain other dangerous ingredients and products that have less than the required amount of the active ingredient.

The FDA advises consumers not to use hand sanitizers produced by the manufacturers identified on the list.[6]

---

[6] "Help Stop the Spread of Coronavirus and Protect Your Family," U.S. Food and Drug Administration (FDA), February 3, 2022. Available online. URL: www.fda.gov/consumers/consumer-updates/help-stop-spread-coronavirus-and-protect-your-family. Accessed December 12, 2022.

Chapter 13 | What to Do If You Were Exposed to COVID-19

If you have tested positive or are showing symptoms of COVID-19, isolate immediately.

ABOUT BEING EXPOSED TO COVID-19

If you were exposed to the virus that causes COVID-19 or have been told by a health-care provider or public health authority that you were exposed, here are the steps that you should take, regardless of your vaccination status or if you have had a previous infection. Learn how COVID-19 spreads and what factors increase or decrease the risk of spread.

AFTER BEING EXPOSED TO COVID-19

Wear a mask as soon as you find out you were exposed. Start counting from day one:
- Day zero is the day of your last exposure to someone with COVID-19.
- Day one is the first full day after your last exposure.

You can still develop COVID-19 up to 10 days after you have been exposed.

Take precautions:
- Wear a high-quality mask or respirator (e.g., N95) any time you are around others inside your home or indoors in public.*
  - Do not go places where you are unable to wear a mask. For travel guidance, see the travel webpage of the Centers for Disease Control and Prevention (CDC; www.cdc.gov/coronavirus/2019-ncov/travelers/index.html#can-i-travel).

Take extra precautions if you will be around people who are more likely to get very sick from COVID-19.

*Masks are not recommended for children under the age of two years and younger or for people with some disabilities. Other prevention actions (such as improving ventilation) should be used to avoid transmission during these 10 days.

Watch for symptoms:
- fever (100.4 °F or greater)
- cough
- shortness of breath
- other COVID-19 symptoms

If you develop symptoms, do the following:
- Isolate immediately.
- Get tested.
- Stay home until you know the result.

Get tested at least five full days after your last exposure. Test even if you do not develop symptoms.

If you test negative, do the following:
- Continue taking precautions through day 10.
  - Wear a high-quality mask when around others at home and indoors in public.
- You can still develop COVID-19 up to 10 days after you have been exposed.

If you test positive, isolate immediately.

What to Do If You Were Exposed to COVID-19

ABOUT NEGATIVE TEST RESULTS

As noted in the U.S. Food and Drug Administration (FDA) labeling for authorized over-the-counter (OTC) antigen tests, negative test results do not rule out severe acute respiratory syndrome coronavirus 2 (SARS-CoV-2) infection and should not be used as the sole basis for treatment or patient management decisions, including infection control decisions.[1]

---

[1] "What to Do If You Were Exposed to COVID-19," Centers for Disease Control and Prevention (CDC), August 24, 2022. Available online. URL: www.cdc.gov/coronavirus/2019-ncov/your-health/if-you-were-exposed.html. Accessed December 12, 2022.

Chapter 14 | What to Do If You or Someone at Home Is Infected with COVID-19

Chapter Contents
Section 14.1—Quarantine and Isolation 181
Section 14.2—Breastfeeding and Caring for Newborns
 If You Have COVID-19 182

Section 14.1 | Quarantine and Isolation

Isolation and quarantine help protect the public by preventing exposure to people who have or may have a contagious disease.
- **Isolation.** It separates sick people with a contagious disease from people who are not sick.
- **Quarantine.** It separates and restricts the movement of people who were exposed to a contagious disease to see if they become sick.

U.S. Quarantine Stations, located at ports of entry and land border crossings, use these public health practices as part of a comprehensive quarantine system that serves to limit the introduction of infectious diseases into the United States and to prevent their spread.[1]

COVID-19 can cause symptoms ranging from mild to very severe. For people who are older or those at high risk of getting very sick from COVID-19, treatment may be available that can reduce the chances of being hospitalized or dying from the disease. Contact a health-care provider right away. Treatment must be started within the first few days to be effective.

CARING FOR SOMEONE SICK AT HOME
Steps to Take When Sick with COVID-19
When to seek emergency medical attention: If someone is showing any emergency warning signs, call 911.
- Stay home and separate from others.
- Improve ventilation (airflow) at home to help prevent COVID-19 from spreading to other people.
- Monitor symptoms and follow health-care provider instructions.
  - Rest, drink fluids, and use over-the-counter (OTC) medicines for fever.

---

[1] "Quarantine and Isolation," Centers for Disease Control and Prevention (CDC), September 29, 2017. Available online. URL: www.cdc.gov/quarantine/index.html. Accessed December 12, 2022.

- Wear a high-quality mask or respirator when around other people.
    - Wear a mask with the best fit, protection, and comfort.
- Practice everyday hygiene and cleaning and avoid sharing personal household items.
    - Wash your hands often.
    - Cover coughs and sneezes.

For Caregivers

If you are caring for someone with COVID-19, do the following:
- Follow everyday preventative actions.
- Wear a high-quality mask when you must be around them.
- Learn what to do after being exposed to COVID-19.[2]

Section 14.2 | Breastfeeding and Caring for Newborns If You Have COVID-19

Current evidence suggests that breast milk is not likely to spread the virus to babies.

COVID-19 vaccination is recommended for people who are pregnant, breastfeeding, or trying to get pregnant now or might become pregnant in the future. In addition, everyone who is eligible, including those who are pregnant, breastfeeding, or trying to get pregnant now or might become pregnant in the future, should get a booster shot. You should always wash your hands with soap and water for 20 seconds before breastfeeding or expressing breast milk, even if you do not have COVID-19. If soap and water are not available, use a hand sanitizer with at least 60 percent alcohol.

---

[2] "If You Are Sick or Caring for Someone," Centers for Disease Control and Prevention (CDC), November 29, 2022. Available online. URL: www.cdc.gov/coronavirus/2019-ncov/if-you-are-sick/index.html. Accessed December 12, 2022.

What to Do If You or Someone at Home Is Infected with COVID-19

If you have COVID-19 and choose to breastfeed, do the following:
- Wash your hands before breastfeeding.
- Wear a mask while breastfeeding and whenever you are within six feet of your baby.

If you have COVID-19 and choose to express breast milk, do the following:
- Use your own breast pump (one not shared with anyone else), if possible.
- Wear a mask as you express breast milk.
- Wash your hands with soap and water for at least 20 seconds before touching any pump or bottle parts and before expressing breast milk.
- Follow recommendations for proper pump cleaning after each use. Clean all parts of the pump that come into contact with breast milk.
- Consider having a healthy caregiver feed the expressed breast milk to the baby. The caregiver should be up-to-date on their COVID-19 vaccines and not be at an increased risk for severe illness from COVID-19. If the caregiver is living in the same home or has been in close contact with you, they might have been exposed.
  - People who have come into close contact with someone with COVID-19 should be tested to check for infection:
    - If you develop symptoms, get tested immediately and isolate until you receive your test results. If you test positive, follow isolation recommendations.
    - If you do not develop symptoms, get tested at least five days after you last had close contact with someone with COVID-19.
    - Self-tests are one of the several options for testing for the virus that causes COVID-19 and may be more convenient than laboratory-based tests and point-of-care tests. Ask your health-care provider

or your local health department if you need help interpreting your test results.
- Any caregiver feeding the baby should wear a mask when caring for the baby for the entire time you are in isolation and during their own quarantine period after you complete isolation.[3]

---

[3] "Breastfeeding and Caring for Newborns If You Have COVID-19," Centers for Disease Control and Prevention (CDC), January 20, 2022. Available online. URL: www.cdc.gov/coronavirus/2019-ncov/if-you-are-sick/pregnancy-breastfeeding.html. Accessed December 12, 2022.

Chapter 15 | Guidance for COVID-19 Prevention and Control in Schools

Schools and early care and education (ECE) programs are an important part of the infrastructure of communities as they provide safe, supportive learning environments for students and children and enable parents and caregivers to be at work. Schools and ECE programs such as Head Start also provide critical services that help mitigate health disparities, such as school lunch programs, and social, physical, behavioral, and mental health services. This guidance can help K-12 schools and ECE programs remain open and help their administrators support safe, in-person learning while reducing the spread of COVID-19. Based on the COVID-19 community levels, this guidance provides flexibility so that schools and ECE programs can adapt to changing local situations, including periods of increased community health impacts from COVID-19.

K-12 schools and ECE programs (e.g., center-based childcare, family childcare, Head Start, or other early learning, early intervention, and preschool/prekindergarten programs delivered in schools, homes, or other settings) should put in place a core set of infectious disease prevention strategies as part of their normal operations. The addition and layering of COVID-19-specific prevention strategies should be tied to the COVID-19 community levels and community- or setting-specific context, such as availability of resources, health status of students, and age of the population served. Enhanced prevention strategies may also be necessary in response to an outbreak in the K-12 or ECE setting. This Centers for Disease Control and Prevention (CDC) guidance is meant to supplement—not replace—any federal, state, tribal, local, or territorial health and safety laws, rules, and regulations with which schools and ECE programs must comply.

Schools and ECE programs play critical roles in promoting equity in learning and health, particularly for groups disproportionately affected by COVID-19. People living in rural areas, people with disabilities, immigrants, and people who identify as American Indian/Alaska Native, Black or African American, and Hispanic or Latino have been disproportionately affected by COVID-19. These disparities have also emerged among children. School and ECE administrators and public health officials can promote equity in learning and health by demonstrating to families, teachers, and staff that comprehensive prevention strategies are in place to keep students, staff, families, and school communities safe and provide supportive environments for in-person learning. Reasonable modifications or accommodations, when necessary, must be provided to ensure equal access to in-person learning for students with disabilities.

Though this guidance is written for COVID-19 prevention, many of the layered prevention strategies described in this guidance can help prevent the spread of other infectious diseases, such as influenza (flu), respiratory syncytial virus (RSV), and norovirus, and support healthy learning environments for all. The next section describes everyday preventive actions that schools and ECE programs can take.

STRATEGIES FOR EVERYDAY OPERATIONS

Schools and ECE programs should take a variety of actions every day to prevent the spread of infectious diseases, including the virus that causes COVID-19. The following set of strategies for everyday operations should be in place at all COVID-19 community levels, including low levels.

Staying Up-to-Date on Vaccinations

Schools, ECE programs, and health departments should promote equitable access to vaccination. Staying up-to-date on routine vaccinations is essential to prevent illness from many different infections. COVID-19 vaccination helps protect eligible people from getting severely ill with COVID-19. For COVID-19, staying up-to-date with COVID-19 vaccinations is the leading public health strategy to prevent severe disease. Not only does it provide individual-level protection, but high vaccination coverage also reduces the burden of COVID-19 on people, schools, health-care systems, and communities. Schools, ECE programs, and health departments can promote vaccination in the following ways:

- Provide information about COVID-19 vaccines and other recommended vaccines. Ensure communication meets the needs of people with limited English proficiency who require language services and individuals with disabilities who require accessible formats.
- Encourage trust and confidence in COVID-19 vaccines.
- Establish supportive policies and practices that make getting vaccinated easy and convenient, for example, a workplace vaccination program or providing paid time off for individuals to get vaccinated or assist family members receiving vaccinations.
- Make vaccinations available on-site by hosting school-located vaccination clinics or connect eligible children, students, teachers, staff, and families to off-site vaccination locations.

Staying Home When Sick

People who have symptoms of respiratory or gastrointestinal infections, such as cough, fever, sore throat, vomiting, or diarrhea, should stay home. Testing is recommended for people with symptoms of COVID-19 as soon as possible after symptoms begin. People who are at risk for getting very sick with COVID-19 and who test positive should consult with a health-care provider right away for possible treatment, even if their symptoms are mild. Staying home when sick can lower the risk of spreading infectious diseases, including COVID-19, to other people.

In accordance with applicable laws and regulations, schools and ECE programs should allow flexible, nonpunitive, and supportive paid sick leave policies and practices. These policies should support workers caring for a sick family member and encourage sick workers to stay home without fear of retaliation, loss of pay, loss of employment, or other negative impacts. Schools should also provide excused absences for students who are sick, avoid policies that incentivize coming to school while sick, and support children who are learning at home if they are sick. Schools and ECE programs should ensure that employees and families are aware of and understand these policies and avoid language that penalizes or stigmatizes staying home when sick.

Ventilation

Schools and ECE programs can optimize ventilation and maintain improvements to indoor air quality (IAQ) to reduce the risk of germs and contaminants spreading through the air. Funds provided through the U.S. Department of Education's Elementary and Secondary Schools Emergency Relief (ESSER) Programs and the Governor's Emergency Education Relief (GEER) Programs and the U.S. Department of Health and Humans Services (HHS) head start and child care American rescue plan can support improvements to ventilation; repairs, upgrades, and replacements in heating, ventilation, and air conditioning (HVAC) systems; purchase of minimum efficiency reporting values 13 (MERV-13) air filters, portable air cleaners, and upper-room germicidal ultraviolet irradiation systems; and the implementation of other public health protocols and CDC guidance. The Clean Air in Buildings Challenge of the U.S. Environmental Protection Agency (EPA) provides specific steps schools and other buildings can take to improve IAQ and reduce the risk of airborne spread of viruses and other contaminants. Ventilation recommendations for different types of buildings can be found in the American Society of Heating, Refrigerating, and Air-Conditioning Engineers (ASHRAE) schools and universities guidance. The CDC does not provide recommendations for, or against, any manufacturer or product.

Guidance for COVID-19 Prevention and Control in Schools

When COVID-19 community levels increase or in response to an outbreak, schools and ECE programs can take additional steps to increase outdoor air intake and improve air filtration. For example, safely opening windows and doors, including on school buses and ECE transportation vehicles, and using portable air cleaners with high-efficiency particulate air (HEPA) filters are strategies to improve ventilation. Schools and ECE programs may also consider holding some activities outside if feasible when the COVID-19 community level is high.

Hand Hygiene and Respiratory Etiquette

Washing hands can prevent the spread of infectious diseases. Schools and ECE programs should teach and reinforce proper handwashing to lower the risk of spreading viruses, including the virus that causes COVID-19. Schools and ECE programs should monitor and reinforce these behaviors, especially during key times in the day (e.g., before and after eating, after using the restroom, and after recess) and should also provide adequate handwashing supplies, including soap and water. If washing hands is not possible, schools and ECE programs should provide hand sanitizer containing at least 60 percent alcohol. Hand sanitizers should be stored up, away, and out of sight of younger children and should be used only with adult supervision for children aged five and under.

Schools and ECE programs should teach and reinforce covering coughs and sneezes to help keep individuals from getting and spreading infectious diseases, including COVID-19.

Cleaning

Schools and ECE programs should clean surfaces at least once a day to reduce the risk of germs spreading by touching surfaces. For more information, see the Cleaning and Disinfecting Your Facility page (www.cdc.gov/coronavirus/2019-ncov/community/disinfecting-building-facility.html). Additionally, ECE programs should follow recommended procedures for cleaning, sanitizing, and disinfection in their setting such as after diapering, feeding, and exposure to bodily fluids.

CONSIDERATIONS FOR PRIORITIZING STRATEGIES

Schools and ECE programs, with help from local health departments, should consider the local context when selecting strategies to prioritize for implementation. Schools and ECE programs should balance the risk of COVID-19 with educational, social, and mental health outcomes when deciding which prevention strategies to put in place. Additional factors to consider are as follows:

- **Age of the population served.** Layered prevention strategies that are most suitable for young children should be given special consideration. Young children may have difficulty wearing a well-fitting mask consistently and correctly, and children under the age of two should not wear masks. For these reasons, layering additional prevention strategies—such as encouraging vaccination among staff and others around unvaccinated children, improved ventilation, and avoiding crowded spaces—should be used.
- **Students with disabilities.** Federal and state disability laws require an individualized approach for working with children and youth with disabilities consistent with the child's individual educational plan (IEP), Section 504 plan, or individualized family service plan (IFSP). Reasonable modifications or accommodations, when necessary, must be provided to ensure equal access to in-person learning for students with disabilities. Administrators should consider additional prevention strategies to accommodate the health and safety of students with disabilities and protect their civil rights and equal access to safe in-person learning. The U.S. Department of Education (ED) provides guidance and resources for schools and ECE programs to ensure students with disabilities continue to receive the services and support they are entitled to so that they have successful in-person educational experiences.
- **People at risk of getting very sick.** Schools and ECE programs should also consider the needs of people

who are at risk of getting very sick with COVID-19 or who have family members at risk of getting very sick with COVID-19. Some students and staff may need additional protections to ensure they can remain safely in the classroom. In addition, people who spend time indoors with individuals at risk for getting very sick with COVID-19 should consider taking extra precautions (e.g., wearing a mask) even when the COVID-19 community level is not high. School districts, schools, ECE programs, and classrooms may choose to implement masking requirements at any COVID-19 community level depending on their community's needs—and especially keeping in mind those for whom these prevention strategies provide critical protection for in-person learning.

- **Equity.** At both the individual and school levels, equity should be considered in all decision-making. Care should be taken so that decisions related to layered prevention strategies and learning options do not disproportionately affect any group of people. For instance, at the health department and school or ECE level, decisions to put in place strategies such as screening testing and contact tracing should be made in a way as to ensure that the same resources are provided to all within the district and community.
- **Resource availability.** Availability of resources, such as funding, personnel, or testing materials, varies by community. Schools or ECE programs may consider prioritizing strategies for responding to an outbreak or ramp strategies up as necessary. Alternatively, they may choose to focus resources on select, at-risk sites within the school or ECE program (such as recommending masking and testing for a classroom in which a student was recently diagnosed with COVID-19). Schools and ECE programs should work with local, state, and federal agencies to identify additional resources to implement strategies, including those provided to

schools and ECE programs through the American rescue plan.
- **Communities served.** The feasibility and acceptability of certain prevention strategies may vary within the community. Schools and ECE programs should consider community context and acceptability when choosing prevention strategies.
- **Pediatric-specific considerations.** Schools and ECE programs should work closely with local health departments to stay updated on the latest science about COVID-19, its impact on the local health-care and hospital system, and any changes to recommended prevention strategies. While children are at a lower risk for getting very sick with COVID-19, some children may still be hospitalized as a result of the infection. When schools and ECE programs are considering increasing the use and number of prevention strategies when the COVID-19 community level is high, schools and ECE programs should take into account the extent to which students are at risk for getting very sick with COVID-19 or have family members at risk for getting very sick with COVID-19.[1]

ADDITIONAL CONSIDERATIONS
Education and Training for School Staff
Provide instructional materials and training to all staff, including substitute teachers and other temporary personnel, about the following:
- symptoms of COVID-19 and how it spreads
- risks for workplace exposures and how teachers and staff can protect themselves
- risk levels for different populations depending on age and medical condition

---

[1] "Operational Guidance for K-12 Schools and Early Care and Education Programs to Support Safe In-Person Learning," Centers for Disease Control and Prevention (CDC), October 5, 2022. Available online. URL: www.cdc.gov/coronavirus/2019-ncov/community/schools-childcare/k-12-childcare-guidance.html. Accessed December 12, 2022.

- proper handwashing
- cleaning and disinfection
- cough and sneeze etiquette
- screen testing overview
- testing strategies for severe acute respiratory syndrome coronavirus 2 (SARS-CoV-2)
- other routine infection control precautions (e.g., putting on or taking off masks, social distancing measures)
- procedures to follow when an employee becomes sick or is exposed to someone who is potentially sick that include the following:
  - Symptomatic people should immediately isolate themselves from other students and staff.
  - Isolate until at least five days have passed since symptoms first appeared (at least 24 hours have passed since the last fever without the use of fever-reducing medications, and symptoms have improved). Isolation may be extended to 10–20 days depending on the severity of the illness or until the national criteria for stopping isolation have been met. Infectiousness peaks around one day before symptom onset and declines within a week of symptom onset, with an average period of infectiousness and risk of transmission between 2–3 days before and eight days after symptom onset. Omicron has a shorter incubation period (2–4 days).

Prevention for Younger Children

Encourage playtime activities that promote prevention strategies:
- Hold playtime and physical activities outdoors as much as possible.
- Supervise children to ensure children do not congregate in large groups.
- Encourage turn-taking activities, such as hopscotch.
- Divide common areas into sections so that more than one child can play at a time but separately, for example, a large sandbox.

- Encourage activities that do not involve physical contact.
- Ensure good hand hygiene following playtime.

Contact Tracing Strategies

Contact tracing with staff and students is an effective strategy to identify and isolate cases and close contacts to reduce COVID-19 transmission. Students, staff, and educators who are not vaccinated and have had close contact with a person diagnosed with COVID-19 are at the greatest risk for infection with SARS-CoV-2. It is important to become familiar with applicable laws, regulations, guidelines, policies, including those relating to privacy, and other resources to support case investigation and contact tracing within schools in an appropriate manner. Contact tracing, in combination with quarantine and isolation, and cleaning and disinfection are also important layers of prevention to keep schools safe.

Contact tracing refers to the process of:
- notifying contacts of exposure to a close contact (someone who has been within six feet of a laboratory-confirmed or probable COVID-19 patient for a cumulative total of 15 minutes or more over a 24-hour period), for example, three individual five-minute exposures for a total of 15 minutes
- referring contacts for SARS-CoV-2 testing
- encouraging contacts to self-quarantine (stay home and away from other people for at least five days and wear a well-fitted mask for 10 full days and take precautions until day 10 of close contact or until they receive a negative test result) or until the national criteria for ending quarantine have been met

Contact tracing strategies can be optimized to maximize the efficient use of limited resources:
- **Case investigation.** It is the process of confirming that the case is aware of their positive test result and then interviewing the case to elicit the names and location

information of close contacts. Case investigation is recommended for:
- probable and confirmed laboratory cases
- contacts with the highest transmission risk (those most likely to become infected)
- notification and quarantine of close contacts, with priority given to those contacts exposed within six days of the case investigation interview to maximize the potential for immediate reduction of further spread of the virus
- **Source investigation.** Also known as "backward contact tracing," it involves looking back over the 14 days prior to the symptom onset or specimen collection date (for asymptomatic cases) to identify people, places, and events or gatherings that might have been the source of the infection for the person with COVID-19.

Additionally, source investigation is useful for:
- identifying additional cases who might be undiagnosed to enhance the detection of clusters (two or more cases that are epidemiologically linked) and outbreaks
- when cases decline significantly and the focus shifts to identifying remaining cases or sources of group transmission

Other considerations are as follows:
- Parents or caregivers should be strongly encouraged to monitor their children for signs of infectious illness including COVID-19 every day.
- Students may rely on school meal programs:
  - If meals or supplementary foods are provided at school, consider distributing packaged meals and supplemental foods.
  - If hot meals are served, have only one person serve the food.

- Food distributors should wear a face mask and wash their hands before putting on gloves.
- When queuing for food, ensure that students maintain physical distance and wear face masks. Ensure that students wash their hands or use alcohol-based hand rubs before eating.
- Have meals in classrooms or outside instead of congregating in cafeterias.[2]

---

[2] "Operational Considerations for Preventing COVID-19 Transmission in Schools in Non-U.S. Settings," Centers for Disease Control and Prevention (CDC), March 15, 2022. Available online. URL: www.cdc.gov/coronavirus/2019-ncov/downloads/Operational-Considerations-for-Schools.pdf. Accessed December 12, 2022.

Chapter 16 | COVID-19 Safety Considerations Related to Music, Arts, and Athletics Programs in Schools

Schools should prioritize in-person learning over in-person extracurricular and athletics programs and activities and should use screening testing in keeping with Centers for Disease Control and Prevention (CDC) recommendations depending on the extent of community transmission of COVID-19. In general, whether occurring as part of instruction or as extracurricular activities, schools should aim to continue to offer music, performing arts, physical education, health education, and athletics programs as part of a well-rounded education for all students during the COVID-19 public health emergency, even if this requires increased screening testing or if some activities may need to be offered virtually or through a hybrid approach.

For music and performing arts, the CDC recommends masks be worn by all students and staff when not playing an instrument that requires the use of their mouth (unless the program is outdoors). When singing, people should wear a mask. Schools can consider holding music and performing arts classes outside or in an open environment or under an open tent, if safe from other hazards, such as heat, cold, and air pollution. If the class is held indoors, then implement as many other prevention strategies as possible, including optimizing ventilation, physical distancing, and cohorting/podding to help minimize class size.

Teachers can use a portable amplifier to keep voices at a low, conversational volume and should limit the exchange (or sharing) of any instruments, parts, music sheets, or any other items. Depending on the instrument, disposable absorbent pads or other receptacles, where possible, should be provided to catch the contents of spit valves. Teachers can consider using "bell covers" for the openings of brass instruments and specially designed bags with hand openings for woodwind instruments to minimize the generation of droplets and aerosols.

The CDC recommends that schools conduct sports activities in ways that reduce the risk of transmission of COVID-19 to players, families, coaches, and communities, which may include establishing a screening testing program and increasing the frequency of screening testing for those engaged in high-risk sports or activities (including unvaccinated coaches or teacher advisors), prioritizing outdoor sports or sports that involve the least physical contact, and wearing a mask.

Where rates of community transmission are high, the CDC recommends that high-risk activities be postponed or conducted virtually. Districts and schools must operate all athletic activities consistent with federal civil rights laws (Title VI of the Civil Rights Act of 1964, Title IX of the Education Amendments of 1972, Section 504 of the Rehabilitation Act of 1973, Title II of the Americans with Disabilities Act) and Part B of the Individuals with Disabilities Education Act. School leaders may need to consult with state and local legal advisors on equity matters.

For high school students in particular, access to athletics can be critical for increasing the options available to students for postsecondary education, specifically as they relate to athletic scholarships. K-12 and higher education athletics leaders should work together to safely preserve these postsecondary education opportunities, consistent with CDC guidance. Districts and schools should consider the following to try to safely maintain student access to

COVID-19 Safety Considerations

athletic programs while ensuring compliance with the nondiscrimination laws:
- Consider community transmission rates in determining if/how to safely continue activities.
  - In areas with low rates of community transmission, the CDC guidelines indicate that extracurriculars such as sports and arts programs may occur with screening testing at least once per week for participants in high-risk sports and activities who are not fully vaccinated.
  - In areas with moderate rates of community transmission, screening testing should be provided at least once per week for unvaccinated students and staff, including those participating in sports or activities.
  - In areas with substantial rates of community transmission, screening testing should be provided at least once per week for unvaccinated students and staff and at least twice per week for those engaged in high-risk sports or activities.
  - In areas with high rates of community transmission, high-risk sports and activities should occur only if all participants are vaccinated or if they can take place virtually, and schools should provide screening testing at least once per week for participants in low- and intermediate-risk sports and activities.
- Organize sports in ways that pose fewer risks. Outdoor sports that allow for physical distancing are safer than indoor sports. Sports that require frequent closeness or contact between players or that involve shared equipment may make it more difficult to maintain physical distancing and, therefore, may present an increased risk for COVID-19 spread. Schools should consider the following:
  - ability to play outdoors
  - ability for participants to wear a mask during the activity

- physical closeness of players during play
- level of intensity of the activity (the risk level increases with higher-intensity sports)
- duration of time (risks to participants, teachers, coaches, and staff increase with longer durations, including time spent traveling to/from a sporting event or other activity, meetings, meals, or other interactions)
- ability to engage in physical distancing while not actively engaged in play, such as when on the bench or sideline
- players' age and ability to comply with physical distancing and other protective actions
- size of the team and field of play
- presence of nonessential visitors or volunteers during practices or games
- travel required outside of the local community

- Limit cross-school transfer for special programs, especially beyond the community.
- Consider eliminating the use of locker rooms if they are small and poorly ventilated or do not allow for physical distancing. Advise students to come to the athletic activity in clothes that are appropriate for participation in the athletic program.
- Limit or prohibit spectators, nonessential visitors, or volunteers and activities involving external groups or organizations as possible—especially with unvaccinated people who are not from the local geographic area (e.g., community, town, city, county).
- Ensure consistent wearing of masks, aligned with guidance for gyms and fitness facilities, indicating that masks should cover the mouth and nose, should be fit to the face, and should be worn during indoor physical conditioning and training or physical education classes (except when showering, at which time students should maintain physical distance). Students should take a break from exercise if any difficulty in breathing is

COVID-19 Safety Considerations

noted and should change their mask or face covering if it becomes wet, sticks to the face, or obstructs breathing. Masks that restrict airflow under heavy exertion are not advised for exercise.
- Use a microphone and speaker and any other needed accommodation as described in a student's Individualized Education Plan (or Program; IEP) or 504 plan when coaches or instructors deliver instructions. The use of face coverings and the need for students to spread out to maintain physical distance might make it more difficult for coaches to be heard.
- Encourage physical distancing during times when players are not actively participating in practice or competition. For example, teams can increase space between players on the sideline, in the dugout, or on the bench. Consider posting signs or visual cues on the ground or walls to indicate appropriate spacing distance. Additionally, coaches can encourage athletes to spread out for individual skill-building work or cardiovascular conditioning, rather than staying clustered together.
- Do not hold indoor practices for outdoor sports and, where feasible, hold practices outdoors for indoor sports.
- Limit or avoid team meetings or social activities or hold such activities virtually.
- Avoid travel to areas with high levels of community transmission and travel when a team is located in an area with high community transmission.[1]

---

[1] "Strategies for Safely Reopening Elementary and Secondary Schools," U.S. Department of Education (ED), August 1, 2021. Available online. URL: www2.ed.gov/documents/coronavirus/reopening.pdf. Accessed December 19, 2022.

Chapter 17 | COVID-19 Control and Prevention at Workplaces

Measures for protecting workers from exposure to and infection with severe acute respiratory syndrome coronavirus 2 (SARS-CoV-2), the virus that causes COVID-19, depend on exposure risk. That risk varies based on the type of work being performed, the potential for interaction (prolonged or otherwise) with people, and contamination of the work environment. Employers should adopt infection prevention and control strategies based on a thorough workplace hazard assessment, using appropriate combinations of engineering and administrative controls, safe work practices, and personal protective equipment (PPE) to prevent worker exposures. Some Occupational Safety and Health Administration (OSHA) standards that apply to preventing occupational exposure to SARS-CoV-2 also require employers to train workers on elements of infection prevention and control, including PPE.

The general guidance below is meant to inform all U.S. workers and employers but does not alter compliance responsibilities for any particular industry. Depending on where their operations fall in the OSHA's exposure risk pyramid, workers and employers should also consult additional, specific guidance for those at either lower (i.e., caution) or increased (i.e., medium, high, or very high) risk of exposure. The exposure risk pyramid and a workplace hazard assessment can help workers and employers identify exposure risk levels commonly associated with various sectors.

All employers should remain alert to and informed about changing outbreak conditions, including as they relate to the community spread of the virus and testing availability, and implement infection prevention and control measures accordingly.

GENERAL GUIDANCE FOR ALL WORKERS AND EMPLOYERS

For all workers, regardless of specific exposure risks, it is always a good practice to do the following:

- Wear cloth face coverings, at a minimum, at all times when around coworkers or the general public. If a respirator, such as an N95 respirator or better, is needed for conducting work activities, then that respirator should be used, and the worker should use their cloth face covering when they are not using the respirator (such as during breaks or while commuting).
- Frequently wash your hands with soap and water for at least 20 seconds. When soap and running water are not immediately available, use an alcohol-based hand sanitizer with at least 60 percent ethanol or 70 percent isopropanol as active ingredients and rub hands together until they are dry. Always wash hands that are visibly soiled.
- Avoid touching your eyes, nose, or mouth with unwashed hands.
- Practice good respiratory etiquette, including covering coughs and sneezes or coughing/sneezing into your elbow/upper sleeve.
- Avoid close contact (within six feet for a total of 15 minutes or more over a 24-hour period) with people who are visibly sick and practice physical distancing with coworkers and the public.
- Stay home if sick.
- Recognize personal risk factors. According to the U.S. Centers for Disease Control and Prevention (CDC), certain people, including older adults and those with underlying conditions such as heart or lung disease, chronic kidney disease requiring dialysis, liver disease,

diabetes, immune deficiencies, or obesity, are at a higher risk for developing more serious complications from COVID-19.

The CDC has also developed interim COVID-19 guidance for businesses and employers. The interim guidance is intended to help prevent workplace exposure to acute respiratory illnesses, including COVID-19. The guidance also addresses considerations that may help employers as community transmission of SARS-CoV-2 evolves. The guidance is intended for non-health-care settings. Health-care workers and employers should consult guidance specific to them, including the information below and on the CDC coronavirus web page. Additional guidance from the Equal Employment Opportunity Commission (EEOC) and other federal agencies may be relevant to both workers and employers.

GUIDANCE FOR JOB TASKS ASSOCIATED WITH A LOWER EXPOSURE RISK

Workers whose jobs do not require contact with people known to have or suspected of having COVID-19, nor frequent close contact with (within six feet for a total of 15 minutes or more over a 24-hour period) the general public or other workers, are at a lower risk of occupational exposure.

As the Hazard Recognition page (https://www.osha.gov/coronavirus/hazards) explains, workers' job duties affect their level of occupational risk, and such risk may change as workers conduct different tasks or circumstances change.

Employers and workers in operations associated with a lower risk of exposure should remain aware of evolving trends in community transmission. Changes in community transmission, or work activities that move employees into higher-risk categories, may warrant additional precautions in some workplaces or for some workers.

Employers should monitor public health communications about COVID-19 recommendations, ensure that workers have access to that information, and collaborate with workers to designate effective means of communicating important COVID-19 information.

GUIDANCE FOR JOB TASKS ASSOCIATED WITH AN INCREASED RISK OF EXPOSURE TO SARS-COV-2

Certain workers are likely to perform job duties that involve medium, high, or very high occupational exposure risks in areas with community transmission of SARS-CoV-2. Many critical sectors depend on these workers to continue their operations. Examples of workers in these exposure risk groups include, but are not limited to, those in health care, emergency response, meat and poultry processing, retail stores (e.g., grocery stores, pharmacies), childcare and schools, and other critical infrastructure or essential operations. These workers and their employers should remain aware of the evolving community transmission risk.

As the Hazard Recognition page (https://www.osha.gov/coronavirus/hazards) explains, workers' job duties affect their level of occupational risk. Employers should assess the hazards to which their workers may be exposed, evaluate the risk of exposure, and select, implement, and ensure workers use controls to prevent exposure. Control measures may include a combination of engineering and administrative controls, safe work practices, and PPE.

All employers should consider developing COVID-19 response plans that use the hierarchy of controls and other tools to address protecting workers who remain in, or will return to, their workplaces during the COVID-19 public health emergency—including as outbreak conditions evolve. This section provides general information about protecting workers whose job tasks are associated with medium, high, and very high risk of exposure to SARS-CoV-2 during the COVID-19 pandemic and is intended to be used in tandem with other industry-specific resources linked above. In addition to considerations discussed in those resources, COVID-19 response plans may need to be addressed.

Worker Screening

Screening workers for COVID-19 signs and/or symptoms (such as through temperature checks) is a strategy that employers may choose to implement as part of their efforts to maintain or resume operations and reopen physical work sites. Employers may consider developing and implementing a screening and monitoring strategy aimed at preventing the introduction of SARS-CoV-2 into the work site.* Those who may be infected with SARS-CoV-2 may not show any signs or symptoms, thus screening and monitoring may have limitations. The complexity of screening will depend on the type of the work site and the risk of a COVID-19 outbreak among staff but, if implemented, should include the following:

- protocols for screening workers before entry into the workplace (which may entail asking workers to take their own temperatures or otherwise perform self-screening measures before reporting to work)
- criteria for the exclusion of sick workers (including asymptomatic workers who have tested positive for SARS-CoV-2 and have not yet been cleared to discontinue isolation)
- criteria for return to work of exposed and recovered employees (those who have had signs or symptoms of COVID-19 but have gotten better)

Because people infected with SARS-CoV-2 can spread the virus even if they do not have signs/symptoms of infection, screening may play a part in a comprehensive program to monitor worker health during the pandemic but may have limited utility on its own. In many workplaces, screening efforts are likely to be most beneficial when conducted at home by individual workers. Employers' temperature screening plans may rely on workers self-monitoring, rather than employers directly measuring, temperatures. Consider implementing such programs in conjunction with sick leave policies that encourage sick workers, including those whose self-monitoring efforts reveal a fever, to stay at home. The Families First Coronavirus Response Act (www.dol.gov/agencies/whd/pandemic/ffcra-employee-paid-leave) requires certain employers to provide employees with paid sick leave or expanded family and medical leave for specified reasons related to COVID-19, eligible for 100 percent reimbursement through employer tax credits.

*Protocols for worker screening must be applied equally, without discrimination based on race, national origin, sex, age, disability, or other protected characteristics.

If employers choose to implement on-site screening or monitoring programs, they may need to be coordinated, as appropriate, with local public health authorities and occupational medicine and health and safety professionals.

Employers implementing on-site screening programs may need to plan for:
- providing verbal screening in appropriate languages to determine whether workers have had new or unexpected symptoms of COVID-19 in the past 24 hours
- checking temperatures of workers at the start of each shift to identify anyone with a fever of 100.4 °F or greater (or reported feelings of feverishness)
- taking measures for testing workers for SARS-CoV-2 and responding to positive test results
- prohibiting employees from remaining in the workplace if they have a fever of 100.4 °F or greater (or report feelings of feverishness) or if screening or testing results indicate that the worker is suspected of having or known to have COVID-19. In such an event, do the following:
  - Encourage workers to self-isolate and contact a health-care provider.
  - Provide information on the employer's return-to-work policies and procedures.
  - Inform human resources, employer health unit (if applicable), bargaining unit representation (if applicable), and supervisor (so the worker can be moved off schedule during illness and a replacement can be assigned, if needed).
  - Conduct contact tracing to identify and inform coworkers or others who may have had exposure.
- taking measures to ensure worker privacy and confidentiality during any screening

Regardless of how employers ultimately decide to implement temperature checks or other health screening measures, they

COVID-19 Control and Prevention at Workplaces

should act cautiously on results. Employers should not presume that individuals who do not have a fever or other symptoms of COVID-19 do not have the virus. Similarly, because of the limitations of current testing capabilities, employers who implement workplace testing strategies should act cautiously on COVID-19 test results. Employers should not presume that individuals who test negative for SARS-CoV-2 infection (i.e., COVID-19) present no hazard to others in the workplace. Employers should ensure that screening protocols are consistent with other labor and disability laws and with collective bargaining agreements where applicable.

Employers should continue to implement universal cloth face coverings, basic hygiene, physical distancing, workplace controls, flexibilities (e.g., sick leave, telework), and employee training described in this and other OSHA and CDC guidance in ways that reflect the risk of community spread of SARS-CoV-2 from the geographical area where the workplace is located.

Identify and Isolate Suspected Cases

In workplaces where exposure to SARS-CoV-2 may occur, prompt identification and isolation of potentially infectious individuals is a critical step in protecting workers, visitors, and others at the work site.

- Wherever feasible, keep infectious people out of the workplace, including through the use of a system for employees to report if they are sick or have symptoms of COVID-19 or through the use of screening measures, as described above.
- If a worker develops signs or symptoms of COVID-19 at the workplace, send the person home to seek medical care. (Similarly, consider asking customers and visitors who develop signs and/or symptoms of COVID-19 at the workplace to leave to avoid infecting others.)
- If the person cannot immediately leave the workplace, isolate the individual in a location away from workers, customers, and other visitors and with a closed door (e.g., in a single occupancy restroom), if possible, until they can go home or leave to seek medical care.

Implement the Hierarchy of Controls

Employers' COVID-19 response plans should utilize the hierarchy of controls, which generally labels and prioritizes controls in the following order from most to least effective: elimination/substitution, engineering controls, administrative controls and safe work practices, and PPE.

Efforts to exclude potentially infectious individuals from the workplace are consistent with the aim of eliminating the hazard.

Engineering controls typically require a physical change to the workplace to isolate workers from a hazard. Examples of engineering controls that employers may find useful for protecting workers from SARS-CoV-2 include the following:

- installing plexiglass, stainless steel, or other barriers between workers, such as on assembly lines, or between workers and customers, such as at points of sale
- using rope and stanchion systems to keep customers/visitors from queuing within six feet of work areas
- adjusting ventilation systems to introduce additional outside air and/or increase air exchange to introduce fresh air (consult a qualified technician if necessary)
- modifying physical workspaces to increase the distance between employees

Administrative controls and safe work practices change policies and procedures for how workers perform job duties to ensure work activities are conducted safely. Examples of administrative controls that employers may find useful for protecting workers from SARS-CoV-2 include the following:

- limiting the number of workers assigned to a particular shift in a facility and ensuring workstations are spaced at least six feet apart
- posting signage, in languages the workers understand, to remind workers, customers, and visitors to maintain a distance of at least six feet between one another and to practice regular hand hygiene
- providing training and information in languages the workers understand

COVID-19 Control and Prevention at Workplaces

- increasing the frequency of cleaning and disinfection within the work site
- encouraging or permitting workers to wear cloth face coverings, if appropriate, to help contain potentially infectious respiratory droplets

PPE protects workers from hazards when engineering and administrative controls are insufficient on their own. The types of PPE that workers may need for protection from exposure to SARS-CoV-2 in areas with community transmission will vary based on work activities, exposure risks, and the results of the employer's hazard assessment. The Additional Considerations for Personal Protective Equipment section provides additional details about PPE selection and use for all employers whose workers have an increased risk of exposure to SARS-CoV-2 during the pandemic. Because of PPE supply chain concerns during the COVID-19 pandemic, employers should consider whether operations that require PPE can be delayed either until PPE is not needed (e.g., because the COVID-19 hazard diminishes) or until PPE supply chains stabilize. Employers should consider accommodations for religious exercise for those employees who, for instance, have or cannot trim facial hair due to religious belief or provide reasonable modifications for persons with disabilities.

Additional Considerations for Personal Protective Equipment

Interim guidance for specific types of workers and employers includes recommended PPE ensembles for various types of activities that workers may perform.
- PPE may be needed when engineering and administrative controls are insufficient to protect workers from exposure to SARS-CoV-2 or other workplace hazards and essential work operations must continue.
- PPE should be selected based on the results of an employer's hazard assessment and workers' specific job duties.

- PPE ensembles should reflect the types of exposures identified in an employer's hazard assessment. Most workers' exposure to SARS-CoV-2 is likely to be through the contact or droplet routes although some workers, including those in health care, postmortem care, and laboratories, may have exposure to aerosols for which higher-level PPE (including an N95 respirator with an assigned protection factor of 10 or better) is needed.
- When disposable gloves are used, workers should typically use a single pair of nitrile exam gloves (unless other gloving protocols are necessary for the work setting or task). Change gloves if they become torn or visibly contaminated with blood or body fluids.
- When both face protection and eye protection are needed, use surgical masks and either goggles or face shields.
  - Personal eyeglasses are not considered adequate eye protection.
  - Cloth face coverings are not acceptable substitutes for PPE intended to prevent worker exposure to droplets or other splashes or sprays of liquids.
- If workers need respirators, they must be used in the context of a comprehensive respiratory protection program that meets the requirements of OSHA's Respiratory Protection standard (29 CFR 1910.134) and includes medical exams, fit testing, and training.
  - Surgical masks are not respirators and do not provide the same level of protection to workers as properly fitted respirators. Cloth face coverings are also not acceptable substitutes for respirators.
  - An OSHA poster (available in 16 languages) and video (Spanish) provide information about how to properly wear and dispose of filtering facepiece respirators.
- If there are shortages of PPE items, such as respirators or gowns, they should be prioritized for high-hazard activities.

COVID-19 Control and Prevention at Workplaces

- Workers need respiratory protection when performing or while present for aerosol-generating procedures, including cardiopulmonary resuscitation (CPR) and intubation.
- Workers must be protected against exposure to human blood, body fluids, other potentially infectious materials, as well as hazardous chemicals and contaminated environmental surfaces.
- The CDC provides strategies for optimizing the supply of PPE, including guidance on extended use and limited reuse of N95 filtering facepiece respirators (FFRs) and methods for decontaminating and reusing disposable filtering facepiece respirators during crises.
  - These guidelines are intended for use in health care but may help employers in other sectors optimize their PPE supplies as well.
- After removing PPE, always wash hands with soap and water, if available, for at least 20 seconds. Ensure that hand hygiene facilities (e.g., sink or alcohol-based hand sanitizer) are readily available at the point of use (e.g., at or adjacent to the PPE removal area).
- Employers should establish and ensure workers follow standard operating procedures for cleaning (including laundering) PPE and items such as uniforms or laboratory coats, as well as for maintaining, storing, and disposing of PPE. When PPE is contaminated with human blood, body fluids, or other potentially infectious materials, employers must follow applicable requirements of the Bloodborne Pathogens standard (29 Case Fatality Rate (CFR) 1910.1030) with respect to laundering. The OSHA's Enforcement Procedures for the Occupational Exposure to Bloodborne Pathogens (Compliance Directives (CPL) 02-02-069) provide additional information.

Employers in all sectors may experience shortages of PPE, including gowns, face shields, face masks, and respirators, as a result of the COVID-19 pandemic. Although employers are always responsible for complying with the OSHA's PPE standards (in the general industry, 29 CFR 1910 Subpart I and in construction, 29 CFR 1926 Subpart E), including the Respiratory Protection standard (29 CFR 1910.134), whenever they apply, the OSHA is providing temporary enforcement flexibility for certain requirements under these and other health standards.

Additional Considerations for Environmental Cleaning and Disinfection

When people touch a surface or object contaminated with SARS-CoV-2, the virus that causes COVID-19, and then touch their own eyes, noses, or mouths, they may expose themselves to the virus.

Early information from the CDC, the National Institutes of Health, and other study partners suggests that SARS-CoV-2 can survive on certain types of surfaces, such as plastic and stainless steel, for 2–3 days. However, because the transmissibility of SARS-CoV-2 from contaminated environmental surfaces and objects is still not fully understood, employers should carefully evaluate whether or not work areas occupied by people suspected to have the virus may have been contaminated and whether or not they need to be disinfected in response.

The CDC provides instructions for environmental cleaning and disinfection for various types of workplaces, including the following:
- health-care facilities, as part of CDC health-care infection control recommendations
- postmortem care facilities, such as autopsy suites
- laboratories
- other non-health-care facilities

Employers operating workplaces during the COVID-19 pandemic should continue routine cleaning and other housekeeping practices in any facilities that remain open to workers or others. Employers who need to clean and disinfect environments potentially contaminated with SARS-CoV-2 should use disinfectants registered with the Environmental Protection Agency (EPA) with label claiming to be effective against SARS-CoV-2. Routine

COVID-19 Control and Prevention at Workplaces

cleaning and disinfection procedures (e.g., using cleaners and water to preclean surfaces before applying an EPA-registered disinfectant to frequently touched surfaces or objects for appropriate contact times as indicated on the product's label) are appropriate for SARS-CoV-2, including in patient care areas in health-care settings in which aerosol-generating procedures are performed.

Workers who conduct cleaning tasks must be protected from exposure to hazardous chemicals used in these tasks. In these cases, the PPE (in the general industry, 29 CFR 1910 Subpart I and in construction, 29 CFR 1926 Subpart E) and Hazard Communication (29 CFR 1910.1200) standards may apply, and workers may need appropriate PPE to prevent exposure to the chemicals. If workers need respirators, they must be used in the context of a comprehensive respiratory protection program that meets the requirements of OSHA's Respiratory Protection standard (29 CFR 1910.134) and includes medical exams, fit testing, and training.

Cleaning chemicals' Safety Data Sheets (www.osha.gov/hazcom) and other manufacturer instructions can provide additional guidance about whether workers need PPE to use the chemicals safely.

Do not use compressed air or water sprays to clean potentially contaminated surfaces, as these techniques may aerosolize infectious material. More information about protecting environmental services workers is included in the worker-specific section below.

Additional Considerations for Worker Training

Train all workers with occupational exposure to SARS-CoV-2 about the sources of exposure to the virus, the hazards associated with that exposure, and appropriate workplace protocols in place to prevent or reduce the likelihood of exposure. Training should include information about how to isolate individuals with suspected or confirmed COVID-19 or other infectious diseases and how to report possible cases. Training must be offered during scheduled work times and at no cost to the employee.

Workers required to use PPE must be trained. This training includes when to use PPE; what PPE is necessary; how to properly don (put on), use, and doff (take off) PPE; how to properly dispose of or disinfect, inspect for damage, and maintain PPE;

and the limitations of PPE. Applicable standards include the PPE (29 CFR 1910.132), Eye and Face Protection (29 CFR 1910.133), Hand Protection (29 CFR 1910.138), and Respiratory Protection (29 CFR 1910.134) standards. The OSHA's website offers a variety of training videos about respiratory protection (www.osha.gov/respiratory-protection/training).

When the potential exists for exposure to human blood, certain body fluids, or other potentially infectious materials, workers must receive the training required by the Bloodborne Pathogens (BBP) standard (29 CFR 1910.1030), including information about how to recognize tasks that may involve exposure and the methods, such as engineering controls, work practices, and PPE, to reduce exposure.

Additional Considerations for Workers with Increased Susceptibility for SARS-CoV-2 Infection or Complications

Consider offering workers who may be at increased susceptibility for SARS-CoV-2 infection or complications from COVID-19 adjustments to their work responsibilities or locations to minimize exposure. Other flexibilities, if feasible, can help prevent potential exposures among workers who have heart or lung disease, chronic kidney disease requiring dialysis, liver disease, diabetes, severe obesity, or immunocompromising health conditions. Employers should be cognizant of the requirements of the Americans with Disabilities Act, the Rehabilitation Act, and the Age Discrimination in Employment Act. The EEOC has issued guidance about COVID-19 and equal employment opportunity laws.

Additional Considerations for Return to Work Planning

The OSHA's guidance on returning to work assists employers in reopening nonessential businesses and their employees returning to work during the evolving coronavirus pandemic. The CDC has issued specific guidelines for returning to work, including after recovering from COVID-19 or having exposure to someone who has COVID-19, for certain sectors (e.g., health care and other critical infrastructure). Return to work guidance for non-healthcare workers may be based on criteria for ending home isolation.

COVID-19 Control and Prevention at Workplaces

The American Industrial Hygiene Association (AIHA) and the National Safety Council (NSC) also provide recommendations to help employers and workers safely return to work.[1]

---

[1] "Control and Prevention," Occupational Safety and Health Administration (OSHA), March 15, 2020. Available online. URL: www.osha.gov/coronavirus/control-prevention. Accessed December 12, 2022.

Chapter 18 | COVID-19 Control Measures and Effectiveness: By Country

The COVID-19 pandemic has caused widespread fear across the globe. Governments implemented strict control measures to slow the spread of the virus. These measures included lockdowns, quarantines, requiring people to wear masks, vaccination requirements, and travel restrictions, among others. However, the effectiveness of these policies has been the subject of much debate and research.

STRINGENCY INDEX
The degree of strictness in government responses to the COVID-19 pandemic can be quantified using a metric called the "stringency index." The Blavatnik School of Government at the University of Oxford manages the Oxford Coronavirus Government Response Tracker (OxCGRT), which collects data for this metric. The stringency index is an overall index derived from a database of nine response indicators, including workplace and school closures, limitations on public gatherings, quarantine requirements, cancellations of public events, and other actions governments have taken in response to the pandemic. The index is presented as a numerical value between 0 and 100, with higher values indicating more stringent COVID-19 response measures implemented by the government, which can be found below (refer to Table 18.1) as of December 31, 2022.

Table 18.1. Stringency Index of the Top 15 Countries by Rank as of December 31, 2022

Country by Rank	Stringency Index
Iran	53.94
Zimbabwe	53.70
China	47.69
Azerbaijan	45.56
Malawi	40.74
Pakistan	40.54
Uganda	38.44
Sierra Leone	37.96
Myanmar	37.04
Guatemala	36.57
Macao	36.11
Austria	35.19
Ghana	33.38
Japan	33.33
Haiti	31.48

(Source: "COVID-19: Stringency Index," Our World in Data.)

Countries with higher stringency indices have seen a slower spread of COVID-19 than those with lower indices. The stringency index is particularly useful because it can be overlaid with countries' death curves to see the effects of government response. For example, countries such as Italy, Spain, and France saw their death curves begin to flatten as they reached their highest stringency, while China's death curve plateaued as it implemented stronger measures.

SCHOOL AND WORKPLACE CLOSURES

One of the critical control measures implemented globally to slow the spread of the virus is the closure of schools and workplaces.

COVID-19 Control Measures and Effectiveness: By Country

This measure aims to reduce the number of people who come into contact with each other, thus slowing the transmission of the virus (refer to Table 18.2).

The closure of schools during the COVID-19 pandemic was initially believed to be necessary as school children were thought to be a significant source of transmission. However, recent research has shown that children are less likely to contract the virus than older individuals. As a result, closing schools for extended periods may not be an effective approach to reducing transmission but could negatively impact students' emotional, mental, and physical health including increased loneliness, academic achievement gaps, reduced physical activity, malnutrition for children who depend on school meals, and increased risk of domestic abuse and violence. However, short-term school suspension may be necessary if physical distancing, enhanced personal hygiene, and other measures are already in place, and the marginal effect of school closure is crucial in achieving the desired control levels.

Table 18.2. School Closure Index of the Top 15 Countries as of December 31, 2022

Country by Rank	School Closures
China	3
Austria	2
Sierra Leone	2
Guatemala	2
Macao	2
Kosovo	2
Poland	1
United States	1
Japan	1
Bahamas	1
Bolivia	1
Bosnia and Herzegovina	1

Table 18.2. Continued

Country by Rank	School Closures
Zimbabwe	1
Singapore	1
Panama	1

(Source: "COVID-19: School and Workplace Closures," Our World in Data.)
0–No measures
1–Closure suggested
2–Closure required (only some categories or levels, e.g., only public schools or only high schools)
3–All levels to be closed

WORKPLACE CLOSURES

Another effective control measure in the spread of COVID-19 is workplace closures. Keeping people at home and reducing the number of people who come into contact with each other reduce the risk of transmission (refer to Table 18.3). However, the overall effectiveness of total workplace closures has negatively impacted the country's economy, and according to available data, countries that implemented workplace closure measures are not necessarily more efficient at controlling the spread of COVID-19 than countries without workplace closures. The data also suggest that relaxed measures tend to be more effective and beneficial to the total economic welfare of the country.

Table 18.3. Workplace Closure Index of the Top 15 Countries as of December 31, 2022

Country by Rank	Workplace Closures
Azerbaijan	3
Angola	2
Austria	2
Egypt	2
Uganda	2

COVID-19 Control Measures and Effectiveness: By Country

Table 18.3. Continued

Country by Rank	Workplace Closures
Sierra Leone	2
Iran	2
Guinea	2
Ghana	2
Kosovo	2
Belgium	1
Italy	1
United States	1
Japan	1
Bahamas	1

(Source: "COVID-19: School and Workplace Closures," Our World in Data.)
0–No measures
1–Closure suggested (or work from home)
2–Specific categories or sectors of workers required to close (or work from home)
3–All, but essential, workplaces required to close (or work from home; e.g., medical professionals or grocery stores)

CANCELLATION OF PUBLIC EVENTS AND GATHERINGS

Canceling significant events and gatherings such as festivals, concerts, conferences, sports, parties, and religious ceremonies prevented large gatherings of people in close contact and helped control the spread of COVID-19 (refer to Table 18.4). However, they have also had negative implications and repercussions such as increased social isolation, particularly for vulnerable populations such as the elderly and people with disabilities affecting their mental health. Public events and gatherings often serve as a way for communities to unite and bond over shared experiences. The cancellation of these events has led to a feeling of disconnectedness for many people.

Table 18.4. Cancellation of Public Events Index of the Top 15 Countries as of December 31, 2022

Country by Rank	Cancellation of Public Events
Azerbaijan	2
Uganda	2
Tunisia	2
Sierra Leone	2
Mali	2
Kenya	2
Iraq	2
Iran	2
Guinea	2
Ghana	2
China	2
Kosovo	2
Japan	1
Austria	1
Bolivia	1

(Source: "COVID-19: Cancellation of Public Events and Gatherings," Our World in Data.)
0–No measures
1–Cancellation recommended
2–Cancellation required

The effectiveness of this measure is based on the fact that the virus is highly contagious and can be easily spread through close contact. Canceling public gatherings limits the number of people who come into contact with each other, thus reducing the risk of transmission. Lower transmission helps reduce the burden on health-care systems by preventing large numbers of people from becoming infected simultaneously (refer to Table 18.5).

COVID-19 Control Measures and Effectiveness: By Country

Table 18.5. Restrictions on Public Gatherings Index of the Top 15 Countries as of December 31, 2022

Country by Rank	Restrictions on Public Gatherings
Tunisia	4
Iran	4
Eritrea	4
Togo	3
Zimbabwe	3
Malawi	3
Haiti	3
Guatemala	3
Ethiopia	3
China	3
Austria	2
Bosnia and Herzegovina	2
Aruba	2
U.S. Virgin Islands	2
Macao	2

(Source: "COVID-19: Cancellation of Public Events and Gatherings," Our World in Data.)
0—No restrictions on gatherings
1—Restrictions on very large gatherings (the limit is above 1,000 people)
2—Restrictions on gatherings of 100–1,000 people
3—Restrictions on gatherings of 10–100 people
4—Restrictions on gatherings of less than 10 people

The cancellation of public events and gatherings hurt the economy, with many businesses and industries suffering as a result.

QUARANTINE RESTRICTIONS

One of the most commonly used measures to slow the virus's spread was quarantine (stay-at-home) restrictions. These required individuals to stay at home and limit their interactions with others to prevent the spread of the virus. These may include mandatory quarantine for individuals who have tested positive for COVID-19 or self-quarantine for individuals who have been exposed to someone who has tested positive.

Having considered one of the most effective means of containing and controlling the spread of COVID-19 further, stay-at-home policies have been linked to varied negative ramifications such as rise in mental health issues, social isolation, financial stress, and uncertainty about the future. Moreover, this has increased domestic violence cases as victims are forced to stay at home with their abusers. Stay-at-home policies have made it harder for victims to seek help, exacerbating the problem. With schools closed and remote learning implemented, students have experienced significant educational disruptions. This has led to concerns about learning loss, particularly for low-income students who may not have access to the technology or resources needed for remote learning. The quarantine restrictions have also resulted in delayed medical care for non-COVID-19-related issues. People are afraid to seek medical attention for fear of contracting the virus, leading to delayed diagnoses and treatments for other health issues. Table 18.6 shows the category of stay-at-home (quarantine) restrictions by country.

Table 18.6. Quarantine Restrictions Index of the Top 15 Countries as of December 31, 2022

Country by Rank	Quarantine Restrictions
Zimbabwe	2
India	2
Myanmar	2
Eritrea	2
Germany	1
Italy	1
United States	1
Japan	1

COVID-19 Control Measures and Effectiveness: By Country

Table 18.6. Continued

Country by Rank	Quarantine Restrictions
Ecuador	1
United Kingdom	0
Ireland	0
France	0
Belgium	0
Netherlands	0
Switzerland	0

(Source: "COVID-19: Stay-at-Home Restrictions," Our World in Data.)
0–No measures
1–Steps against leaving the house recommended
2–Leaving the house except for grocery shopping, daily exercise, and "essential" trips prohibited
3–Only a few exceptions for leaving the house (e.g., only one person can leave at a time, allowed to leave only once every few days, etc.)

RESTRICTIONS ON TRAVEL

COVID-19 has significantly impacted global travel, with many countries implementing strict control measures to limit the spread of the virus (refer to Table 18.7). These measures have included restrictions on local and international travel for individuals coming from high-risk areas by closing borders and prohibiting traveling altogether. Overall, the effectiveness of these travel control measures has varied depending on the country and the strictness with which they were implemented.

Table 18.7. Restrictions on Local Travel Index of the Top 15 Countries as of December 31, 2022

Country by Rank	Restrictions on Local Travel
Azerbaijan	2
Brazil	2
Iran	2

Table 18.7. Continued

Country by Rank	Restrictions on Local Travel
India	2
Myanmar	2
Guinea	2
Democratic Republic of Congo	2
United States	1
Japan	1
Zimbabwe	1
United Kingdom	0
Ireland	0
France	0
Belgium	0
Netherlands	0

(Source: "Restrictions on Internal Movement," Our World in Data.)
0—No measures
1—Movement restriction recommended
2—Movement restricted

TESTING AND CONTACT TRACING

Tests, such as reverse transcription-polymerase chain reaction (RT-PCR) antigen and serological tests, allow identification of the virus in infected individuals (refer to Table 18.8). Contact tracing allows government and public health agencies to notify individuals who have been in close contact with an infected person (refer to Table 18.9) and track the status of those infected. Together, these measures help identify and isolate individuals who may have been exposed to the virus, reducing the risk of further spread.

COVID-19 Control Measures and Effectiveness: By Country

Table 18.8. Testing Policy Index of the Top 15 Countries as of December 31, 2022

Country by Rank	Testing Policy
France	3
Belgium	3
Netherlands	3
Germany	3
Italy	3
Russia	3
United States	3
Algeria	3
Andorra	3
Argentina	3
Austria	3
Azerbaijan	3
Bahrain	3
Barbados	3
Belarus	3

(Source: "COVID-19: Testing and Contact Tracing," Our World in Data.)
0—No testing policy
1—Only those who (a) have symptoms and (b) meet specific criteria are eligible (e.g., key workers, admitted to hospital, came into contact with a known case, returned from overseas)
2—Testing anyone who exhibits COVID-19 symptoms
3—Open public testing (e.g., "drive through" testing for asymptomatic people)

Table 18.9. Contact Tracing Index of the Top 15 Countries as of December 31, 2022

Country by Rank	Contact Tracing
Belgium	2
Netherlands	2

Table 18.9. Continued

Country by Rank	Contact Tracing
Germany	2
Italy	2
Austria	2
Bahamas	2
Bangladesh	2
Bolivia	2
Brunei	2
Togo	2
Vietnam	2
Singapore	2
Senegal	2
Rwanda	2
Puerto Rico	2

(Source: "COVID-19: Testing and Contact Tracing," Our World in Data.)
0–No contact tracing
1–Limited contact tracing—not carried out in all cases
2–Comprehensive contact tracing—done for all cases

VACCINATION POLICY

Vaccination is the most effective measure implemented globally to control the virus's spread. According to the OxCGRT (refer to Table 18.10), more than 13 billion doses of the COVID-19 vaccine have been administered worldwide, covering close to 70 percent of the world's total population, with 26 percent of people in low-income countries receiving at least one dose of the vaccine and 700,144 doses given every day on a weekly average as of February 24, 2023.

The vaccination policy aims to ensure that the vaccines are distributed fairly and equitably and administered to those who need them most. The World Health Organization (WHO) has

COVID-19 Control Measures and Effectiveness: By Country

recommended that priority be given to essential workers, healthcare workers, the elderly, and people with underlying comorbid health conditions. Many countries have adopted this approach.

Further research is needed to assess the effectiveness of public health measures after adequate vaccination coverage has been achieved, and controlling the pandemic depends on high vaccination coverage and ongoing adherence to effective public health measures.

Table 18.10. Total Number of Vaccinations of the Top 15 Countries as of December 31, 2022

Country	Total Vaccinations
China	3.47 billion
India	2.2 billion
United States	666.15 million
Brazil	480.33 million
Indonesia	443.17 million
Japan	373 million
Mexico	225.06 million
Germany	191.58 million
Russia	183.88 million
France	153.44 million
United Kingdom	151.24 million
Italy	143.36 million
South Korea	129.64 million
Spain	104.18 million
Canada	96.3 million

(Source: "Coronavirus (COVID-19) Vaccinations," Our World in Data.)

REPORTING OF POLICIES

Government health organizations, such as the WHO and the Centers for Disease Control and Prevention (CDC), report COVID-19 control measures and effectiveness indices through official websites, press releases, and other publications. These reports often include information on the current number of cases, deaths, and recoveries, as well as the latest updates on testing and tracing programs, social distancing guidelines, and other measures.

Effective reporting of policies and COVID-19 control measures is essential to evaluate their impact and improve their efficacy. Public health authorities and governments should provide regular updates on these policies, analyzing their impact on the overall control. Clear communication and transparency of data sources and methods are also crucial for building trust and ensuring accountability.

Overall, COVID-19 control measures and effectiveness indices are essential tools for understanding the impact of government actions on the spread of the virus and for making informed decisions about public health. However, it is essential to remember that while these measures and indicators are significantly important, they are just a part of the broader response to controlling and containing the COVID-19 spread. It is crucial to take into account other factors such as the accessibility of health-care resources and the general health of the population. Local public and health authorities need to consider specific health and sociocultural needs of communities when implementing public health measures and weigh the overall effectiveness of these measures for the general welfare of people.

References

Adams-Prassl, Abi; Boneva, Teodora; Golin, Marta and Rauh, Christopher. "Inequality in the Impact of the Coronavirus Shock: Evidence from Real Time Surveys," Science Direct, September 2020. Available online. URL: www.sciencedirect.com/science/article/pii/S0047272720301092. Accessed December 22, 2022.

Alfano, Vincenzo and Ercolano, Salvatore. "The Efficacy of Lockdown against COVID-19: A Cross-Country Panel Analysis," Springer Nature, June 3, 2020. Available online. URL: https://link.springer.com/article/10.1007/s40258-020-00596-3. Accessed January 19, 2023.

"Considerations for Implementing and Adjusting Public Health and Social Measures in the Context of COVID-19," World Health Organization (WHO), June 14, 2021. Available online. URL: www.who.int/publications/i/item/considerations-in-adjusting-public-health-and-social-measures-in-the-context-of-covid-19-interim-guidance. Accessed December 22, 2022.

"Coronavirus (COVID-19) Vaccinations," Our World in Data, May 10, 2021. Available online. URL: https://ourworldindata.org/covid-vaccinations. Accessed January 19, 2023.

"Country Policy Responses (COVID-19 and the World of Work)," International Labour Organization (ILO), April 6, 2020. Available online. URL: www.ilo.org/global/topics/coronavirus/regional-country/country-responses/lang--en/index.htm. Accessed January 18, 2023.

"COVID-19 Government Response Tracker," University of Oxford, March 18, 2020. Available online. URL: www.bsg.ox.ac.uk/research/covid-19-government-response-tracker. Accessed January 18, 2023.

"COVID Data Tracker," Centers for Disease Control and Prevention (CDC), March 10, 2022. Available online. URL: https://covid.cdc.gov/covid-data-tracker/#datatracker-home. Accessed December 22, 2022.

Fuss, Franz Konstantin; Weizman, Yehuda & Tan, Adin Ming. "COVID-19 Pandemic: How Effective Are Preventive Control Measures and Is a Complete Lockdown Justified? A Comparison of Countries and States," Multidisciplinary Digital Publishing Institute (MDPI), December 30, 2021. Available online. URL: www.mdpi.com/2673-8112/2/1/3. Accessed January 19, 2023.

Hakobyan, Shushanik; Rawlings, Henry and Yao, Jiaxiong. "Equitable Access to Vaccines: Myth or Reality?"

International Monetary Fund (IMF), December 16, 2022. Available online. URL: www.imf.org/en/Publications/WP/Issues/2022/12/16/Equitable-Access-to-Vaccines-Myth-or-Reality-527070. Accessed January 19, 2023.

"Impact of the Stringency of Lockdown Measures on COVID-19: A Theoretical Model of a Pandemic," National Center for Biotechnology Information (NCBI), 2021. Available online. URL: www.ncbi.nlm.nih.gov/pmc/articles/PMC8491873. Accessed February 24, 2022.

Kuhfeld, Megan; Soland, James; Tarasawa, Beth; Johnson, Angela; Ruzek, Erik and Liu, Jing. "Projecting the Potential Impact of COVID-19 School Closures on Academic Achievement," American Educational Research Association (AERA), October 28, 2020. Available online. URL: https://journals.sagepub.com/doi/10.3102/0013189X20965918. Accessed December 22, 2022.

"Low-Income Country Debt Rises to Record $860 Billion in 2020," The World Bank Group, October 11, 2021. Available online. URL: www.worldbank.org/en/news/press-release/2021/10/11/low-income-country-debt-rises-to-record-860-billion-in-2020. Accessed January 18, 2023.

Mathieu, Edouard; Ritchie, Hannah; Rodés-Guirao, Lucas; Appel, Cameron; Gavrilov, Daniel; Giattino, Charlie; Hasell, Joe; Macdonald, Bobbie; Dattani, Saloni; Beltekian, Diana; Ortiz-Ospina, Esteban and Roser, Max. "Policy Responses to the Coronavirus Pandemic," Our World In Data, March 5, 2020. Available online. URL: https://ourworldindata.org/policy-responses-covid?country=~USA. Accessed January 19, 2023.

Miller, Korin. "Study Shows Which COVID-19 Policies Are Most Effective," Verywell Health, January 9, 2021. Available online. URL: www.verywellhealth.com/most-effective-covid-19-safety-policies-5094599. Accessed January 19, 2023.

Talic, Stella. "Effectiveness of Public Health Measures in Reducing the Incidence of COVID-19, SARS-CoV-2

Transmission, and COVID-19 Mortality: Systematic Review and Meta-Analysis," BMJ Publishing Group Ltd, November 18, 2021. Available online. URL: www.bmj.com/content/375/bmj-2021-068302. Accessed January 19, 2023.

"What Is Stringency Index?" Civilsdaily, May 9, 2020. Available online. URL: www.civilsdaily.com/news/what-is-stringency-index. Accessed January 19, 2023.

"WHO Releases First Data on Global Vaccine Market since COVID-19," World Health Organization (WHO), November 9, 2022. Available online. URL: www.who.int/news/item/09-11-2022-who-releases-first-data-on-global-vaccine-market-since-covid-19. Accessed January 18, 2023.

Part 3 | Clinical Care and Treatment Information for COVID-19

Chapter 19 | Clinical Spectrum of SARS-CoV-2 Infection

Patients with severe acute respiratory syndrome coronavirus 2 (SARS-CoV-2) infection can experience a range of clinical manifestations, from no symptoms to critical illness. In general, adults with SARS-CoV-2 infection can be grouped into the following severity of illness categories; however, the criteria for each category may overlap or vary across clinical guidelines and clinical trials, and a patient's clinical status may change over time.

- **Asymptomatic or presymptomatic infection.** Individuals test positive for SARS-CoV-2 using a virologic test (i.e., a nucleic acid amplification test (NAAT) or an antigen test) but have no symptoms that are consistent with COVID-19.
- **Mild illness.** Individuals have any of the various signs and symptoms of COVID-19 (e.g., fever, cough, sore throat, malaise, headache, muscle pain, nausea, vomiting, diarrhea, and loss of taste and smell) but do not have shortness of breath, dyspnea, or abnormal chest imaging.
- **Moderate illness.** Individuals show evidence of lower respiratory disease during clinical assessment or imaging and have an oxygen saturation (SaO_2) measured by pulse oximetry (SpO_2) ≥94 percent on room air at sea level.

- **Severe illness.** Individuals have SpO_2 <94 percent on room air at sea level, a ratio of arterial partial pressure of oxygen to fraction of inspired oxygen (PaO_2/FiO_2) <300 mm Hg, a respiratory rate >30 breaths/min, or lung infiltrates >50 percent.
- **Critical illness.** Individuals who have respiratory failure, septic shock, and/or multiple organ dysfunction.

SpO_2 is a key parameter for defining the illness categories listed above. However, pulse oximetry has important limitations. Clinicians who use SpO_2 when assessing a patient must be aware of those limitations and conduct the assessment in the context of that patient's clinical status.

Patients who are aged ≥65 years are at a higher risk of progressing to severe COVID-19. Other underlying conditions associated with a higher risk of severe COVID-19 include asthma, cancer, cardiovascular disease, chronic kidney disease, chronic liver disease, chronic lung disease, diabetes, advanced or untreated human immunodeficiency virus (HIV) infection, obesity, pregnancy, cigarette smoking, and being a recipient of immunosuppressive therapy or a transplant. Health-care providers should closely monitor patients with these conditions until they achieve clinical recovery.

The initial evaluation for patients may include chest imaging (e.g., x-ray, ultrasound, or computed tomography (CT) scan) and an electrocardiogram. Laboratory testing should include a complete blood count with differential and a metabolic profile, including liver and renal function tests. Although inflammatory markers such as C-reactive protein (CRP), D-dimer, and ferritin are not routinely measured as part of standard care, results from such measurements may have prognostic value.

The definitions for the severity of illness categories also apply to pregnant patients. However, the threshold for certain interventions is different for pregnant patients and nonpregnant patients. For example, oxygen (O_2) supplementation for pregnant patients is generally used when SpO_2 falls below 95 percent on room air at sea level to accommodate the physiologic changes in O_2 demand during pregnancy and to ensure adequate O_2 delivery to the fetus.

Clinical Spectrum of SARS-CoV-2 Infection

If laboratory parameters are used for monitoring pregnant patients and making decisions about interventions, clinicians should be aware that normal physiologic changes during pregnancy can alter several laboratory values. In general, leukocyte cell count increases throughout gestation and delivery and peaks during the immediate postpartum period. This increase is mainly due to neutrophilia. D-dimer and CRP levels also increase during pregnancy and are often higher in pregnant patients than nonpregnant patients. Detailed information on treating COVID-19 in pregnant patients can be found in special considerations in pregnancy and in the pregnancy considerations subsections in the guidelines (www.covid19treatmentguidelines.nih.gov/special-populations/pregnancy).

In pediatric patients, radiographic abnormalities are common and, for the most part, should not be the only criteria used to determine the severity of illness. The normal values for respiratory rate also vary with age in children; therefore, hypoxemia should be the primary criterion used to define severe COVID-19, especially in younger children. In a small subset of children and young adults, SARS-CoV-2 infection may be followed by the severe inflammatory condition multisystem inflammatory syndrome in children (MIS-C).

CLINICAL CONSIDERATIONS FOR THE USE OF PULSE OXIMETRY

During the COVID-19 pandemic, the use of pulse oximetry to assess and monitor patients' oxygenation status increased in hospital, outpatient health-care facility, and home settings. Although pulse oximetry is useful for estimating blood oxygen levels, pulse oximeters may not accurately detect hypoxemia under certain circumstances. To avoid delays in recognizing hypoxemia, clinicians who use pulse oximetry to assist with clinical decisions should keep these limitations in mind.

Pulse oximetry results can be affected by skin pigmentation, thickness, or temperature. Poor blood circulation or the use of tobacco or fingernail polish also may affect results. The U.S. Food and Drug Administration (FDA) advises clinicians to refer to the label or manufacturer website of a pulse oximeter or sensor to ascertain its accuracy. The FDA also advises using pulse oximetry only as an estimate of blood oxygen saturation because an SpO_2 reading represents a range of arterial SaO_2. For example, an SpO_2 reading of 90 percent may represent a range of SaO_2 from 86 to 94 percent.

Several published reports have compared measurements of SpO_2 and SaO_2 in patients with and without COVID-19. The studies demonstrated that occult hypoxemia (defined as SaO_2 <88% despite SpO_2 >92%) was more common in patients with darker skin pigmentation, which may result in adverse consequences. The likelihood of error was greater in the lower ranges of SpO_2. In two studies, greater incidences of occult hypoxemia were observed in patients who were Black, Hispanic, or Asian than in patients who were White. In one of these studies, occult hypoxemia was associated with more organ dysfunction and hospital mortality.

A five-hospital registry study of patients evaluated in the emergency department or hospitalized for COVID-19 found that 24 percent were not identified as eligible for treatment due to overestimation of SaO_2. The majority of patients (55%) who were not identified as eligible were Black. The study also examined the amount of time delay patients experienced before their treatment eligibility was identified. The median delay for patients who were Black was one hour longer than for those who were White.

In pulse oximetry, skin tone is an important variable, but accurately measuring oxygen saturation is a complex process. One observational study in adults was unable to identify a consistently predictable difference between SaO_2 and SpO_2 over time for individual patients. Factors other than skin pigmentation (e.g., peripheral perfusion, pulse oximeter sensor placement) are likely involved.

Despite the limitations of SpO_2, an FDA-cleared pulse oximeter for home use can contribute to an assessment of a patient's overall clinical status. Practitioners should advise patients to follow the manufacturer's instructions for use, place the oximeter on the index or ring finger, and ensure the hand is warm, relaxed, and held below the level of the heart. Fingernail polish should be removed before testing. Patients should be at rest, indoors, and breathing quietly without talking for several minutes before testing. Rather than accepting the first reading, patients or caretakers should observe the readings on the pulse oximeter for ≥30 seconds until a steady number is displayed. Patients should inform their health-care provider if the reading is repeatedly below a previously specified value (generally 95% on room air at sea level). SpO_2 has been widely adopted as a remote patient monitoring tool, but when the use of pulse oximeters is compared with close monitoring of clinical progress via video consultation, telephone calls, text messaging, or home visits, there is insufficient evidence that it improves clinical outcomes.

Not all commercially available pulse oximeters have been cleared by the FDA. SpO_2 readings obtained through non-FDA-cleared devices, such as over-the-counter (OTC) sports oximeters or mobile phone applications, lack sufficient accuracy for clinical use. Abnormal readings on these devices should be confirmed with an FDA-cleared device or an arterial blood gas analysis.

Regardless of the setting, SpO_2 should always be interpreted within the context of a patient's entire clinical presentation. A patient's signs and symptoms (e.g., dyspnea, tachypnea, chest pain, changes in cognition or attentional state, cyanosis) should be given greater weight than an SpO_2 result.

ASYMPTOMATIC OR PRESYMPTOMATIC INFECTION

Asymptomatic SARS-CoV-2 infection can occur although the percentage of patients who remain truly asymptomatic throughout the course of infection is variable and incompletely defined. It is unclear what percentage of individuals who present with asymptomatic infection progress to clinical disease. Some asymptomatic individuals have been reported to have objective radiographic findings consistent with COVID-19 pneumonia.

MILD ILLNESS

Patients with mild illness may exhibit a variety of signs and symptoms (e.g., fever, cough, sore throat, malaise, headache, muscle pain, nausea, vomiting, diarrhea, and loss of taste and smell). They do not have shortness of breath, dyspnea on exertion, or abnormal imaging. Most patients who are mildly ill can be managed in an ambulatory setting or at home through telemedicine or telephone visits. No imaging or specific laboratory evaluations are routinely indicated in otherwise healthy patients with mild COVID-19. Older patients and those with underlying comorbidities are at higher risk of disease progression; therefore, health-care providers should monitor these patients closely until clinical recovery is achieved.

MODERATE ILLNESS
Moderate illness is defined as evidence of lower respiratory disease during clinical assessment or imaging, with SpO_2 ≥94 percent on room air at sea level. Given that pulmonary disease can progress rapidly in patients with COVID-19, patients with moderate disease should be closely monitored. If bacterial pneumonia is suspected, administer empiric antibiotic treatment, reevaluate the patient daily, and deescalate or stop antibiotics if further testing indicates the patient does not have a bacterial infection.

SEVERE ILLNESS
Patients with COVID-19 are considered to have severe illness if they have SpO_2 <94 percent on room air at sea level, PaO_2/FiO_2 <300 mm Hg, a respiratory rate >30 breaths/min, or lung infiltrates >50 percent. These patients may experience rapid clinical deterioration. Oxygen therapy should be administered immediately using a nasal cannula or a high-flow oxygen device. If bacterial pneumonia or sepsis is suspected, administer empiric antibiotics, reevaluate the patient daily, and deescalate or stop antibiotics if further testing indicates the patient does not have a bacterial infection.

CRITICAL ILLNESS
SARS-CoV-2 infection can cause acute respiratory distress syndrome (ARDS), virus-induced distributive (septic) shock, cardiac shock, an exaggerated inflammatory response, thrombotic disease, and exacerbation of underlying comorbidities.

Successful clinical management of a patient with COVID-19, as with any patient in the intensive care unit (ICU), includes treating

Clinical Spectrum of SARS-CoV-2 Infection

both the medical condition that initially resulted in ICU admission as well as other comorbidities and nosocomial complications.

INFECTIOUS COMPLICATIONS IN PATIENTS WITH COVID-19

Some patients with COVID-19 may have additional infections when they present for care or that develop during the course of treatment. These coinfections may complicate treatment and recovery. Older patients or those with certain comorbidities or immunocompromising conditions may be at higher risk for these infections. The use of immunomodulators such as dexamethasone, interleukin-6 inhibitors (e.g., tocilizumab, sarilumab), or Janus kinase inhibitors (e.g., baricitinib, tofacitinib) to treat COVID-19 may also be a risk factor for infectious complications; however, when these therapies are used appropriately, the benefits outweigh the risks. Infectious complications in patients with COVID-19 can be categorized as follows:

- **Coinfections at presentation**. Although most individuals present with only SARS-CoV-2 infection, concomitant viral infections, including influenza and other respiratory viruses, have been reported. Community-acquired bacterial pneumonia has also been reported, but it is uncommon, with a prevalence that ranges from zero to six percent of people with SARS-CoV-2 infection. Antibacterial therapy is generally not recommended unless additional evidence for bacterial pneumonia is present (e.g., leukocytosis, the presence of a focal infiltrate on imaging).
- **Reactivation of latent infections**. There are case reports of underlying chronic hepatitis B virus (HBV) and latent tuberculosis infections reactivating in patients with COVID-19 who receive immunomodulators as treatment although the data are currently limited. Reactivation of herpes simplex virus and varicella zoster virus infections have also been reported. Cases of severe and disseminated strongyloidiasis have been reported in patients with COVID-19 during treatment with tocilizumab and

corticosteroids. Many clinicians would initiate empiric treatment (e.g., with the antiparasitic drug ivermectin), with or without serologic testing, in patients who are from areas where strongyloides is endemic (i.e., tropical, subtropical, or warm temperate areas).
- **Nosocomial infections.** Hospitalized patients with COVID-19 may acquire common nosocomial infections, such as hospital-acquired pneumonia (including ventilator-associated pneumonia), line-related bacteremia or fungemia, catheter-associated urinary tract infection, and *Clostridioides difficile*–associated diarrhea. Early diagnosis and treatment of these infections are important for improving outcomes in these patients.
- **Opportunistic fungal infections.** Invasive fungal infections, including aspergillosis and mucormycosis, have been reported in hospitalized patients with COVID-19. Although these infections are relatively rare, they can be fatal, and they may be seen more commonly in patients who are immunocompromised or receiving mechanical ventilation. The majority of mucormycosis cases have been reported in India and are associated with diabetes mellitus or the use of corticosteroids. The approach for managing these fungal infections should be the same as the approach for managing invasive fungal infections in other settings.

SARS-COV-2 REINFECTION AND BREAKTHROUGH INFECTION

As seen with other viral infections, reinfection after recovery from prior infection has been reported for SARS-CoV-2. Reinfection may occur as initial immune responses to the primary infection wane over time. The true prevalence of reinfection is not known and likely varies depending on the circulating variants. A national database study in Qatar estimated that previous infection prevented reinfection with the Alpha, Beta, and Delta variants of concern (VOCs), with 90, 86, and 92 percent effectiveness,

Clinical Spectrum of SARS-CoV-2 Infection

respectively. Protection against reinfection with the Omicron VOC was about 56 percent effective. Furthermore, an investigation of Omicron infection after Delta infection in four U.S. states identified 10 cases of reinfection that occurred <90 days after a symptomatic infection (one reinfection required hospitalization). The majority of reinfection cases (70%) occurred in people who were unvaccinated. Fewer patients were symptomatic during reinfection than during the initial infection. Among patients who were symptomatic, the median duration of symptoms was shorter with reinfection than with the initial infection.

Breakthrough SARS-CoV-2 infections (i.e., infection in people who completed the primary vaccine series) have been reported. Breakthrough SARS-CoV-2 infection appears to be less likely to lead to severe illness than infection in people who are unvaccinated. An analysis of electronic health record data from a large U.S. sample of 664,722 patients seen from December 2020 to September 2021 found that full vaccination was associated with a 28 percent reduction in the risk of a breakthrough infection. That study also found that the time to breakthrough infection was shorter for patients with immunocompromising conditions (i.e., people with HIV or solid organ or bone marrow transplant recipients) than for those with no immunocompromising conditions. In addition, guidelines for the diagnosis and evaluation of suspected SARS-CoV-2 reinfection or breakthrough infection are provided by the Centers for Disease Control and Prevention (CDC).

Although data are limited, no evidence suggests that the treatment of suspected or documented SARS-CoV-2 reinfection or breakthrough infection should be different from the treatment used during the initial infection, as outlined in Therapeutic Management of Nonhospitalized Adults with COVID-19 (www.covid19treatmentguidelines.nih.gov/management/clinical-management-of-adults/nonhospitalized-adults--therapeutic-management) and Therapeutic Management of Hospitalized Adults with COVID-19 (www.covid19treatmentguidelines.nih.gov/management/clinical-management-of-adults/hospitalized-adults--therapeutic-management).

PERSISTENT SYMPTOMS AND OTHER CONDITIONS AFTER ACUTE COVID-19

Some patients may experience persistent symptoms or other conditions after acute COVID-19. Adult and pediatric data on the incidence, natural history, and etiology of these symptoms and organ dysfunction are emerging. However, reports on these data have several limitations, including differing case definitions. In addition, many reports only included patients who attended post-COVID clinics, and the studies often lack comparator groups. No specific treatments for persistent effects of COVID-19 have been shown to be effective although general management strategies have been proposed, including interim guidance from the CDC, the American Academy of Physical Medicine and Rehabilitation (AAPMR; www.aapmr.org/members-publications/covid-19/multidisciplinary-quality-improvement-initiative), and the U.K.'s COVID-19 rapid guideline (www.nice.org.uk/guidance/ng188/chapter/Recommendations).

The nomenclature for this phenomenon is evolving, and no clinical terminology has been established. It has been referred to as post-COVID condition, post-COVID syndrome, post-acute sequelae of SARS-CoV-2, or, colloquially, "long COVID." Affected patients have been referred to as "long-haulers." MIS-C and multisystem inflammatory syndrome in adults (MIS-A) are serious postinfectious complications of acute COVID-19.

The CDC has defined post-COVID conditions as new, returning, or ongoing symptoms that people experience four weeks or more after being infected with SARS-CoV-2. In October 2021, the World Health Organization (WHO) published a clinical case definition that described the post-COVID clinical condition as usually occurring three months after the onset of COVID-19 with symptoms that last for two months or more and cannot be explained by an alternative diagnosis.

Persistent Symptoms

The prevalence of persistent post-COVID clinical signs and symptoms remains unclear. In a systematic review of 25 observational cohort studies, prevalence varied widely (from 5% to 80%) and likely reflected differences in study populations, case definitions, and data resources. Another large, systematic review found a similar prevalence of post-COVID symptoms six months after initial infection between studies from high-income or low- and middle-income countries and between studies in which >60 percent or <60 percent of the patients were hospitalized.

A prospective study conducted at the University of Washington investigated mostly outpatients with laboratory-confirmed SARS-CoV-2 infection (150 participants had mild illness; 11 had no symptoms; and 11 had moderate or severe disease that required hospitalization). Participants completed a follow-up questionnaire 3–9 months after illness onset; 33 percent of outpatients and 31 percent of hospitalized patients reported one or more than one persistent symptoms. Persistent symptoms were reported by 27 percent of the patients aged 18–39 years, 30 percent of those aged 40–64 years, and 43 percent of those aged ≥65 years.

In these and other studies, the most commonly reported non-neurologic, persistent symptoms included fatigue or muscle weakness, joint pain, chest pain, palpitations, shortness of breath, and cough. From January 2020 to April 2021, the CDC conducted an Internet-based survey of 3,135 noninstitutionalized adults who self-reported receiving either a positive or negative SARS-CoV-2 test result. The study found that fatigue, shortness of breath, and cough were commonly reported symptoms lasting four weeks or more after onset. The prevalence of these symptoms among participants with a positive test result versus the prevalence among participants with a negative test result was 22.5 percent versus 12 percent for fatigue, 15.5 percent versus 5.2 percent for shortness of breath, and 14.5 percent versus 4.9 percent for cough.

Some of the reported symptoms overlap with postintensive care syndrome symptoms that have been described for patients without COVID-19. Prolonged symptoms and disabilities after COVID-19 have also been reported in patients with milder illness, including outpatients.

Patients who had breakthrough infection after COVID-19 vaccination are less likely to report symptoms that persist 28 days or more than patients with SARS-CoV-2 infection who are unvaccinated. The COVID Symptom Study, conducted from December 2020 to July 2021, included participants who used a mobile application to report symptoms after breakthrough infections or reinfection.

The investigators found that the odds of reporting symptoms for 28 days or more were reduced by about half among participants who received two vaccine doses when compared with participants who received one or zero vaccine doses.

A study of electronic health record data from 59 health-care organizations, primarily in the United States, compared the records of people who did not receive any vaccine doses with records of people who received two vaccine doses. In the six months after infection, those who received two vaccine doses had a lower risk for some, but not all, long COVID outcomes, such as fatigue, muscle weakness, loss of the sense of smell, or hair loss.

Cardiopulmonary Injury

A U.S. Department of Veterans Affairs (VA) study of a national health-care database compared 153,760 veterans who survived the first 30 days of COVID-19 to contemporary and historical control cohorts that had no evidence of SARS-CoV-2 infection. When compared with the control cohorts, patients with history of COVID-19 had a greater incidence of post-acute cardiovascular outcomes (e.g., cerebrovascular disorder, dysrhythmia, inflammatory heart disease, ischemic heart disease, heart failure, thromboembolic disease) at 12 months.

A prospective study of pulmonary function examined longitudinal data from the adult Copenhagen General Population Study and found that pulmonary function declined faster for the 107 patients with mostly mild COVID-19 than for a matched sample from the general population.

Neuropsychiatric Impairment

Neuropsychiatric impairments have been reported among patients who have recovered from acute COVID-19. Reported persistent neurologic symptoms include headaches, vision changes, hearing loss, impaired mobility, numbness in extremities, restless legs syndrome, tremors, memory loss, cognitive impairment, sleep difficulties, concentration problems, mood changes, and loss of smell or taste.

Clinical Spectrum of SARS-CoV-2 Infection

One study in the U.K. administered cognitive tests to 84,285 participants who had recovered from suspected or confirmed SARS-CoV-2 infection. These participants had worse performances across multiple domains than would be expected for people with the same ages and demographic profiles; this effect was observed even among those who had not been hospitalized. However, the study authors did not report when the tests were administered in relation to the diagnosis of COVID-19.

A retrospective cohort study examined the electronic health records of 273,618 patients from 59 health-care organizations, primarily in the United States. The study reported that cognitive dysfunction (defined using International Classification of Diseases, Tenth Revision codes) 3–6 months after diagnosis was worse for people with COVID-19 than for people with influenza. Other studies have reported high rates of anxiety and depression among patients who evaluated their psychiatric distress using self-report scales. Reports also show that patients aged ≤60 years experienced more psychiatric symptoms than patients aged >60 years.

Metabolic Perturbations

There have been reports of new-onset diabetes after COVID-19. A study of a VA national health-care database analyzed the records of 181,280 people who survived the first 30 days of COVID-19 and compared them to a contemporary control cohort that had no evidence of SARS-CoV-2 infection. People with a history of COVID-19 had a 40 percent greater risk of diabetes 12 months after infection than people in the control cohort. A CDC study of people aged <18 years reported that those with a history of COVID-19 had an increased risk of diabetes >30 days after SARS-CoV-2 infection when compared with those with no history of infection.

Research on persistent symptoms and other conditions after COVID-19 is ongoing, including the RECOVER initiative (recovercovid.org) of the National Institutes of Health (NIH) which aims to better characterize the prevalence, characteristics, and pathophysiology of postacute sequelae of SARS-CoV-2 and inform potential therapeutic strategies.

CONSIDERATIONS IN PREGNANCY

Minimal data are available on differences or unique characteristics of postacute sequelae of SARS-CoV-2 among pregnant patients. Persistent symptoms after acute COVID-19 have been reported in pregnant people. In a prospective cohort study of 594 patients (95% of whom were outpatients) with SARS-CoV-2 infection who were pregnant or recently pregnant, 25 percent had persistent symptoms eight weeks or more after symptom onset. The most commonly reported persistent symptoms among this cohort were fatigue, shortness of breath, and loss of smell or taste. For pregnant patients and their children, as well as for all patients affected by post-acute sequelae of SARS-CoV-2, more research is needed to understand any unique long-term effects of COVID-19. The RECOVER initiative plans to enroll and longitudinally follow pregnant patients and their children to better understand any long-term effects of COVID-19.[1]

---

[1] COVID-19 Treatment Guidelines, "Clinical Spectrum of SARS-CoV-2 Infection," National Institutes of Health (NIH), September 26, 2022. Available online. URL: www.covid19treatmentguidelines.nih.gov/overview/clinical-spectrum. Accessed December 13, 2022.

Chapter 20 | Interim COVID-19 Treatment in Outpatients

There is strong scientific evidence that antiviral treatment of outpatients at risk for severe COVID-19 reduces their risk of hospitalization and death. The antiviral drugs nirmatrelvir with ritonavir (Paxlovid) and remdesivir (Veklury) are the preferred treatments for eligible adult and pediatric patients who are at high risk for progression to severe COVID-19. Clinicians should consider COVID-19 treatment in patients with mild-to-moderate COVID-19 who have one or more risk factors for severe COVID-19. Treatment must be started early to be effective.

RISK FACTORS FOR SEVERE COVID-19
Severe outcomes of COVID-19 are defined as hospitalization, intensive care, ventilatory support, or death. There may be other medical conditions associated with severe COVID-19 not listed here, and clinical judgment is needed.

Risk factors for severe COVID-19 include the following:
- being aged over 50, with risk increasing substantially at age 65 or older
- being unvaccinated or not being up-to-date on COVID-19 vaccinations
- having specific medical conditions and behaviors

Some people from racial and ethnic minority groups are at risk of being disproportionately affected by COVID-19 from many factors, including limited access to vaccines and health care. Healthcare providers can consider these factors when evaluating the risk for severe COVID-19 and the use of outpatient therapeutics.

OUTPATIENT TREATMENTS FOR COVID-19
Oral Nirmatrelvir with Ritonavir (Paxlovid)

In a clinical trial, Paxlovid reduced the risk of hospitalization and death by 89 percent in unvaccinated outpatients with COVID-19 at higher risk of severe disease. Serious adverse events are uncommon with Paxlovid treatment. Paxlovid is given twice daily for five days, starting as soon as possible and within five days of symptom onset, and is approved for use in adult and pediatric patients (12 years of age and older weighing at least 40 kg). Clinicians should be aware of the eligibility criteria and the potential for drug interactions with the use of Paxlovid that may preclude Paxlovid use or may require temporary discontinuation of other medications.

COVID-19 rebound has been reported to occur in a small percentage of patients between two and eight days after initial recovery and is characterized by recurrent but milder symptoms and viral detection after having tested negative.

Intravenous Remdesivir (Veklury)

Remdesivir (Veklury) reduced the risk of hospitalization and death by 87 percent in unvaccinated outpatients with COVID-19 at higher risk of severe disease. A three-day course of intravenous (IV) remdesivir initiated within seven days of symptom onset is the second preferred treatment option after Paxlovid for adults and pediatric patients (age >28 days and weight >3 kg).

Alternative Therapies

When Paxlovid or remdesivir are not accessible or clinically appropriate, the oral antiviral molnupiravir can be used. Clinicians can use the link below to review details on eligibility and indication.

Interim COVID-19 Treatment in Outpatients

The U.S. Food and Drug Administration (FDA) has also issued an Emergency Use Authorization (EUA) to permit the emergency use of COVID-19 convalescent plasma with high titers of anti-SARS-CoV-2 antibodies for the treatment of COVID-19 in patients with the immunosuppressive disease or receiving immunosuppressive treatment, in either the outpatient or inpatient setting.

Symptomatic Management
All patients with symptomatic COVID-19 should be offered symptom management with over-the-counter antipyretics, analgesics, or antitussives for fever, headache, myalgias, and cough.[1]

MANAGE YOUR COVID-19 SYMPTOMS AT HOME
If you are sick with COVID-19 or think you might have COVID-19, follow the steps given at www.cdc.gov/coronavirus/2019-ncov/if-you-are-sick/index.html?CDC_AA_refVal=https%3A%2F%2Fwww.cdc.gov%2Fcoronavirus%2F2019-ncov%2Fif-you-are-sick%2Fsteps-when-sick.html to care for yourself and help protect other people in your home and community.

OUT-OF-HOSPITAL ANTIVIRAL TREATMENT OPTIONS FOR COVID-19
The FDA authorized two antivirals, Pfizer's Paxlovid and Merck's molnupiravir, for the treatment of COVID-19 in certain patients.[2]

---

[1] "Interim Clinical Considerations for COVID-19 Treatment in Outpatients," Centers for Disease Control and Prevention (CDC), December 16, 2022. Available online. URL: www.cdc.gov/coronavirus/2019-ncov/hcp/clinical-care/outpatient-treatment-overview.html. Accessed January 6, 2023.
[2] "COVID-19 Treatments and Therapeutics," U.S. Department of Health and Human Services (HHS), December 23, 2022. Available online. URL: www.hhs.gov/coronavirus/covid-19-treatments-therapeutics/index.html. Accessed January 6, 2023.

Chapter 21 | COVID-19 Treatment in Hospital

Chapter Contents
Section 21.1—Medical Management of COVID-19 259
Section 21.2—Critical Care Management of COVID-19 263

Section 21.1 | Medical Management of COVID-19

TEST TO TREAT LOCATIONS

There are now locations where you can get tested, and if you test positive for COVID-19, you may also be eligible to receive treatment. If you test positive at a different location or with an at-home test, you can also go to these Test to Treat locations to receive a prescription from a qualified health-care provider and treatment on the spot if eligible. Some Test to Treat sites also have telehealth options available.

HOSPITAL TREATMENTS FOR COVID-19

There are treatments for hospitalized patients with severe cases of COVID-19 that have been approved or authorized for emergency use by the U.S. Food and Drug Administration (FDA).
- Remdesivir is an antiviral drug approved by the FDA for the treatment of COVID-19 in hospitalized adults and hospitalized pediatric patients at least 12 years of age. It works by stopping severe acute respiratory syndrome coronavirus 2 (SARS-CoV-2) from spreading in the body.
- The FDA has authorized additional treatments for emergency use, including convalescent plasma, monoclonal antibodies, and other treatment combinations.
- Health-care providers and scientists are investigating other drugs and treatments that may slow or reduce the virus' growth and spread in the body, as well as enhance breathing, provide disease-fighting antibodies, and help with other symptoms.

ENSURING THE SAFETY AND EFFECTIVENESS OF TREATMENTS

After a public health emergency was declared for the COVID-19 pandemic, it was determined that the FDA could authorize the

emergency use of tests, treatments, and vaccines to reduce suffering and loss of life and restore the health and security of your country.
- The FDA has approved the use of one antiviral drug Veklury (remdesivir) to treat COVID-19.
- The FDA has also issued emergency use authorizations (EUAs) to allow health-care providers to use products that are not yet approved, or that are approved for other uses, to treat patients with COVID-19 if certain legal requirements are met.
- The National Institutes of Health (NIH) is leading and supporting research on safe and effective treatments to fight COVID-19.[1]

KNOW YOUR TREATMENT OPTIONS FOR COVID-19

Patients today have more treatment options in the battle against COVID-19. The FDA has approved two drug treatments for COVID-19 and has authorized others for emergency use during this public health emergency. In addition, many more therapies are being tested in clinical trials to evaluate whether they are safe and effective in combating COVID-19.

Here is a closer look at some of the available COVID-19 treatments and how to get more information about them and others. Talk to your health-care provider about available treatment options if you have COVID-19. Your provider will know the best option for you, based on your symptoms, risks, and health history.

WHAT TREATMENTS ARE AVAILABLE FOR COVID-19?

The FDA has approved the antiviral drug Veklury (remdesivir) for adults and certain pediatric patients with COVID-19. This is an intravenous (IV) therapy. The FDA has also approved the immune modulator Olumiant (baricitinib) for certain hospitalized adults with COVID-19.

During public health emergencies, the FDA may authorize the use of unapproved drugs or unapproved uses of approved drugs

---

[1] "COVID-19 Treatments and Therapeutics," U.S. Department of Health and Human Services (HHS), December 23, 2022. Available online. URL: www.hhs.gov/coronavirus/covid-19-treatments-therapeutics/index.html. Accessed January 4, 2023.

under certain conditions. This is called an "EUA." Therapeutic products authorized under an EUA are listed on the FDA's EUA web page (www.fda.gov/emergency-preparedness-and-response/mcm-legal-regulatory-and-policy-framework/emergency-use-authorization#coviddrugs). These products are not a substitute for vaccination against COVID-19.

For example, the FDA has issued EUAs for several monoclonal antibody treatments for COVID-19 for the treatment, and in some cases prevention (prophylaxis), of COVID-19 in adults and pediatric patients. Monoclonal antibodies are laboratory-made molecules that act as substitute antibodies. They can help your immune system recognize and respond more effectively to the virus, making it more difficult for the virus to reproduce and cause harm.

There are also two oral antiviral pills, Paxlovid and Lagevrio (molnupiravir), authorized for patients with mild-to-moderate COVID-19, with strong scientific evidence they can reduce the risk of progressing to severe disease, including hospitalization and death. If you have a positive COVID-19 test and symptoms, contact your health-care provider to see if these treatment options are right for you.

The FDA is continually monitoring how authorized and approved treatments for COVID-19 are affected by changing variants. If data shows the authorized dose of a treatment is unlikely to be effective against a current variant, the FDA may announce that the therapy is no longer authorized for use at this time. When that happens, the U.S. government recommends that the product be stored in case that treatment works on a future variant.

The FDA continues to work with developers, researchers, manufacturers, the NIH, and other partners to help expedite the development and availability of therapeutic drugs and biological products to prevent or treat COVID-19. To check whether a drug is approved by the FDA, search the database of approved drugs by visiting the Drugs@FDA database (www.accessdata.fda.gov/scripts/cder/daf/).

Researchers are studying drugs that are already approved for other health conditions as possible treatments for COVID-19. Additionally, the FDA created the Coronavirus Treatment Acceleration Program (CTAP) to use every available means to assess new treatments and move them to patients as quickly as possible.

WHAT SHOULD YOU DO IF YOU HAVE, OR THINK YOU HAVE, COVID-19?

The Centers for Disease Control and Prevention (CDC) have recommendations for people who are sick with COVID-19 or think they might have COVID-19.

In general, most people have mild illnesses and can recover at home. If you think you have been exposed to COVID-19, notify your doctor, monitor your symptoms, and get emergency medical care immediately for emergency warning signs, such as trouble breathing.

If you think you need a COVID-19 diagnostic test, you can find a community testing site in your state. You can also use an FDA-authorized at-home COVID-19 diagnostic test, which gives you the option of self-testing where it is convenient for you. Be aware that COVID-19 diagnostic tests are authorized for specific uses. For example, some tests can be used by people with and without symptoms, and other tests are only for people with symptoms. Also, laboratory-based tests, such as polymerase chain reaction (PCR) tests, are generally more accurate than at-home tests.

HOW CAN YOU ACCESS THESE TREATMENTS?

Depending on your medical history, risks, and symptoms, your health-care provider can help you determine whether a therapy that is FDA-approved, or available under an EUA, is right for you. Also, the U.S. government maintains a locator tool for COVID-19 therapeutics.

HOW CAN YOU KNOW WHAT DRUGS ARE SAFE?

Always check that your information is from a trusted source. If you have questions about any medication, contact the FDA's Division of Drug Information at 301-796-3400 or druginfo@fda.hhs.gov.

COVID-19 Treatment in Hospital

HOW CAN YOU PARTICIPATE IN A COVID-19-RELATED CLINICAL TRIAL?

Talk to your health-care provider about possibly enrolling in a clinical trial in your area. For information about clinical trials for COVID-19 treatments, visit clinicaltrials.gov and the COVID-19 Prevention Network (www.coronaviruspreventionnetwork.org).[2]

Section 21.2 | Critical Care Management of COVID-19

COVID-19 can progress to critical illness, including hypoxemic respiratory failure, acute respiratory distress syndrome (ARDS), septic shock, cardiac dysfunction, thromboembolic disease, hepatic and/or renal dysfunction, central nervous system disease, and exacerbation of underlying comorbidities in both adults and children. In addition, a multisystem inflammatory syndrome in adults (MIS-A) can occur several weeks or months after severe acute respiratory syndrome coronavirus 2 (SARS-CoV-2) infection, which can lead to critical illness.

Many of the initial recommendations for the management of critically ill adults with COVID-19 in these guidelines were extrapolated from experience with other causes of sepsis and respiratory failure. However, there is now a rapidly growing body of evidence regarding the management of critically ill patients with COVID-19.

Treating patients with COVID-19 in the intensive care unit (ICU) often requires managing underlying illnesses or COVID-19-related morbidities. As with any patient who is admitted to the ICU, clinicians also need to focus on preventing ICU-related complications.

---

[2] "Know Your Treatment Options for COVID-19," U.S. Food and Drug Administration (FDA), May 19, 2022. Available online. URL: www.fda.gov/consumers/consumer-updates/know-your-treatment-options-covid-19. Accessed January 4, 2023.

SELECTED CLINICAL MANIFESTATIONS OF COVID-19 CRITICAL ILLNESS
Inflammatory Response due to COVID-19 in Adults

Patients with COVID-19 may express increased levels of proinflammatory cytokines and anti-inflammatory cytokines, which has previously been referred to as "cytokine release syndrome" or "cytokine storm." However, these terms are both imprecise and misnomers because the magnitude of cytokine elevation in many patients with COVID-19 is modest compared to that in patients with many other critical illnesses, such as sepsis and ARDS. In addition, some patients with elevated cytokine levels have no specific pathology that can be attributed to the elevated levels.

Patients with COVID-19 and severe pulmonary involvement often manifest extrapulmonary disease and exhibit laboratory markers of acute inflammation. Patients with these manifestations of the severe pulmonary disease typically progress to critical illness 10–12 days after the onset of COVID-19 symptoms.

Multisystem Inflammatory Syndrome in Adults

There are case reports describing patients who had evidence of acute or recent SARS-CoV-2 infection (confirmed by a nucleic acid amplification test (NAAT) or an antigen or antibody test) with minimal respiratory symptoms but with laboratory markers of severe inflammation (e.g., elevated levels of C-reactive protein (CRP), ferritin, D-dimer, cardiac enzymes, liver enzymes, and creatinine) and various other symptoms, including fever and shock. These patients also had signs of cardiovascular, gastrointestinal, dermatologic, and neurologic disease. This constellation of signs and symptoms has been designated MIS-A. To date, most adults with MIS-A have survived. This syndrome is similar to the multisystem inflammatory syndrome in children (MIS-C), which is much more well-described.

The current case definition for MIS-A from the Centers for Disease Control and Prevention (CDC) states that patients must be aged 21 or more, be hospitalized for 24 or more hours, or have an illness that results in death and meet the clinical and laboratory criteria outlined below. The patient should not have a likely

COVID-19 Treatment in Hospital

alternative diagnosis for the illness (e.g., bacterial sepsis, exacerbation of a chronic medical condition).

CLINICAL CRITERIA

Patients must have a subjective or documented fever (≥38.0 °C) for 24 or more hours prior to a hospitalization or within the first three days of hospitalization and at least three of the following clinical criteria, which must have occurred prior to a hospitalization or within the first three days of hospitalization. At least one must be a primary clinical criterion.

- primary clinical criteria:
  - severe cardiac illness, which includes myocarditis, pericarditis, coronary artery dilatation/aneurysm, new-onset right or left ventricular dysfunction (left ventricular ejection fraction <50%), second- or third-degree atrioventricular block, or ventricular tachycardia (cardiac arrest alone does not meet this criterion)
  - rash and nonpurulent conjunctivitis
- secondary clinical criteria:
  - new-onset neurologic signs and symptoms that include encephalopathy in a patient without prior cognitive impairment, seizures, meningeal signs, or peripheral neuropathy (including Guillain-Barré syndrome (GBS))
  - shock or hypotension that is not attributable to medical therapy (e.g., sedation, renal replacement therapy)
  - abdominal pain, vomiting, or diarrhea
  - thrombocytopenia (platelet count <150,000 cells/μL)

LABORATORY CRITERIA

- the presence of laboratory evidence of inflammation and SARS-CoV-2 infection
- elevated levels of at least two of the following:
  - CRP
  - ferritin

- interleukin 6 (IL-6)
- erythrocyte sedimentation rate
- procalcitonin
- a positive SARS-CoV-2 test result for current or recent infection using a reverse transcription polymerase chain reaction, serology, or antigen test

These criteria must be met by the end of day three of hospitalization, where the date of hospital admission is day zero.

Because there is no specific diagnostic test for MIS-A, diagnosis of this inflammatory syndrome is one of exclusion after other causes (e.g., bacterial sepsis) have been eliminated. Although there are currently no controlled clinical trial data in patients with MIS-A to guide treatment of the syndrome, case reports have described the use of intravenous immunoglobulin, corticosteroids, or anti-IL-1 receptor antagonist therapy.

COVID-19-Induced Cardiac Dysfunction, Including Myocarditis

The published literature describes cardiac injury or dysfunction in up to 24 percent of adults who are hospitalized with COVID-19. COVID-19 may be associated with an array of cardiovascular complications, including acute coronary syndrome, myocarditis, stress (Takotsubo) cardiomyopathy, arrhythmias, and thromboembolic disease.

Thromboembolic Events and COVID-19

Critically ill adults with COVID-19 have been observed to have a prothrombotic state and higher rates of venous thromboembolic disease. In some studies, thromboemboli have been diagnosed even in patients who received chemical prophylaxis with heparinoids. Autopsy studies provide additional evidence of both thromboembolic disease and microvascular thrombosis in patients with COVID-19. Some authors have called for "routine surveillance" of ICU patients for venous thromboembolism.

Renal and Hepatic Dysfunction due to COVID-19

Although SARS-CoV-2 is primarily a pulmonary pathogen, renal and hepatic dysfunction are consistently described in adults with severe COVID-19. In a 2020 multicenter cohort study of critically ill adults in the United States, 20.6 percent of patients developed acute kidney injury (AKI) that was treated with renal replacement therapy (RRT). In a cohort of critically ill adults in Brazil, the development of an AKI that required RRT was associated with poor prognosis.

Other Complications Related to Intensive Care Unit

When treating patients with COVID-19, clinicians also need to minimize the risk of conventional ICU complications. Patients who are critically ill with COVID-19 are at risk for nosocomial infections, such as ventilator-associated pneumonia, hospital-acquired pneumonia, catheter-related bloodstream infections, and other complications of critical illness care.

Critically ill patients with COVID-19 may also experience prolonged delirium and/or encephalopathy. The risk factors that are associated with delirium include the use of mechanical ventilation, restraints, benzodiazepines, opioids, vasopressors, and antipsychotics. Neurological manifestations of COVID-19 have been described in a significant proportion of hospitalized patients and are more frequent in patients with severe disease. Autopsy studies have reported both macrovascular and microvascular thrombosis with evidence of hypoxic ischemia. Adequate management of critically ill patients with COVID-19 includes paying careful attention to the best sedation practices and monitoring for stroke.

IMPORTANT CONSIDERATIONS IN THE CARE OF CRITICALLY ILL PATIENTS WITH COVID-19

Interactions between Drugs Used to Treat COVID-19 and Drugs Used to Treat Comorbidities

All ICU patients should be routinely monitored for drug–drug interactions. The potential for drug–drug interactions between investigational medications or medications that are used off-label to treat COVID-19 and concurrent drugs should be considered.

Sedation Management in Adults with COVID-19

International guidelines provide recommendations on the prevention, detection, and treatment of pain, sedation, and delirium in ICU patients. Sedation management strategies, such as maintaining a light level of sedation (when appropriate) and minimizing sedative exposure, have shortened the duration of mechanical ventilation and the length of stay in the ICU for patients without COVID-19.

The ICU liberation campaign of the Society of Critical Care Medicine (SCCM) promotes the ICU Liberation Bundle (A–F) to improve post-ICU patient outcomes. The A–F Bundle includes the following elements:
- assessing, preventing, and managing delirium
- assessing, preventing, and managing pain
- both spontaneous awakening and breathing trials
- choice of analgesia and sedation
- early mobility and exercise
- family engagement and empowerment

The A–F Bundle also provides frontline staff with practical application strategies for each element. The A–F Bundle should be incorporated using an interprofessional team model. This approach helps standardize communication among team members, improves survival, and reduces long-term cognitive dysfunction in patients. Despite the known benefits of the A–F Bundle, its impact has not been directly assessed in patients with COVID-19; however, the use of the bundle should be encouraged, when appropriate, to improve ICU patient outcomes. Prolonged mechanical ventilation of COVID-19 patients, coupled with deep sedation and potentially neuromuscular blockade, increases the workload of ICU staff. Additionally, significant drug shortages may force clinicians to use older sedatives with prolonged durations of action and active metabolites, impeding the routine implementation of SCCM's PADIS guidelines (www.sccm.org/ICULiberation/

Guidelines). This puts patients at additional risk for ICU and post-ICU complications.

Postintensive Care Syndrome

Post-intensive care syndrome (PICS) is a spectrum of cognitive, psychiatric, and/or physical disability that affects survivors of critical illness and persists after a patient leaves the ICU. Patients with PICS may present with varying levels of impairment, including profound muscle weakness (ICU-acquired weakness), problems with thinking and judgment (cognitive dysfunction), and mental health problems, such as problems sleeping, post-traumatic stress disorder (PTSD), depression, and anxiety. ICU-acquired weakness affects 33 percent of all patients who receive mechanical ventilation, 50 percent of patients with sepsis, and ≤50 percent of patients who remain in the ICU for one week or more. Cognitive dysfunction affects 30–80 percent of patients discharged from the ICU. About 50 percent of ICU survivors do not return to work within one year after discharge. Although no single risk factor has been associated with PICS, there are opportunities to minimize the risk of PICS through medication management (using the A–F Bundle), physical rehabilitation, follow-up clinics, family support, and improved education about the syndrome. PICS also affects family members who participate in the care of their loved ones. In one study, a third of family members who had major decision-making roles experienced mental health problems, such as depression, anxiety, and PTSD.

Some patients with COVID-19 who have been treated in the ICU express manifestations of PICS. Although specific therapies for COVID-19-induced PICS are not yet available, physicians should maintain a high index of suspicion for cognitive impairment and other related problems in survivors of severe or critical COVID-19 illness.

Advance Care Planning and Goals of Care

The advance care plans and the goals of care for all critically ill patients must be assessed at hospital admission and regularly thereafter. This is an essential element of care for all patients. Information on palliative care for patients with COVID-19 can be found on the National Coalition for Hospice and Palliative Care website (www.nationalcoalitionhpc.org).

To guide shared decision-making in cases of serious illness, advance care planning should include identifying existing advance directives that outline a patient's preferences and values. Values and care preferences should be discussed, documented, and revisited regularly for patients with or without prior directives. Specialty palliative care teams can facilitate communication between clinicians and surrogate decision-makers, support frontline clinicians, and provide direct patient care services when needed.

Surrogate decision-makers should be identified for all critically ill patients with COVID-19 at hospital admission. Infection-control policies for COVID-19 often create communication barriers for surrogate decision-makers, and most surrogates will not be physically present when discussing treatment options with clinicians. Many decision-making discussions will occur via telecommunication.[3]

---

[3] COVID-19 Treatment Guidelines, "Introduction to Critical Care Management of Adults with COVID-19," National Institutes of Health (NIH), May 31, 2022. Available online. URL: www.covid19treatmentguidelines.nih.gov/management/critical-care-for-adults/introduction-to-critical-care-for-adults. Accessed December 13, 2022.

Chapter 22 | Care of Post-COVID Conditions

For most patients, the goal of medical management of post-COVID conditions is to optimize function and quality of life. Ideally, health-care professionals, in consultation with the relevant specialists, should develop a comprehensive management plan based on their patients' presenting symptoms, underlying medical and psychiatric conditions, personal and social situations, and their treatment goals.

- Setting achievable goals through shared decision-making can be beneficial.
- Transparency is important for the process of goal setting; health-care professionals should advise patients that post-COVID conditions are not yet well understood and assure them that support will continue to be provided as new information emerges.
- Health-care professionals and patients should continue to discuss progress and challenges and reassess goals as needed.
- Symptoms not explained by, or out of proportion to, objective findings are not uncommon after COVID-19 and should not be dismissed, even if there is not yet a full understanding of their etiology or their expected duration.

Effective post-COVID care might include the following:
- Provide holistic patient-centered management approaches to improve patient's quality of life and

function and partner with patients to identify achievable health goals.
- Facilitate standardized, trauma-informed approaches to assessing symptoms and conditions.
- Set expectations with patients and their families that outcomes from post-COVID conditions differ among patients. Some patients may experience symptom improvement within the first three months, whereas others may continue to experience prolonged or worsening of symptoms.
- Continue follow-up over the course of illness, with considerations of broadening the testing and management approach over time if symptoms do not improve or resolve while remaining transparent that there is much more to learn about post-COVID conditions.
- Establish partnerships with specialists for physical and mental health care, when needed, which may include comprehensive rehabilitation services.
- Connect patients to social services when available, including assistance for other hardships (e.g., financial, family illness, bereavement, caregiving) and resources on disability and reasonable accommodations for work or school and connections to patient support groups.

SYMPTOM MANAGEMENT APPROACHES

Many post-COVID conditions can be improved through already-established symptom management approaches (e.g., breathing exercises to improve symptoms of dyspnea). Creating a comprehensive rehabilitation plan may be helpful for some patients and might include physical and occupational therapy, speech and language therapy, or vocational therapy, as well as neurologic rehabilitation for cognitive symptoms. A conservative physical rehabilitation plan might be indicated for some patients (e.g., persons with post-exertional malaise), and consultation with physiatry for cautious initiation of exercise and recommendations about pacing may be useful. Gradual return to activity as tolerated could be helpful for most patients.

Care of Post-COVID Conditions

Optimizing the management of underlying medical conditions might include counseling on lifestyle components such as nutrition, sleep, and stress reduction (e.g., meditation). COVID-19 vaccination should be offered to all eligible people, regardless of their history of severe acute respiratory syndrome coronavirus 2 (SARS-CoV-2) infection.

Patient diaries and calendars might be useful to document changes in health conditions and symptom severity—especially in relation to potential triggers such as exertion (physical and cognitive), foods, menstruation, and treatments or medications. Such diaries and calendars can provide greater insight into patients' symptoms and lived experience for health-care providers. Health-care providers should encourage patients to report any new or changing symptoms and to discuss any changes in activities or routines.

Patients with post-COVID conditions may share some of the symptoms that occur in patients who experience:
- myalgic encephalomyelitis/chronic fatigue syndrome
- fibromyalgia
- posttreatment Lyme disease syndrome
- dysautonomia
- mast cell activation syndrome (MCAS)

Symptom management approaches that have been helpful for these disorders may also benefit some patients with post-COVID conditions (e.g., activity management (pacing) for post-exertionalmalaise).

MEDICATIONS

Medications approved by the U.S. Food and Drug Administration (FDA) or over-the-counter medications, as well as vitamin or electrolyte supplements, may be helpful for indicated illnesses (e.g., headache, anxiety) or documented deficiencies (e.g., vitamin deficiency) after carefully weighing the benefits and risks of pharmaceutical interventions. Some treatments have been offered that lack evidence of efficacy or effectiveness and could be harmful to patients. Health-care providers should inquire about any unprescribed medications, herbal remedies, supplements, or other treatments that patients may be taking for their post-COVID conditions and evaluate for drug interactions.

Follow-up visits with a health-care professional might be considered every 2–3 months, with the frequency adjusted up or down depending on the patient's condition and illness progression. Continuity of care is important in the management of post-COVID conditions.

HOLISTIC SUPPORT FOR PATIENTS WITH POST-COVID CONDITIONS

Evidence indicates that holistic support for the patient throughout their illness course can be beneficial.

Recognizing and validating the impact of illness on quality of life should be part of the ongoing health-care professional and patient interaction. Health-care professionals can provide information on peer support resources (e.g., patient support groups, online forums). Support groups are connecting individuals, providing support, and sharing resources for persons affected by COVID-19. When material, employment, or other social support needs are identified, health-care professionals should consider referral themselves (if they are knowledgeable and able) and engaging a social worker, caseworker, community health worker, or similarly trained professional to assist.

PATIENT GROUPS WITH SPECIAL CONSIDERATIONS

People who belong to racial and ethnic minority populations have experienced a higher burden of COVID-19—in part because of structural racism and long-standing disparities in social determinants of health—which has led to a higher incidence of post-COVID conditions in some of these same populations.

- At the same time, people in these groups might have less access to the primary health care and treatment options that are needed by people suffering from post-COVID conditions.
- Furthermore, since people from racial and ethnic minority groups are disproportionately affected by some

chronic conditions that have characterized post-COVID conditions, new or worsening symptoms from these conditions might not be recognized as post-COVID conditions, leading to underestimation of post-COVID conditions prevalence in these populations.
- Tools for cross-cultural communication and language access, including translated materials on post-COVID conditions and interpreter services, could help address health literacy and improve communication effectiveness.
- Deploying resources to these communities can help ensure disproportionately affected residents are aware of post-COVID conditions and have access to needed services.

People with Disabilities

People with disabilities may require close follow-up related to functional limitations. Many adults with disabilities already experience challenges in accessing health services, and they may need different clinical management of their symptoms after SARS-CoV-2 infection, especially if their long-term symptoms are difficult to distinguish from their underlying chronic conditions.

People Experiencing Homelessness and People in Correctional Facilities

People experiencing homelessness or housing instability as well as people in correctional facilities may also experience challenges accessing health care and other support services. People with pre-existing substance use disorder may be at risk for relapse.

People with Barriers to Accessing Health Care

People with barriers to accessing health care due to lack of health insurance, access to health-care professionals who accept their health insurance, or lack of transportation, childcare, or paid sick leave may face additional challenges accessing health care. Telehealth visits may be helpful for such patients with access to broadband.

Lastly, patient advocacy groups have raised concerns that some post-COVID conditions have been either misdiagnosed as or misattributed to psychiatric causes or deconditioning, particularly among persons who belong to groups that have been marginalized or disproportionately impacted. Sensitivity to and awareness of stigma, completing a full clinical evaluation, and maintaining an attitude of empathy and understanding can help address these concerns.[1]

---

[1] "Post-COVID Conditions: Information for Health-Care Providers," Centers for Disease Control and Prevention (CDC), December 16, 2022. Available online. URL: www.cdc.gov/coronavirus/2019-ncov/hcp/clinical-care/post-covid-conditions.html#management. Accessed January 3, 2023.

Chapter 23 | Managing Health-Care Operations during COVID-19

Chapter Contents
Section 23.1—Case Investigation and Contact Tracing 279
Section 23.2—Surveillance and Data Analytics 283
Section 23.3—Optimizing Personal Protective
　　　　　　　Equipment Supplies 286
Section 23.4—Community Mitigation 291
Section 23.5—CDC Strategy for Global
　　　　　　　Response to COVID-19 (2020–2023) 301

Section 23.1 | Case Investigation and Contact Tracing

Case investigation and contact tracing have been used for decades to slow or stop the spread of infectious diseases and are essential in controlling the transmission of infectious diseases, including COVID-19. In nearly all countries, the number of COVID-19 cases and contacts has outpaced the capacity of the public health system to quickly notify and isolate all cases and quarantine all contacts.

WHAT IS THE DIFFERENCE BETWEEN CASE INVESTIGATION AND CONTACT TRACING?

Case investigation is part of the process of supporting patients with suspected or confirmed infection and includes a discussion to help patients recall everyone with whom they had close contact during the time frame in which they may have been infectious.

Contact tracing lets people know they may have been exposed to an infectious agent and what to do next for their own health and the health of others.

Case investigation and contact tracing involve getting the names of all relevant contacts and following up with them. Case investigation and contact tracing programs for COVID-19 should be tailored to local resources and needs.

HOW DOES CONTACT TRACING HELP STOP THE SPREAD OF COVID-19?

Contact tracing slows the spread of COVID-19 by letting people know they may have been exposed to the coronavirus because they were in close contact with someone who tested positive for the severe acute respiratory syndrome coronavirus 2 (SARS-CoV-2), the virus that causes COVID-19. Therefore, they should stay home for 14 days. Public health authorities may consider options to reduce quarantine.

ARE THERE DIFFERENT WAYS TO CONDUCT CONTACT TRACING?

- **Traditional contact tracing (also called "forward contact tracing")**. Programs may choose to focus their efforts on traditional contact tracing, where the emphasis is on people who were exposed to/had contact with a person who tested positive.
    - Ask the infected person who they were in contact with beginning from two days before their symptoms started or before the date of their positive test if they did not have symptoms.
    - Prioritize case investigation of those people who were recently infected with COVID-19 to rapidly identify infection in those they may have exposed while infectious. Isolating these newly infected people prevents them from spreading the virus to others.
- **Source investigation (also called "backward contact tracing")**. Programs may choose to focus on or include source investigation during case investigation. Source investigation places the emphasis on identifying the source of exposure of the person who tested positive.
    - Ask the infected person who they have been with and where they have been during the period 2–14 days before their symptoms started or before the date of their positive test if they did not have symptoms.
    - Probability of being infected as part of a cluster is greater than the probability of infecting someone, so it may be more efficient to identify the setting(s) where the infected person could have gotten COVID-19.

Source investigation may be more efficient than traditional contact tracing when the number of cases and contacts outpaces the capacity of the public health system to quickly notify and isolate all cases and quarantine all contacts.

SAMPLE CASE STUDY

A student develops symptoms on December 1. The case investigator asks the student about her contacts (who she was in contact

with) starting two days before her symptoms began, to find people she may have exposed to SARS-CoV-2, the virus that causes COVID-19.
- Contact tracer finds 155 total contacts
- Through contact tracing, all contacts were told to quarantine and get tested.
- No contacts develop symptoms or test positive.
- No new cases were identified.

SOURCE INVESTIGATION

The case investigator asks the student about her activities and contacts 2–14 days before her symptoms started, between November 17 and 29, to find where she may have been infected and ultimately who else might be infected.

The case investigator determines the following:
- The student attended a birthday party on November 21.
- The student's family hosted a celebration on November 26.
- About 15 family members from three different cities attended.
- Total of 21 people attended the family celebration.

The case investigator cross-references the names of birthday party and family celebration attendees and finds the following:
- Nobody at the birthday party was identified as a COVID-19 case.
- Two people identified at the family celebration had already tested positive for COVID-19.
- Through contact tracing and source investigation, all 21 people who attended the family celebration are notified that they are close contacts of a case. They go into quarantine and are tested.
- This leads to five more people testing positive for COVID-19.

FINAL RESULT

Eight people, including the student who was the first to test positive on December 1, were identified through the family celebration as infected cases.

CONTACT TRACING AND SOURCE INVESTIGATION TIMELINE

- The student's family hosted a celebration on November 26 (refer to Figure 23.1).
- Fifteen family members traveled from three different cities to attend dinner that happened in a fourth city.
- Total of 21 people attended the family celebration.
- Two people who attended the family celebration tested positive for COVID-19.
- Source investigation identified five more people who attended the family celebration on November 26. They also tested positive for COVID-19.
- The final result is that eight people including the student were identified through case investigation.[1]

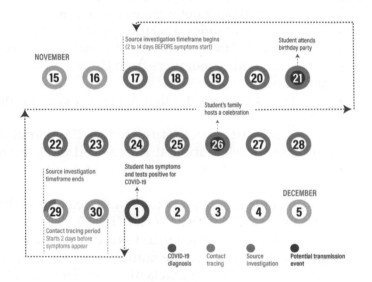

Figure 23.1. Contact Tracing and Source Investigation Timeline

Centers for Disease Control and Prevention (CDC)

---

[1] "Case Investigation and Contact Tracing," Centers for Disease Control and Prevention (CDC), July 12, 2021. Available online. URL: www.cdc.gov/coronavirus/2019-ncov/global-covid-19/case-investigation-contact-tracing.html. Accessed December 13, 2022.

Section 23.2 | Surveillance and Data Analytics

This section provides information and resources to help public health departments and laboratories investigate and report COVID-19 cases.

- **Report COVID-19 cases**. The Centers for Disease Control and Prevention (CDC) has developed a form that provides a standardized approach to reporting COVID-19 cases (individuals with at least one respiratory specimen that tested positive for the virus that causes COVID-19). These data are needed to track the impact of the outbreak and inform public health response.
- **Monitor COVID-19 cases**. COVID-19 surveillance draws from a combination of data sources from existing influenza and viral respiratory disease surveillance, syndromic surveillance, case reporting, commercial lab reporting, ongoing research platforms, and other new systems designed to answer specific questions. These systems combined create an updated, accurate picture of severe acute respiratory syndrome coronavirus 2 (SARS-CoV-2) spread and its effects in the United States and provide data used to inform the U.S. national public health response to COVID-19.

RESOURCES FROM THE CENTERS FOR DISEASE CONTROL AND PREVENTION

For surveillance of COVID-19 and its cause, SARS-CoV-2, in the United States, the CDC is using multiple surveillance systems run in collaboration with state, local, and territorial health departments; public health; commercial and clinical laboratories; vital statistics offices; health-care providers; emergency departments; and academic partners to monitor COVID-19 disease in the United States.

COVID Data Tracker Weekly Review
At www.cdc.gov/coronavirus/2019-ncov/covid-data/covidview/index.html, the CDC report provides a weekly summary and interpretation of key indicators that have been adapted to track the COVID-19 pandemic in the United States.

Cases in the United States
The page https://covid.cdc.gov/covid-data-tracker/#cases_new-caserateper100k is updated daily. Numbers close out at 4 p.m. the day before reporting.

Hospitalization Rates
Through https://gis.cdc.gov/grasp/covidnet/COVID19_3.html, the CDC monitors lab-confirmed COVID-19 hospitalizations, risk factors, and outcomes of those hospitalized each week.

Mortality Reporting
At www.cdc.gov/nchs/nvss/covid-19.htm, the CDC provides provisional death counts for COVID-19 and pneumonia based on death certificates with updates Monday–Friday.

Information for Reporting Cases
To prevent the further spread of SARS-CoV-2 and to collect information to better understand the virus and its impact on health outcomes, the CDC has developed a form (www.cdc.gov/coronavirus/2019-ncov/php/hd-breakthrough.html) that provides a standardized approach to reporting COVID-19 cases (individuals with at least one respiratory specimen that tested positive for the virus that causes COVID-19).

Information for Reporting Cases in Fully Vaccinated People (Vaccine Breakthrough Cases)
At www.cdc.gov/coronavirus/2019-ncov/php/reporting-pui.html, the CDC characterizes the SARS-CoV-2 lineages responsible for COVID-19 cases in fully vaccinated people, including variants.

CDC encourages local health departments, health-care providers, and clinical laboratories that identify COVID-19 cases to request a respiratory specimen and report the case to the state health department.

COVID-NET Interactive

Interactive and downloadable data available at https://gis.cdc.gov/grasp/covidnet/COVID19_3.html are used to estimate age-specific hospitalization rates on a weekly basis and describe characteristics of persons hospitalized with COVID-19.

CDC COVID-19 Information Management Resources (VADS)

At https://phinvads.cdc.gov/vads/SearchVocab.action, the CDC develops and maintains the COVID-19 data interoperability standards and regulations repository that is based on communication and collaboration with standard development and standard implementation organizations.

eCR Now: COVID-19 Electronic Case Reporting

Electronic Case Reporting (eCR; www.cdc.gov/coronavirus/2019-ncov/php/electronic-case-reporting.html) is the automated generation and transmission of case reports from the electronic health record (EHR) to public health agencies for review and action.

Calculating Percent Positivity

For federal COVID-19 response reporting purposes, laboratory test percent positivity (https://public4.pagefreezer.com/browse/CDC%20Covid%20Pages/16-07-2022T13:36/https://www.cdc.gov/coronavirus/2019-ncov/lab/resources/calculating-percent-positivity.html) represents the percentage of all real-time reverse transcriptase-polymerase chain reaction (RT-PCR) tests conducted that are positive.[2]

---

[2] "Surveillance and Data Analytics," Centers for Disease Control and Prevention (CDC), March 26, 2021. Available online. URL: www.cdc.gov/coronavirus/2019-ncov/php/surveillance-data-analytics.html. Accessed December 14, 2022.

Section 23.3 | Optimizing Personal Protective Equipment Supplies

Personal protective equipment (PPE) is used every day by healthcare personnel (HCP) to protect themselves, patients, and others when providing care. PPE helps protect HCP from many hazards encountered in health-care facilities.

The greatly increased need for PPE caused by the COVID-19 pandemic has caused PPE shortages, posing a tremendous challenge to the U.S. health-care system. Health-care facilities are having difficulty accessing the needed PPE and are having to identify alternative ways to provide patient care.

Surge capacity refers to the ability to manage a sudden increase in patient volume that would severely challenge or exceed the present capacity of a facility. While there are no commonly accepted measurements or triggers to distinguish surge capacity from daily patient care capacity, surge capacity is a useful framework to approach a decreased supply of PPE during the COVID-19 response. To help health-care facilities plan and optimize the use of PPE in response to COVID-19, the Centers for Disease Control and Prevention (CDC) has developed a PPE Burn RateCalculator (www.cdc.gov/coronavirus/2019-ncov/hcp/ppe-strategy/burn-calculator.html). The following are the three general strata that have been used to describe surge capacity and can be used to prioritize measures to conserve PPE supplies along the continuum of care and (refer to Table 23.1):

- **Conventional capacity.** It includes measures consisting of engineering, administrative, and PPE controls that should already be implemented in general infection prevention and control plans in health-care settings.
- **Contingency capacity.** It includes measures that may be used temporarily during periods of anticipated PPE shortages. Contingency capacity strategies should only be implemented after considering and implementing conventional capacity strategies. While the current supply may meet the facility's current or anticipated utilization rate, there may be uncertainty if future supply will be adequate and, therefore, contingency capacity strategies may be needed.

- **Crisis capacity.** It includes strategies that are not commensurate with U.S. standards of care but may need to be considered during periods of known PPE shortages. Crisis capacity strategies should only be implemented after considering and implementing conventional and contingency capacity strategies. Facilities can consider crisis capacity strategies when the supply is not able to meet the facility's current or anticipated utilization rate.

The CDC's optimization strategies for PPE offer a continuum of options for use when PPE supplies are stressed, running low, or exhausted. Contingency and then crisis capacity measures augment conventional capacity measures and are meant to be considered and implemented sequentially. As PPE availability returns to normal, health-care facilities should promptly resume standard practices.

Decisions to implement contingency and crisis strategies are based on the following assumptions:
- Facilities understand their current PPE inventory and supply chain.
- Facilities understand their PPE utilization rate.
- Facilities are in communication with local health-care coalitions and federal, state, and local public health partners (e.g., public health emergency preparedness and response staff) to identify additional supplies.
- Facilities have already implemented conventional capacity measures.
- Facilities have provided HCP with required education and training, including having them demonstrate competency with donning and doffing, with any PPE ensemble that is used to perform job responsibilities, such as the provision of patient care.

HCP and facilities—along with their health-care coalitions, local and state health departments, and local and state partners—should work together to develop strategies that identify and extend PPE supplies so that recommended PPE will be available when needed most. When using PPE optimization strategies, training on PPE

Table 23.1. Summary Strategies to Optimize the Supply of Personal Protective Equipment

PPE Type	Conventional	Contingency	Crisis
All PPE	• Use physical barriers and other engineering controls. • Limit number of patients going to hospital or outpatient settings. • Use telemedicine whenever possible. • Limit all HCP not directly involved in patient care. • Limit face-to-face HCP encounters with patients. • Limit visitors to the facility to those essential for patients' physical or emotional well-being. • Cohort patients and/or HCP.	• Selectively cancel elective and nonurgent procedures and appointments for which PPE is typically used by HCP. • Decrease length of hospital stay for medically stable patients with an infectious diagnosis for whom PPE use is recommended during their care.	• Cancel all elective and nonurgent procedures and appointments for which PPE is typically used by HCP.
N95 respirators	• Implement just-in-time fit testing. • Limit respirators during training. • Implement qualitative fit testing. • Use alternatives to N95 respirators such as other filtering facepiece respirators, elastomeric respirators, and powered air-purifying respirators.	• Temporarily suspend annual fit testing. • Use N95 respirators beyond the manufacturer-designated shelf life for training and fit testing. • Extend the use of N95 respirators by wearing the same N95 for repeated close contact encounters with several different patients.	• Use respirators beyond the manufacturer-designated shelf life for health care delivery. • Use respirators approved under standards used in other countries. • Implement limited reuse of N95 respirators. During times of crisis, it may be needed to practice limited reuse on top of extended use. • Use additional respirators beyond the manufacturer-designated shelf life that have not been evaluated by the National Institute for Occupational Safety and Health (NIOSH). • Prioritize the use of N95 respirators and face masks by activity.

Table 23.1. Continued

PPE Type	Conventional	Contingency	Crisis

Face masks	• Use face masks according to product labeling and local, state, and federal requirements.
	• In health-care settings, face masks are used by HCP as follows:
	  • PPE to protect their nose and mouth from exposure to splashes, sprays, splatter, and respiratory secretions (e.g., for patients on droplet precautions)
	  • source control to cover their mouth and nose to prevent the spread of respiratory secretions when they are talking, sneezing, or coughing
		• Remove face masks from facility entrances and other public areas.
		• Implement extended use of face masks as PPE.
		• Restrict face masks for use only by HCP when needed as PPE. Patients and HCP requiring only source control may use a cloth mask.
			• Use face masks beyond the manufacturer-designated shelf life during patient care activities.
			• Implement limited reuse of face masks with extended use.
			• Prioritize face masks for HCP for selected activities such as essential surgeries, activities where splashes and sprays are anticipated, and contact with an infectious patient, for whom face mask use is recommended.
			• When no respirators or face masks are available: use a face shield that covers the entire front (that extends to the chin or below) and sides of the face with no face mask.

Gowns	• Use isolation gown alternatives that offer equivalent or higher protection including reusable (i.e., washable) gowns. • *Note:* In general, CDC does not recommend the use of more than one isolation gown at a time when providing care to confirmed or suspected COVID-19 patients.	• Consider the use of coveralls. • Use gowns beyond the manufacturer-designated shelf life for training. • Use gowns or coveralls conforming to international standards.	• Extend the use of isolation gowns. • Prioritize gowns for activities where splashes and sprays are anticipated, during high-contact patient care, and for patients colonized or infected with emerging highly-resistant organisms. • Consider using gown alternatives that have not been evaluated as effective. • Reuse of isolation gowns is not recommended (risks of transmission among HCP and patients likely outweigh any potential benefits).

Table 23.1. Continued

PPE Type	Conventional	Contingency	Crisis
Eye protection	• Use eye protection according to product labeling and local, state, and federal requirements. • Shift eye protection supplies from disposable to reusable devices.	• Extend the use of eye protection.	• Use eye protection devices beyond the manufacturer-designated shelf life. • Prioritize eye protection for activities where splashes and sprays are anticipated or prolonged face-to-face or close contact with a potentially infectious patient is unavoidable. • Consider using safety glasses that cover the sides of the eyes.
Gloves	• Continue providing patient care as in usual infection control practice. • *Note:* The CDC does not recommend double gloves when providing care to suspected or confirmed COVID-19 patients.	• Use gloves past their manufacturer-designated shelf life for training activities. • Use gloves conforming to other U.S. and international standards.	• Use gloves past their manufacturer-designated shelf life for health care delivery. • Consider non-health-care glove alternatives. • Extend the use of disposable medical gloves.

(Source: "Summary for Healthcare Facilities: Strategies for Optimizing the Supply of PPE during Shortages," Centers for Disease Control and Prevention (CDC).)

use, including proper donning and doffing procedures, must be provided to HCP before they carry out patient care activities.[3]

Section 23.4 | Community Mitigation

COMMUNITY MITIGATION MEASURES FOR LOWER-RESOURCE COUNTRIES

Community mitigation measures are actions taken to prevent the further spread of infectious diseases and protect all people, especially groups of people at increased risk for severe illness, disproportionally affected groups, and essential workers. The goal for using mitigation strategies in countries that are experiencing community transmission of COVID-19 is to decrease transmission overall while minimizing the negative social or economic effects of strategies such as isolation, quarantine, or closing of businesses, schools, and other public, congregate settings.

Governments, individuals, communities, businesses, and health-care providers contribute to an overall community mitigation strategy to minimize illness and death rates as well as the social and economic impact of COVID-19. Countries should consider community mitigation measures and choose which ones to put in place to prepare for and respond to community transmission of COVID-19.

Signs of ongoing community transmission include:
- detection of confirmed cases of COVID-19 with no epidemiologic link to known cases
- more than three generations of local transmission

Implementation of community mitigation measures is based on:
- encouraging personal responsibility to follow recommended actions

---

[3] "Optimizing Supply of PPE and Other Equipment during Shortages," Centers for Disease Control and Prevention (CDC), July 16, 2020. Available online. URL: www.cdc.gov/coronavirus/2019-ncov/hcp/ppe-strategy/general-optimization-strategies.html. Accessed December 14, 2022.

- emphasizing government and community responsibility to make sure people have access to information and resources required to follow recommended actions
- ensuring government, community institutions (schools, places of worship, marketplaces, childcare providers), businesses, and households put recommended actions in place, with a focus on actions that protect those at increased risk of severe illness, those who are disproportionately impacted, and first responders
- focusing on settings that provide critical infrastructure or services to minimize their risk of disruption
- minimizing disruptions to daily life, to the extent possible
- adapting interventions supported by existing public health programs to address immediate community mitigation needs
- promoting government and community responsibility to pass setting- and population-specific policies endorsing recommended actions

FACTORS TO CONSIDER WHEN DETERMINING COMMUNITY MITIGATION STRATEGIES
Epidemiology
- level of transmission and disease dynamics
- number, setting (e.g., schools, workplaces), and source (e.g., community gathering points, events) of outbreaks
- impact of outbreaks on delivery of health-care or other critical infrastructure or services
- epidemiology of COVID-19 in surrounding communities, districts, provinces, and neighboring countries

Community Characteristics
- size of community and population density
- level of community engagement and public support for public health initiatives
- size and characteristics of disproportionately affected populations

Managing Health-Care Operations during COVID-19

- access to health care
- access to potable water and sanitation
- transportation (e.g., public, walking)
- planned large events or mass gatherings
- how connected the community is to other communities or countries (e.g., transportation hub, market, or industrial center)

Health-Care Capacity
- health-care workforce
- number of health-care facilities (including ancillary facilities)
- volume of testing activity (based on protocols and eligibility for testing)
- capacity to provide intensive care
- availability of personal protective equipment

Public Health Capacity
- public health workforce
- testing capacity (materials, equipment, staff)
- availability of resources to implement mitigation strategies
- ability to monitor and evaluate implementation and impact of strategies
- available support from other government agencies and partner organizations

TRANSMISSION SCENARIOS

Countries or subnational areas will have to respond rapidly to one or more of the following transmission scenarios:
- no cases
- one or more cases, imported or locally detected (sporadic cases)
- clusters of cases all linked by time, geographic location, and common exposures
- larger outbreaks of local transmission (community transmission)

Global experience with COVID-19 has demonstrated that in many regions with seemingly low levels of COVID-19 transmission, aggressive testing strategies focused on people with symptoms of respiratory infections may reveal additional underlying community transmission. Such a scenario may result in a rapid progression to substantial, uncontrolled transmission in the community. It is critical that countries prepare aggressively for future transmission scenarios, even if they are currently experiencing minimal community transmission. Once cases are identified, ministries of health, subnational public health authorities, and other implementing partners should be prepared to respond rapidly to varying levels of disease spread. Transmission scenarios, adopted by the World Health Organization (WHO), are outlined in Table 23.2.

Table 23.2. Transmission Scenarios, Adopted by the World Health Organization (WHO)

Level of Community Transmission	Community Characteristics and Description	Level of Mitigation
Scenario 1: No active cases	No new cases detected for at least 28 days (two times the maximum incubation period) in the presence of a robust surveillance system. This implies a near-zero risk of infection for the general population.	Low mitigation (providing guidance and educational materials, updating mitigation and prevention strategies)
Scenario 2: Imported or sporadic cases	Cases detected in the past 14 days all imported, sporadic (e.g., laboratory-acquired or zoonotic), or linked to imported or sporadic cases, and there are no clear signals of further locally acquired transmission. This implies minimal risk of infection for the general population.	Moderate mitigation (encouraging physical distancing and source control measures in public places, initiating contact tracing activities)

Managing Health-Care Operations during COVID-19

Table 23.2. Continued

Level of Community Transmission	Community Characteristics and Description	Level of Mitigation
Scenario 3: Clusters of cases	Cases detected in the past 14 days predominantly limited to well-defined clusters that are not directly linked to imported cases, but which are all linked by time, geographic location, and common exposures. Several unidentified cases are assumed to be in the area. This implies a low risk of infection to others in the wider community if exposure to these clusters is avoided.	Moderate mitigation (encouraging physical distancing and source control measures in public places, initiating contact tracing activities)
Scenario 4: Community transmission		
Level 1	Low incidence of locally acquired, widely dispersed cases detected in the past 14 days, with many of the cases not linked to specific clusters. Transmission may be focused on certain population subgroups. This implies low risk of infection for the general population.	Significant mitigation (mask mandates in public places, schools closed or virtual instruction, only essential businesses open)
Level 2	Moderate incidence of locally acquired, widely dispersed cases detected in the past 14 days. Transmission is less focused on certain population subgroups. This implies a moderate risk of infection for the general population.	Significant mitigation (mask mandates in public places, schools closed or virtual instruction, only essential businesses open)

Table 23.2. Continued

Level of Community Transmission	Community Characteristics and Description	Level of Mitigation
Level 3	High incidence of locally acquired, widely dispersed cases in the past 14 days. Transmission is widespread and not focused on population subgroups. This implies a high risk of infection for the general population.	Significant mitigation (mask mandates in public places, schools closed or virtual instruction, only essential businesses open)
Level 4	Very high incidence of locally acquired, widely dispersed cases in the past 14 days. This implies very high risk of infection for the general population.	Stay-at-home orders or shelter-in-place measures

COMMUNITY MITIGATION ACTIVITIES BY EPIDEMIOLOGIC SCENARIO
Community Action Plans

Community action plans can be developed by a wide variety of community groups (faith organizations, residential units, businesses) to provide setting-specific guidance to community members for various transmission scenarios. This includes planning for the provision of services and supplies when close contact and group gatherings are not allowed, limiting travel, and related measures.

DURING ALL TRANSMISSION SCENARIOS
- Create setting-specific action plans in case of illness in the community or disruption of daily activities due to COVID-19 (physical distancing, securing supplies, special considerations for populations at high risk).

DURING SCENARIOS 2–4
- Implement the established action plan and adjust as needed, based on the epidemiologic situation.

- Provide guidance for the provision of services and supplies to people at increased risk of severe disease (medical care, food, and water) while limiting close contact and group gatherings.
- Establish screening (for temperature, respiratory symptoms, loss of taste or smell, and exposure history) of persons entering community settings.
- Limit nonessential travel (personal and work-related).
- Limit social gatherings or community events and adapt to disruptions in routine activities (school, work, business closures) according to guidance from local officials.

DURING SCENARIO 4 (ALL LEVELS)
- Cancel nonessential travel and nonessential gatherings.
- Limit or restrict the number of people allowed to visit community settings (e.g., marketplaces, transportation hubs).
- Provide services and supplies to people required to shelter in place (medical care, food, and water) while limiting close contact or group settings and exposures.

Personal Protective Measures
The best way to prevent illness is to avoid being exposed to the virus that causes COVID-19 by using personal protective measures such as handwashing, mask use, physical distancing, and ventilation. Provide guidance on how to wear a face mask and wash hands properly and inform the community how to safely attend small gatherings and large events. Governments should encourage community members to continue practicing personal protective measures during all transmission scenarios.

DURING ALL TRANSMISSION SCENARIOS
- Provide guidance on protective measures (handwashing, mask use, physical distancing, and ventilation).

DURING SCENARIOS 2–4
- Implement physical distancing measures, including reducing large gatherings and altering schedules to reduce crowding.
- Provide guidance on source control measures (face masks) and consider requiring the use of source control in public settings.
- Provide guidance on proper ventilation in indoor settings to reduce the risk of transmission.
- Encourage both small and large gatherings to be held outdoors when possible.
- Provide guidance on home-based care for sick individuals.

Water, Sanitation, Hygiene (WASH), and Cleaning

While the virus that causes COVID-19 is primarily spread through respiratory droplets, the transmission may still occur through touching shared surfaces. It is important for community members to have continuous, safe access to clean water for the purposes of washing hands and cleaning surfaces at all stages of transmission. At stages of minimal transmission, supplies should be procured, and guidance should be shared with the community to ensure access to needed public goods and facilities for washing hands and cleaning surfaces. Handwashing and cleaning practices should be implemented in both public and private settings.

DURING ALL TRANSMISSION SCENARIOS
- Identify mechanisms to supply water, soap, and cleaning supplies to the public.
- Identify communities at risk and ensure supply chains to support handwashing measures.
- Provide guidance on cleaning frequently touched surfaces and the importance of ensuring water, soap, and cleaning supplies are readily available.

DURING SCENARIOS 2–4
- Prioritize the availability of handwashing and cleaning supplies to the public.
- Provide guidance for establishing handwashing stations.
- Require every person to wash their hands before entering community settings.
- Require thorough cleaning of community settings.
- Provide guidance on how to clean a home when someone is sick.

Contact Tracing

Contact tracing helps contain an outbreak by identifying those people who may have been exposed to a sick individual. Necessary adaptations to contact tracing programs will depend on the setting and will need to adapt to best suit the current epidemiology as the outbreak evolves. Contact tracing may be most feasible when there are few cases or a limited number of clusters. As cases rise, contact tracing resources may need to be directed toward high-priority settings. Community trust is critical for contact tracing to be successful. Community buy-in, ownership, and active participation are essential to successfully implementing contact tracing for COVID-19. Below are considerations for when to implement contact tracing efforts.

DURING ALL TRANSMISSION SCENARIOS
- Train and recruit staff to conduct contact tracing activities.
- Develop guidance for monitoring close contacts and implementing quarantine and isolation.
- Identify methods to optimize contact tracing through simplified data collection, monitoring, and additional staffing.
- Conduct contact tracing and managing and monitoring of contacts as advised in MoH guidance.

- Monitor close contacts through culturally appropriate and community-based efforts.
- Isolate laboratory-confirmed COVID-19 cases until cases are no longer considered infectious.

DURING SCENARIO 4 (ALL LEVELS)
- Prioritize contact tracing activities and resources for high-risk settings (critical infrastructure, populations at risk for severe disease).

Schools and Workplaces
Schools and workplace settings are at risk for COVID-19 transmission due to people from different households interacting for prolonged periods of time. Modifying activities in schools and workplaces should be considered to keep community members safe while still meeting essential educational and economic needs. Precautions that can support the mitigation of COVID-19 transmission should be implemented, including mask use, increased ventilation, physical distancing, and moving activities to outdoor settings when possible.

DURING ALL TRANSMISSION SCENARIOS
- Educate community members on the need to stay home from school or work when they feel ill with any type of symptoms.
- Educate administrators on the need for sick leave allowance and provision of distance learning or working from home, if possible.

DURING SCENARIOS 3 AND 4
- Provide guidance to implement short-term closures (for cleaning, disinfecting, and contact tracing, as needed).
- Instruct administrators to implement distance learning or work-from-home arrangements, when possible, for people at increased risk of severe illness or those with close family or household members at increased risk of severe illness.

Managing Health-Care Operations during COVID-19

DURING SCENARIO 4 (ALL LEVELS)
- Instruct administrators to implement broader or longer-term closures.
- Direct administrators to implement extended distance learning and work-from-home arrangements, when possible, or ensure appropriate physical distancing between staff at workplaces deemed essential.
- Direct administrators to ensure flexible leave or work schedules for those who need to stay home due to school closures or childcare dismissals or to care for elderly or ill persons.[4]

Section 23.5 | CDC Strategy for Global Response to COVID-19 (2020–2023)

This section provides an overarching framework for the global response of the U.S. Centers for Disease Control and Prevention (CDC) to the COVID-19 pandemic. The CDC strategy aligns with the U.S. government (USG) strategy and the U.S. National Security Strategic goals to protect the American people and ensure U.S. health security by mitigating the spread of infectious disease threats abroad, ending the pandemic, and building resilience and readiness for future pandemics. The updated CDC strategy also aligns with the U.S. COVID-19 Global Response and Recovery Framework (www.whitehouse.gov/wp-content/uploads/2022/09/U.S.-COVID-19-GLOBAL-RESPONSE-RECOVERY-FRAME-WORK-_clean_9-14_7pm.pdf) released in September 2022. The updated U.S. framework has three main objectives.

U.S. GOVERNMENT GLOBAL COVID-19 OBJECTIVES
- Accelerate widespread, sustained, and equitable access to and delivery of safe and effective COVID-19 vaccinations

---

[4] "Framework for Implementation of COVID-19 Community Mitigation Measures for Lower-Resource Countries," Centers for Disease Control and Prevention (CDC), July 20, 2021. Available online. URL: www.cdc.gov/coronavirus/2019-ncov/global-covid-19/community-mitigation-measures.html. Accessed December 14, 2022.

and integrate COVID-19 vaccination into health systems while minimizing disruptions to other routine immunizations and health services.
- Strengthen health systems to facilitate prevention, detection, and response to COVID-19, including through widespread, sustained, and equitable access to diagnostics and therapeutics and integrate COVID-19 management into health systems while minimizing disruptions to other essential health services.
- Strengthen the global health security architecture to prevent, detect, and respond to COVID-19 and future pandemic threats.

CDC activities align most closely with objectives, accelerate access to safe and effective COVID-19 vaccinations, strengthen health systems to facilitate response to COVID-19, and strengthen international global health security architecture.

The updated CDC strategy defines the agency's priorities and guides the development of criteria for monitoring and evaluating public health achievements and the agency's impact on health security at home and abroad. The strategy also addresses the urgent need to prioritize our global response work to reduce the global burden of COVID-19 and build global public health capacity to prevent, prepare for, and control future pandemics. The CDC's response work focuses on working with local and global partners to address the COVID-19 pandemic. The agency provides global public health leadership that furthers evidence-based science and strengthens COVID-19 technical expertise.

The CDC will focus on mitigating the global impacts of COVID-19 and using its scientific and technical expertise to support your global health platform and program successes. In alignment with the USG strategy principle of transparency and accountability, the CDC remains committed to seeking the best data and analyzing scientific findings to improve decision-making and approaches for delivering public health interventions. The CDC will implement activities using a phased approach that accounts for short- and long-term public health needs, including anticipating and preparing for future global public health emergencies.

STRATEGIC OBJECTIVES
- Strengthen capacity to plan for and deliver COVID-19 vaccines and therapeutics and to evaluate vaccines and vaccination and treatment programs using timely and accurate data.
- Strengthen capacity at the country and regional levels to prevent, detect, and respond to COVID-19 cases and future pandemic threats by strengthening the global public health workforce; supporting approaches to prevention and treatment; strengthening surveillance and laboratory systems for severe acute respiratory syndrome coronavirus 2 (SARS-CoV-2), other respiratory viruses, and emerging threats; and modernizing data systems to ensure that timely and accurate data are available to inform public health decision-making.
- Prevent and mitigate COVID-19 transmission across borders, in communities, in health-care facilities, and among health-care workers and minimize disruptions to essential health services to protect critical public health programs.
- Contribute to the scientific understanding of COVID-19, other pandemics, and emerging threats and address critical unknowns regarding mutations, clinical severity, modes of transmission, and long-term sequelae and immunity.
- Strengthen the global health architecture by working with multilateral and multisectoral partners to augment surveillance, laboratories, alert systems, and capacities for early and effective prevention, detection, and response to potential health emergencies.

KEY ACTIVITIES
Note. This list demonstrates examples of activities for each strategic objective. The list is not comprehensive and does not imply funding support for any specific activity.
- Strengthen capacity to plan for and deliver COVID-19 vaccines and to evaluate vaccines and vaccination programs using timely and accurate data.

- Accelerate global COVID-19 vaccinations through Global VAX, a whole-of-USG effort to turn vaccines in vials into vaccinations in arms around the world.
- Support and strengthen national immunization advisory groups in evidence-based policy-making.
- Support vaccine program planning, including microplanning.
- Provide technical expertise and resources to strengthen the capacity of the immunization workforce to deliver COVID-19 vaccines.
- Strengthen systems for reporting data on vaccinations and for detecting, reporting on, and responding to adverse events following immunization.
- Improve vaccine confidence and demand for COVID-19 vaccines.
- Evaluate the effectiveness of vaccines, including in different combinations and in different contexts and as viruses evolve and mutate.
- Evaluate the quality and effectiveness of vaccination programs.
- Strengthen capacity at country and regional levels to prevent, detect, and respond to COVID-19 cases and future pandemic threats by strengthening the global public health workforce; strengthening surveillance and laboratory systems for SARS-CoV-2, other respiratory viruses, and emerging threats; and modernizing data systems to ensure that timely and accurate data are available to inform public health decision-making.
  - Increase capacity to detect, investigate, report, and respond to COVID-19 transmission.
  - Provide technical support to partner governments through their Ministries of Health, other relevant ministries, international or national organizations, and agencies responsible for human health, animal health, and public health emergency preparedness to reduce the impact of COVID-19 on groups disproportionately affected.

- Increase the capacity of national- and local-level surveillance and laboratory systems, including strengthening existing respiratory disease surveillance platforms, to detect and report priority pathogens and perform appropriate genetic sequence analysis.
- Support countries' development and deployment of health information systems to facilitate the timely collection, management, analysis, and sharing of critical public health data.
- Support training of critical field epidemiologists to analyze and interpret surveillance data and to investigate, track, and contain outbreaks.
- Support critical training of laboratorians to ensure timely and accurate laboratory diagnosis and reporting.
- Support training and capacity building of data scientists who can analyze and interpret epidemiology and laboratory data to inform decision-making.
- Support countries' timely sharing of surveillance and epidemiologic data across all relevant sectors to rapidly identify and disseminate knowledge and build upon the evidence base for successful intervention.
- Support country capacity to prioritize, administer, and monitor adverse reactions to and efficacy of therapeutic agents.
- Strengthen border health security, planning, and surveillance at ports of entry.
- Support countries to develop and implement public health policies, laws, and regulations necessary—including quarantine, isolation, and mitigation measures—to prevent, detect, and respond to health threats.
- Promote international coordination as regulatory frameworks are evaluated to ensure responsiveness to emerging and reemerging infectious diseases.

- Improve coordination and management of the COVID-19 response through a One Health approach that strengthens preparedness activities across human, animal, and environmental health sectors.
- Strengthen animal health surveillance systems, including reporting and linkage to human health programs to prevent unnecessary spillover.
- Identify risks associated with zoonotic disease transmission (e.g., occupation, animal ownership, livestock, place of residence near wildlife).
- Collaborate with international partners to identify animal species involved in COVID-19 spillover to humans (reservoir host or intermediate host).
- Assess virus prevalence in various species of animals (reservoirs(s) and possible intermediate host(s)).
- Identify and describe possible transmission modes of COVID-19 between animals and humans.
- Develop risk reduction strategies for preventing disease transmission between animals and humans, as well as between different animal species.
- Support global animal health partners for the development of animal diagnostic tests, including serological tests for animal population screening.
- Support the development and use of integrated One Health surveillance systems for reporting and responding to animals infected with SARS-CoV-2 (and with other pathogens).
- Support global One Health partners, including the Food and Agriculture Organization (FAO), the World Organization for Animal Health (OIE), and the World Health Organization (WHO) Tripartite in developing guidance and building capacity on the human–animal–environment aspects of COVID-19 and other zoonotic diseases.
- Support training and capacity building in the animal health workforce and strengthen linkages with the human health sector.

- Prevent and mitigate COVID-19 transmission across borders, in the community, in health-care facilities, and among health-care workers and minimize disruptions to essential health services to protect critical public health programs.
  - Mitigate COVID-19 transmission in communities.
  - Facilitate activities to reduce the spread of COVID-19 within communities.
  - Support contact tracing activities.
  - Support mitigation activities that address those at higher risk for serious illness from COVID-19.
  - Support risk and media communications addressing misinformation and disinformation, particularly reaching populations with low adherence to mitigation recommendations.
  - Support water, sanitation, and hygiene activities, targeting groups experiencing limited access to clean water.
  - Support the development and implementation of appropriate mitigation activities for refugees, displaced persons, and other underresourced communities.
  - Provide direct assistance to country governments to support screening operations and bolster border health systems at priority points of entry (POE).
  - Map and analyze trends in population mobility to anticipate and respond to COVID-19 and other infectious disease outbreaks through targeted interventions.
  - Evaluate the impact and adherence levels of recommended mitigation measures and share lessons learned across countries.
  - Evaluate the impact of nonpharmaceutical interventions to support the development of evidence-based recommendations.
  - Support critical needs of health-care facilities, health-care workers, and public health personnel

and minimize disruptions to essential health services.
- Develop and implement approaches to rapidly identify, triage, and isolate suspected and confirmed COVID-19 among patients, health-care workers, and visitors to reduce health-care-associated virus spread.
- Provide practical laboratory platforms, including genetic sequencing, and point-of-care/point-of-need diagnostics to improve the detection and differential diagnosis of SARS-CoV-2 infection and other respiratory viruses.
- Strengthen infection prevention and control policies and procedures in rural and urban health-care settings.
- Build on existing infection prevention and control to coordinate and accelerate implementation.
- Improve situational awareness of critical information in the health-care system, such as preparedness, supplies, equipment, and capacity.
- Facilitate the safe and respectful management of human remains.
- Support and evaluate clinical mitigation activities to keep health services from being overwhelmed by COVID-19 patients.
- Develop operational guidance for maintaining essential health services and public health activities during the COVID-19 pandemic.
- Communicate with essential public health service recipients about the safety and importance of continuing to seek and receive health services.
- Secure commodities including personal protective equipment (PPE) and laboratory diagnostics to maintain health services and public health programs.
- Coordinate closely between essential health services—such as diagnostic and curative services for malaria and neglected tropical diseases,

immunization services, HIV/TB programs, maternal and child health programs, and COVID-19 programs—during activity planning to modify strategies that ensure COVID-19 precautions, implement protocols for protecting health workers, and apply mitigation measures for targeted communities.
- Develop infection prevention and control guidance for health-care providers, including vaccinators and TB service providers on how to safely undertake patient-centered work in the COVID-19 environment.
- Expand differentiated service delivery models to increase access to lifesaving medical countermeasures—such as antiretroviral treatment for people living with HIV or combination antibiotic regimens for people with active TB cases—through multi-month medication dispensing, community-based delivery options, and increasing clinic hours.
- Use effective online modules to continue workforce training and expand telehealth services.
- Develop and implement strategies to ensure access to critical health services (multi-month dispensing, passes that allow attendance at clinic appointments).
- Promote vaccination and provide training and supplies to health-care workers to reduce the occupational risk of COVID-19.
- Support clear health communications that facilitate appropriate care seeking.
- Monitor progress in critical health programs and the impact of the COVID-19 pandemic on such programs.
- Contribute to the scientific understanding of COVID-19, other pandemics, and emerging threats and address critical unknowns regarding mutations, clinical severity, modes of transmission, and long-term sequelae and immunity.

- Collaborate with partner countries and organizations to study transmission and conduct modeling to guide prevention and control measures and build research capacity.
- Conduct and participate in therapeutic and vaccine clinical trials as appropriate.
- Collect and report data to provide critical information on the clinical course and outcomes of COVID-19 and use that information to improve clinical care.
- Support countries' timely sharing of research data.
- Evaluate and assess mitigation measures, strengthen surveillance, and use evaluations to improve programs and surveillance systems.
- Evaluate the impact of preventive or protective interventions.
- Improve pathogen identification and characterization using next-generation sequencing and other advanced molecular technologies.
- Monitor long-term impacts for people infected with SARS-CoV-2.
- Collaborate with partner countries and organizations to identify approaches to minimize the impact of COVID-19 on critical public health programs.
- Contribute to the scientific understanding of COVID-19 and address crucial unknowns regarding clinical severity, extent, and pathways of transmission and infection with support for special investigations (see the CDC Science Agenda (www.cdc.gov/coronavirus/2019-ncov/science/science-agenda-covid19.html) for key priority areas).
- Minimize or mitigate misinformation and disinformation that undermines scientific evidence, understanding, and trust between communities and local public health authorities.
- Strengthen the global health architecture, working with multilateral and multisectoral partners to augment

surveillance, laboratories, alert systems, and capacities for early and effective prevention, detection, and response to potential health emergencies.
- Broaden global respiratory surveillance activities by building on and enhancing the Global Influenza Surveillance and Response System (GISRS) in collaboration with the WHO.
- Address gaps in core public health systems by developing sustainable, systems-based approaches through the National Public Health Institutes.
- Support the WHO and other international organizations as they provide guidance for building International Health Regulations (IHRs) core capacities.
- Participate in the development of a new pandemic preparedness instrument and strengthen IHRs reporting to improve early and effective prevention, detection, and response to health emergencies.
- Support the development and implementation of tools to assess health security gaps and plans/approaches to address gaps following the assessment.
- Provide technical expertise through bilateral partnerships and international efforts that support the country's efforts to build health security capacity.[5]

---

[5] "CDC Strategy for Global Response to COVID-19 (2020-2023)," Centers for Disease Control and Prevention (CDC), November 10, 2022. Available online. URL: www.cdc.gov/coronavirus/2019-ncov/global-covid-19/global-response-strategy.html. Accessed December 14, 2022.

Chapter 24 | Beware of Fraudulent Coronavirus Tests, Vaccines, and Treatments

While the U.S. Food and Drug Administration (FDA) remains vigilant to protect families and communities from COVID-19, some people might be tempted to buy or use questionable products that claim to help diagnose, treat, cure, and even prevent coronavirus disease. Vaccination is one of the best ways to protect everyone, who is eligible, from COVID-19. The FDA has approved two vaccines for the prevention of COVID-19 and issued emergency use authorizations (EUAs) for others.

The FDA continues to work with vaccine and drug manufacturers, developers, and researchers to help facilitate the development and availability of medical products—such as additional vaccines, antibodies, and medicines—to prevent or treat COVID-19. Meanwhile, some people and companies are trying to profit from this pandemic by selling unproven and illegally marketed products that make false claims, such as being effective against the coronavirus. Unlike the products approved or authorized by the FDA, fraudulent products that claim to cure, treat, or prevent COVID-19 have not been evaluated by the agency for safety and effectiveness and might be dangerous to you and your family.

The FDA is particularly concerned that these deceptive and misleading products might cause people to delay or stop appropriate medical treatment for COVID-19, leading to serious and life-threatening harm. It is likely that the products do not do what they claim, and the ingredients in them could cause adverse effects and could interact and potentially interfere with medications to treat many underlying medical conditions. The FDA has also seen unauthorized fraudulent test kits for COVID-19 being sold online. You will risk unknowingly spreading COVID-19 or not getting treated appropriately if you use an unauthorized test.

TREATMENTS FOR COVID-19

The FDA is working with medical product developers to rapidly facilitate the development of vaccines and treatments for COVID-19 to help make them available. So far, the FDA has approved only one treatment for COVID-19 and has issued EUAs for others. Fraudulent COVID-19 products can come in many varieties, including dietary supplements and other foods, as well as products claiming to be tests, drugs, medical devices, or vaccines. The FDA has been working with retailers to remove dozens of misleading products from store shelves and online. The agency will continue to monitor social media and online marketplaces promoting and selling fraudulent COVID-19 products.

For example, the FDA and the Federal Trade Commission (FTC) issued warning letters to companies for selling fraudulent COVID-19 products. The products cited include teas, essential oils, tinctures, and colloidal silver. The FDA is actively monitoring for any firms marketing products with fraudulent COVID-19 diagnostic, prevention, and treatment claims. The FDA is exercising its authority to protect consumers from firms selling unauthorized products with false or misleading claims. The FDA may send warning letters or pursue seizures or injunctions against people, products, or companies that violate the law. The FDA is also increasing enforcement at ports of entry to ensure that fraudulent products do not enter the country through borders. In addition, the FDA is monitoring complaints of fake coronavirus treatments, vaccines, and tests. Consumers and health-care professionals can help by reporting suspected fraud to the FDA's health fraud program or the office of criminal investigations.

Beware of Fraudulent Coronavirus Tests, Vaccines, and Treatments

TAKING DRUGS INTENDED FOR ANIMALS IS DANGEROUS

Products marketed for veterinary use, or "for research use only" or otherwise not for human consumption, have not been evaluated for safety and should never be used by humans. They may have adverse effects, including serious illness and death when taken by people.

The FDA has received multiple reports of people who have needed medical attention, including hospitalization, after self-medicating with ivermectin intended for livestock. The FDA has not authorized or approved ivermectin for use in preventing or treating COVID-19 in humans or animals. The FDA is also aware of people trying to prevent COVID-19 by taking chloroquine phosphate, which is sold to treat parasites in aquarium fish.

HOW TO PROTECT YOURSELF AND YOUR FAMILY FROM CORONAVIRUS FRAUD

The FDA advises consumers to be cautious of websites and stores selling products that claim to prevent, treat, or cure COVID-19. Here are some tips to identify false or misleading claims:

- Be suspicious of products that claim to treat a wide range of diseases.
- Personal testimonials are no substitute for scientific evidence.
- Few diseases or conditions can be treated quickly, so be suspicious of any therapy claimed as a "quick fix."
- If it seems too good to be true, it probably is.
- "Miracle cures," which claim scientific breakthroughs or contain secret ingredients, are likely a hoax.

If you have symptoms of COVID-19, follow the guidelines of the Centers for Disease Control and Prevention (CDC) and speak to your medical provider. Your health-care provider will advise you about whether you should get tested and the process for being tested in your area. If you have a question about a treatment or test found online, talk to your health-care provider or doctor. If you have a question about a medication, call your pharmacist or the FDA. The FDA's Division of Drug Information (DDI) will answer almost any drug question.

The DDI pharmacists are available by email, druginfo@fda.hhs.gov, and by phone, 855-543-3784 (DRUG) and 301-796-3400. The sale of fraudulent COVID-19 products is a threat to public health. The best way to prevent COVID-19 is to get vaccinated. If you are concerned about COVID-19, talk to your health-care provider and follow the advice of the FDA's federal partners about how to prevent the spread of this illness.[1]

---

[1] "Beware of Fraudulent Coronavirus Tests, Vaccines and Treatments," U.S. Food and Drug Administration (FDA), February 3, 2022. Available online. URL: www.fda.gov/consumers/consumer-updates/beware-fraudulent-coronavirus-tests-vaccines-and-treatments. Accessed December 13, 2023.

Chapter 25 | COVID-19 and Alternative Treatments

Some people have sought "alternative" remedies to prevent or treat COVID-19. Some of these purported remedies include teas, essential oils, tinctures, herbal therapies such as oleander/oleandrin, and silver products such as colloidal silver. The Office of Dietary Supplements at the National Institutes of Health (NIH) has detailed fact sheets for consumers and health professionals about specific dietary supplements and COVID-19. But there is no scientific evidence that any of these alternative remedies can prevent or cure COVID-19. In fact, some of them may not be safe to consume. It is important to understand that although many herbal or dietary supplements (and some prescription drugs) come from natural sources, "natural" does not always mean that a product is a safer or better option for your health. Most people with COVID-19 have mild illnesses and can recover at home. If you are worried about your symptoms, the coronavirus self-checker can assist in the decision to seek care.

COVID-19 vaccination helps protect people from getting sick or severely ill with COVID-19, but some people who are fully vaccinated still get COVID-19, and some have been hospitalized with COVID-19. The Centers for Disease Control and Prevention (CDC) and the U.S. Food and Drug Administration (FDA) have information on the vaccines that are approved and authorized in the United States to prevent COVID-19.

For people who are more likely to get very sick from COVID-19 infection, treatments are available that can reduce the chances of being hospitalized or dying from the disease. Medications to treat COVID-19 must be prescribed by a health-care provider and started as soon as possible after diagnosis to be effective. For people at high risk of getting very sick from COVID-19, contact a health-care provider right away to determine if you are eligible for treatment, even if your symptoms are mild.[1]

---

[1] "COVID-19 and 'Alternative' Treatments: What You Need To Know," National Center for Complementary and Integrative Health (NCCIH), June 2022. Available online. URL: www.nccih.nih.gov/health/covid-19-and-alternative-treatments-what-you-need-to-know. Accessed December 20, 2022.

Chapter 26 | Spiritual and Psychosocial Support for People with COVID-19 at Home

Many people who get sick or lose a family member want their spiritual leader to provide spiritual support. During the COVID-19 pandemic, the safest means of providing spiritual and psychological support is by phone, over a video call, or through private social media chat platforms. Spiritual leaders may pray, share theological and scriptural reflections, and share messages of hope.

If in-person spiritual support is needed, this chapter provides guidance so that it can be done as safely as possible:
- Get vaccinated for COVID-19 and continue using other methods to decrease your risk of getting COVID-19.
- Maintain at least a distance of two arm's lengths (two meters) from others, including when distributing food or praying.
- Wear a mask to prevent the spread of COVID-19.
- Consider meeting outside where it is easier to keep people apart and where there is more ventilation.

If you must enter the home of a sick person:
- When in the home, open windows and doors to allow in fresh air (natural ventilation).

- Do not open windows and doors if doing so poses a safety or health risk to children or other family members (e.g., risk of falling or triggering asthma symptoms).
- Wash your hands before entering and after leaving the home; for visits lasting a number of hours, wash hands often while in the home.
  - Scrub hands for 20 seconds to remove harmful germs.
  - If soap and water are not readily available, you can use an alcohol-based hand sanitizer that contains at least 60 percent alcohol.

Spend a few minutes speaking with others in the household about how they can minimize their risk of getting COVID-19. Tell members of the household that a person with mild symptoms should:
- isolate themselves from other family members, if possible
- follow government guidance for COVID-19 if it is not possible to safely isolate from others, which may include wearing a mask or going to a community isolation center

While visiting the family, do the following:
- Offer words of hope.
- It is best not to touch anyone while praying for them to prevent the risk of contracting or spreading COVID-19.
- If the sick family member is having trouble breathing, chest pain, or confusion, someone should call the COVID-19 hotline, contact the nearest health clinic, or call an ambulance.
- Wash your hands before you leave the house. Wash your hands before and after you remove your mask. Wash your hands for 20 seconds with water and soap, a diluted chlorine solution, or an alcohol-based hand rub to help prevent getting COVID-19 or spreading it in the community.

CHECKLIST OF ITEMS TO REVIEW OR BRING WITH YOU BEFORE VISITING HOMES
- a mask
- alcohol-based hand rub with at least 60 percent alcohol
- tissues
- home-based care kit: paracetamol, disposable gloves, washcloth, calling card, disinfectant, soap, mask
- list of local COVID-19 information and updates (e.g., list of isolation centers)
- list of social support services available (e.g., a prayer phone line, email communication, a private social media prayer group)
- list of preventive actions to emphasize (see below)

PREVENTIVE ACTIONS TO EMPHASIZE DURING AN IN-PERSON VISIT
- Stay home when sick (except when you need emergency care for a health condition or medical care).
- Wear a face mask if you leave your home or if you cannot isolate yourself from other family members at home.
- Cover coughs and sneezes with a tissue or use the inside of your elbow. Throw the tissue away in a trash bin immediately and wash your hands.
- Wash your hands often with soap and water for at least 20 seconds.
- Clean and disinfect frequently touched surfaces in the home.
- Limit as much as possible close contact with others in the home who are sick or show symptoms (keep at least two arm's length or two meters away). Anyone sick or infected should separate themselves from others by staying in a specific "sick room" or area (if available).
- Open windows and doors to allow in fresh air (natural ventilation).
  - Do not open windows and doors if doing so poses a safety or health risk to children or other family

members (e.g., risk of falling or triggering asthma symptoms).
- You are responsible for helping keep your community safe by following recommended preventive actions:
  - Avoid touching your face with unwashed hands, especially your eyes, nose, or mouth.
  - Know and share only facts about COVID-19 and help prevent the spread of rumors and stigma in your community.

Check with health authorities for information and recommendations on community actions designed to prevent and limit exposure to COVID-19.[1]

---

[1] "Providing Spiritual and Psychosocial Support to People with COVID-19 at Home (Non-U.S. Settings)," Centers for Disease Control and Prevention (CDC), February 3, 2022. Available online. URL: www.cdc.gov/coronavirus/2019-ncov/global-covid-19/providing-spiritual-support.html. Accessed December 15, 2022.

Chapter 27 | Palliative Care and COVID-19

WHAT IS PALLIATIVE CARE?

Palliative care offers care and support from a team of health providers such as doctors, nurses, and social workers. Palliative care is not just for those who are nearing the end of life. In fact, it is for anyone at any age who has a serious illness—and their family caregivers.

Jeri Miller, Ph.D., leads research on end-of-life and palliative care at the National Institute of Nursing Research. As people face serious illnesses, including COVID-19, Dr. Miller explains how a palliative care team can help.

HOW DOES PALLIATIVE CARE WORK?

Palliative care is specialized care for people living with a serious illness. You can receive palliative care at the same time you are receiving treatments for your serious illness. What palliative care does is provide relief from symptoms such as pain, shortness of breath, fatigue, and others. It also helps you with practical needs, manage the medical treatments you are receiving, improve your quality of life, and provide help to your family.

WHEN DO PEOPLE GET PALLIATIVE CARE?

Some people receive palliative care for a long time; others do not. It is based not on your prognosis but on your needs. Hospice is a special form of palliative care for individuals in the last stages of an illness or advanced disease. After someone passes away, palliative care teams can help support family members who may be grieving that loss.

WHO PROVIDES PALLIATIVE CARE?

It is provided by a specially trained team of doctors, nurses, social workers, and others who work with you and your own doctor. They work together to make sure that your care is coordinated with your providers and that they listen to your preferences for care to help you understand your treatment options and choices. They make sure to provide expert symptom management when you are seriously ill.

CURRENT AREAS OF RESEARCH IN PALLIATIVE CARE

Much of the research centers on discovering better ways to manage pain and symptoms that occur in a serious illness. The focus is not just on the ill individual but also on the impact of an illness on family caregivers who, together with their ill loved one, are experiencing the challenges of a serious illness. Researchers are also trying to understand the unique needs of palliative care in underserved and vulnerable populations. That is so important right now because palliative care is for everyone, everywhere.[1]

---

[1] MedlinePlus, "What Is Palliative Care?" National Institutes of Health (NIH), October 27, 2020. Available online. URL: https://magazine.medlineplus.gov/article/what-is-palliative-care. Accessed December 21, 2022.

Chapter 28 | Coronavirus and Your Health Coverage

UPDATES FROM MEDICARE
- **Telehealth**. During COVID-19, Medicare expanded access to telehealth services. This includes common office visits, mental health counseling, and preventive screenings. This way doctors and other providers can offer services without patients going to the office.
- **Lab tests for COVID-19**. You pay no out-of-pocket costs.
- **All medically necessary hospitalizations**. This includes if you are diagnosed with COVID-19 and need to stay in the hospital under quarantine instead of being discharged from the hospital after an inpatient stay.

Remember: If you need to see your doctor, please call them first. If you develop emergency warning signs for COVID-19, get medical attention immediately.

WHAT IS COVERED?
- If you already have coverage through the Marketplace, the coverage for coronavirus is generally the same as any other viral infection.
- Read more about what Marketplace plans cover at www.healthcare.gov/coverage/what-marketplace-plans-cover.

Check with your health insurance company for specific benefits and coverage policies.

REMINDERS
- All Marketplace plans are prohibited from excluding coverage because of preexisting conditions.
- Plans cannot end coverage due to a change in health status.
- Log in to update your information if you have changes in address, household income, job, or household size.
- You may be able to change your plan if certain situations apply.

SPECIAL ENROLLMENT PERIODS
Some life changes can allow you to enroll in a plan for the first time or change your plan.

Here are a few common life changes:
- loss of health coverage
- change in household income
- getting married
- having a baby
- changes in the household (dependents, death, divorce)
- changes in address
- released from incarceration
- gained citizenship or lawful presence in the United States

WATCH OUT FOR SCAMS
Protect Your Identity from Scammers!
It is easy to get distracted and let your guard down during these uncertain times. Scammers may try to steal your personal information. They might lie about sending you coronavirus vaccines, tests, masks, or other items in exchange for your personal information.
- Only share your information with your care provider's office, pharmacy, hospital, health insurer, or other trusted health-care provider.
- Check your claims summary forms or explanation of benefits for errors.

Coronavirus and Your Health Coverage

- It is important to always guard your insurance card like a credit card.

Remember, Medicare will never call you to ask for or check your Medicare number.[1]

---

[1] "Coronavirus and Your Health Coverage: Get the Basics," Centers for Medicare & Medicaid Services (CMS), November 2021. Available online. URL: www.cms.gov/files/document/c2c-covid-overview.pdf. Accessed December 14, 2022.

Chapter 29 | Ongoing Research on COVID-19

Chapter Contents
Section 29.1—Chronic Viral Infection and Long COVID 331
Section 29.2—How Breathing Activates the Lungs' Defenses against Coronavirus 332
Section 29.3—Role of Technology during the Pandemic 334

Chapter 29 | Ongoing Research on COVID-19

Section 29.1 | Chronic Viral Infection and Long COVID

In a small study supported by the National Institute of Allergy and Infectious Diseases (NIAID), researchers found that chronic viral infections may influence the likelihood of someone developing long COVID. They also found that different chronic infections were associated with the development of different long COVID symptoms.

WHAT DID THE RESEARCHERS DO?

Some viruses cause underlying chronic infections. These viruses stay inactive in your body without making you sick and can then reactivate if the body is dealing with another infection or if it is under stress. The reactivated virus can produce symptoms, especially in people with weakened immune systems. Viruses that can cause chronic infections include human immunodeficiency virus (HIV), herpesviruses such as cytomegalovirus (CMV), and Epstein-Barr virus (EBV).

Researchers wanted to see whether people with these underlying chronic infections were likely to develop long COVID, especially if these viruses had reactivated or infected someone around the same time they developed COVID-19. They interviewed 280 people who had long COVID and took blood samples to determine whether they had a chronic infection and whether that infection would have been active at the same time they were infected with severe acute respiratory syndrome coronavirus 2 (SARS-CoV-2).

The likelihood of someone developing long COVID was influenced by the underlying chronic infection they had, researchers found. For example, people with a reactivated EBV infection were likely to develop long COVID, while people with a reactivated CMV infection were less likely to develop severe long COVID (defined as having five or more symptoms associated with long COVID).

The researchers also found that different symptoms of long COVID seemed to be related to different underlying infections. For example, people with HIV were likely to develop memory and concentration issues, while people who had reactivation of one of the herpesviruses were likely to show fatigue. People with CMV were less likely to have memory and concentration symptoms.

WHY IS THIS RESEARCH IMPORTANT?
The results of this study are preliminary, but the research may show that there are distinct types of long COVID and that a person's biological makeup could influence whether they develop long-term symptoms and what kinds of symptoms they have after SARS-CoV-2 infection. Future studies of long COVID and chronic viral immune responses will be needed to fully understand how these conditions influence each other.[1]

Section 29.2 | How Breathing Activates the Lungs' Defenses against Coronavirus

Scientists researching viruses such as influenza or severe acute respiratory syndrome coronavirus 2 (SARS-CoV-2), the virus that causes COVID-19, have often had to study how diseases work and test drugs using animals or cell cultures, a technique in which cells are removed from living organs and grown under controlled conditions. However, using animals or cell cultures to predict how effective a drug can be in the human respiratory tract poses challenges. Drugs that may seem to be safe and effective in these experiments can be harmful or ineffective in humans.

This prompted a research team led by Dr. Donald Ingber at the Wyss Institute at Harvard University to develop "lung-on-a-chip" models that may help you better understand diseases, test drugs, and develop new therapies. The chips are based on techniques from the computer industry and tissue chip engineering. About

---
[1] COVID-19, "The Relationship between Chronic Viral Infection and Long COVID," National Institutes of Health (NIH), November 22, 2022. Available online. URL: https://covid19.nih.gov/news-and-stories/relationship-between-chronic-viral-infection-and-long-covid. Accessed January 3, 2023.

the size of a memory stick, they model human organs such as the liver, heart, and lungs.

In a study supported in part by the National Heart, Lung, and Blood Institute of the National Institutes of Health (NIH), researchers used this technology to learn how the lung's mechanical breathing motions help boost immunity in the organ's tissue against viral infection.

WHAT DID THE RESEARCHERS DO?

In prior studies, the team used a chip to model viral infection and to observe immune responses in the human upper airway, the area between the nose or mouth and the windpipe.

For this study, researchers used a new lung alveolus chip—named for the tiny cup-shaped cavities that take in the oxygen you breathe. They wanted to see how the motion of breathing affects infection in the deepest parts of the lung. The chip has a flexible membrane that mimics a tiny set of alveoli. By applying suction to the chip, researchers made the membrane stretch and relax rhythmically, like the alveoli in your lungs do during breathing.

The new study used the influenza A virus subtype H3N2 (A/H3N2) strain of the influenza virus, a leading cause of lung infections, hospitalizations, and deaths. When it was added to the chip, the virus caused tissue damage and cell death. In response, the tissue activated an injury and repair process to combat the virus.

The team compared the lung chip's response with and without breathing movements. They found that genes involved in the immune response to the virus were more active in the lung tissue when the alveoli moved, as in breathing.

WHY IS THIS RESEARCH IMPORTANT?

The human alveolus chip can model not only the breathing motions of the lung but also immune responses to infection. This allows researchers to look at the deep parts of the lung where infections are often more severe and can lead to hospitalizations and death.

Research using this kind of experimental lung model can help scientists repurpose existing drugs, understand disease pathology, and develop new lifesaving therapies to face the current COVID-19 pandemic as well as other respiratory viruses with highly infectious capabilities.[2]

Section 29.3 | Role of Technology during the Pandemic

ROLE OF TELEHEALTH AND TELEMEDICINE DURING COVID-19

The World Health Organization (WHO) "pulse survey," implemented over one year into the COVID-19 pandemic, reports substantial disruptions persist in continued essential health services. In 2020, countries reported that on average, about half of essential health services were disrupted. In the first three months of 2021, however, countries reported progress, with just over one-third of services now being disrupted. WHO developed guidance (https://apps.who.int/iris/bitstream/handle/10665/332240/WHO-2019-nCoV-essential_health_services-2020.2-eng.pdf) for maintaining essential health services during the COVID-19 outbreak and another guidance to assess each facility's readiness to continue frontline service during the COVID-19 pandemic. For continued essential services assessment, facilities can use the WHO facility assessment tool. This assessment includes health-care provider readiness training on personal protective equipment (PPE) and facility infection disease prevention and control (IPC).

To reduce staff and patient exposure to sick people, preserve PPE, and minimize the impact of patient surges on facilities, telehealth services help provide necessary care to patients while minimizing the transmission risk of SARS-CoV-2, the virus that causes COVID-19, to health-care workers and patients. The way health care is delivered during the COVID-19 pandemic has changed. Health-care systems may need to adjust the way they triage,

---

[2] COVID-19, "How Breathing Activates the Lung's Defenses against COVID-19," National Institutes of Health (NIH), August 8, 2022. Available online. URL: https://covid19.nih.gov/news-and-stories/how-breathing-activates-lung-defenses-covid-19#:~:text=In%20response%2C%20the%20tissue%20activated,alveoli%20moved%2C%20as%20in%20breathing. Accessed January 3, 2023.

evaluate, and care for patients using methods that do not rely on in-person encounters:

- **Pan American Health Organization (PAHO)**. The PAHO highlights teleconsultations as a safe and effective way to assess suspected COVID-19 cases and to guide the patient's diagnosis and treatment, minimizing the risk of disease transmission. Telemedicine enables many of the key clinical services to continue to operate regularly and without interruption in the course of a public health emergency. PAHO also developed COVID-19 and telemedicine tools for assessing the maturity level or readiness of health institutions to implement telemedicine services.
- **The American College of Obstetricians and Gynecologists (ACOG)**. The ACOG, for example, developed and published telehealth recommendations including access to technology, equipment, patient privacy, payment modality, and licensing. The WHO also published a guidance document (www.who.int/publications/i/item/9789240038073) on how to plan and conduct telehealth consultations with children, adolescents, and their families, encouraging telehealth among children and their families. The guidance document encourages and informs facility managers developing telehealth systems.

TELEHEALTH

Telehealth is remote patient care and monitoring. It allows direct transmission of a patient's clinical measurements from a distance to their health-care provider and may or may not be in real time. The telehealth session may also be facilitated by a health-care professional (to other health-care professionals), Village Health Volunteer (VHV), a Community Health Worker (CHW) visiting the patient, or the patient herself/himself, a parent, or a legal guardian. Telehealth can be any combination of health-care services including telemedicine. Some health-care specialties default to "referring to all of such services" as telehealth. "TeleCOVID-19" care is Telemedicine.

Examples of telehealth care are as follows:
- screening for COVID-19, testing recommendations, and guidance on isolation or quarantine
- general health care (i.e., wellness visits, blood pressure control, advice about certain nonemergency illnesses, such as common rashes)
- nonemergency follow-up clinics
- prescriptions for medication
- nutrition counseling
- mental health counseling
- physical therapy exercise
- teleradiology
- tele intensive care (in infectious disease hospitalizations)
- telemedicine

Telehealth decreases contact with health-care facilities, other patients, and health-care staff in order to reduce the risk of COVID-19 spread in the community.

Generally, telehealth modalities are as follows:
- **Synchronous**. Real-time telephone or live audio–video interaction, typically with a patient, using a smartphone, tablet, or computer.
  - For example: In some cases, peripheral medical equipment (e.g., digital stethoscopes, otoscopes, ultrasounds) can be used by another health-care provider (e.g., nurse, medical assistant) physically with the patient, while the consulting medical provider conducts a remote evaluation.
- **Asynchronous**. The provider and patient communication does not happen in real time.

For example, "store and forward" technology allows messages, images, or data to be collected at one point in time and interpreted or responded to later. Patient portals can facilitate this type of communication between provider and patient through secure messaging. Other examples of telehealth modalities developed/

used by the American College of Obstetricians and Gynecologists include the following:
- Live, two-way (or real-time) synchronous audio and video allow specialists, local physicians, and patients to see and hear each other in real time to discuss conditions, for example, via phone or computer.
- Store-and-forward telemedicine, also referred to as "asynchronous telemedicine," sends medical imaging such as x-rays, photos, ultrasound recordings, or other static and video medical imaging to remote specialists for analysis and future consultation.
- Remote patient monitoring collects personal health and medical data from a patient in one location and electronically transmits the data to a physician in a different location for use in care and related support.
- mHealth is a general term for self-managed patient care using mobile phones or other wireless technology and does not necessarily involve monitoring by a physician. It is most commonly used to deliver or reinforce patient education about preventive care and provide medication reminders, appointment reminders, and other essential self-care steps that patients should undertake to maintain their optimal obstetric health.

TELEMEDICINE

Telemedicine is the use of electronic information and telecommunication technology to get needed health care while practicing physical distancing. This encourages the meaningful use of patient health measures to help guide the engagement of patients in care.

Telemedicine goals for developing countries should include, but not be limited to, the following:
- **Remote diagnosing and teleconsulting* system**. Data (including signals and images) are locally (patient-side) acquired and stored and then forwarded to the main hospital, where physicians can analyze those data. The remote (physician-side) hospital will then send back the diagnosis.

- **Remote diagnosis performed with patient assisted by nurses.** If no physician is in the neighborhood: such a situation typically occurs in rural locations of developing countries, and in some cases, a preliminary diagnosis is locally performed by the aid of a decision support system (DSS).
- **Remote monitoring system.** The patient is monitored in a remote location; her/his signals are continuously acquired, forwarded to the main hospital, and, possibly, locally analyzed by a DSS. Alarms are remotely detected and transmitted back to the patient side. The monitoring system can be managed and locally controlled by a physician or by a nurse.
- **Remote intervention system.** The patient enters the operating room, the intervention is performed through a local (patient-side) robot that is remotely controlled by a physician in the main hospital. The remote intervention requires that some local assistance is performed by a physician or by a nurse.
- **Remote education (e-learning) system.** Students or caregivers (mostly physicians, nurses, and technicians) attend classes taught from remote academic institutions and possibly by bidirectional communication interact with the teacher by making up questions. Remote education can be locally assisted by a local tutor, during and/or after the classes.

*Teleconsulting, that is, expert second opinion, is performed among physicians, where a nonspecialist physician requires a remote consultation with one or more specialist physicians: Typically, such a situation occurs in emergency centers of rural locations, in minor hospitals in developed countries, or in any location of developing countries.

POTENTIAL USES OF TELEMEDICINE DURING COVID-19 PANDEMIC
Triaging and Screening for COVID-19 Symptoms

Telehealth can be used to screen for COVID-19 symptoms and assess patients for potential exposure. Phone screening, online screening tools, mobile applications, or virtual telemedicine visits can be used to evaluate patients for COVID-19 symptoms, assess the severity of their symptoms, and decide whether the patient needs to be seen for evaluation, needs to be admitted to the hospital, or can be managed at home. Screening algorithms can be used in telehealth communication.

For patients who may need to be hospitalized, mobile phones and tablets or other telehealth technology can be used for home-based evaluation for hospital care by mobile home health-care units, community health volunteers/workers, or emergency services to communicate with health-care providers at a health facility. Health-care providers can use telehealth to conduct a remote evaluation of the patient's medical condition and determine if the patient needs to be in a regular hospital bed or in an intensive care unit. Making this decision remotely can avoid rushing the patient through the emergency room upon arrival at the hospital, limiting the exposure of emergency department personnel and other health-care workers and preserving PPE.

Telehealth can also be used to screen patients before they visit the health-care facility for non-COVID-19 care. If COVID-19 symptoms are reported during the telehealth interview, patients could be advised to delay nonemergent care and first seek testing for COVID-19.

Contact Tracing

Telehealth, especially via phone, can be used to interview patients with COVID-19 to determine who they were in contact with during the time they were potentially infectious and to follow up with their contacts to inform them of the need to quarantine, assess whether they have any symptoms, and tell them what to do if symptoms develop.

Monitoring COVID-19 Symptoms

Patients with mild or moderate COVID-19 symptoms can isolate in a community isolation center or be monitored at home to avoid overcrowding in health-care facilities and save hospital beds for more severe cases. Using telemedicine technology (e.g., phones or apps), health-care providers can check in with patients frequently to monitor their condition, provide advice, and determine if the patient's condition is deteriorating and if they need to be evaluated for in-person care, such as hospitalization.

Providing Specialized Care for Hospitalized Patients with COVID-19

Patients who are hospitalized with COVID-19 may require care from a diverse team (e.g., nurses, respiratory therapists, physicians). One member of the team can enter the patient's room and consult with the rest of the team using telehealth technology (tablets, phones) to assess the condition of the patient, adjust therapies or treatment plans, and manage complications.

In addition, health facilities can use telehealth to consult with physicians who have specialized training or expertise in respiratory infections such as COVID-19. Tele-intensive care unit platforms, which consist of real-time audio, visual, and electronic connections between remote critical care teams (intensivists and critical care nurses) and patients in distant intensive care units (ICUs), can also be used to monitor critically ill patients and provide expert guidance for care.

Tele-radiology can also be used to consult with radiologists at remote locations. Telehealth can also be used to provide online training on COVID-19 for medical professionals and health-care workers.

Providing Access to Essential Health Care for Non-COVID-19 Patients

Telehealth can be used as a strategy to maintain continuity of care, to the extent possible, to avoid negative consequences from preventive, chronic, or routine care that might otherwise be delayed due to COVID-19 concerns. Telehealth visits can help determine when it is reasonable to defer an in-person visit or service.

Follow-up visits can be conducted by phone or Internet to reduce the number of in-person visits and overcrowding in outpatient settings. Providers can use Internet-based drug prescriptions and provide multi-month dispensing of medications to further reduce the need for in-person encounters.

Remote access to other telehealth modalities can also help assure health-care access when an in-person visit is not practical or feasible due to COVID-19 concerns. To mitigate stress during COVID-19, mental and behavioral health services can be provided to the population through hotlines or virtual provider-patient visits.

Monitoring Recovering COVID-19 Patients

After COVID-19 patients are discharged from the hospital, health-care providers can use telehealth technology to follow up with those who might need to continue isolation at home or be monitored for any sudden deterioration or long-term health effects due to COVID-19.

STEPS TO TAKE WHEN SETTING UP A TELEMEDICINE PRACTICE

The American Medical Association (AMA) Telehealth Implementation Playbook gives a step-by-step guide (www.ama-assn.org/system/files/2020-04/ama-telehealth-implementation-playbook.pdf) on the implementation of a digital health solution. In order to set up a telehealth practice, the aim of continuity of care, license needed and the approved reimbursement process, for the local location of the practice has to be in place. The 12 steps to implementation are as follows:

- Identify the need for telemedicine.
- Create a telemedicine team.
- Develop a clear definition of what a successful telemedicine practice is.
- Evaluate digital technology vendors to be engaged throughout the process.
- Make a case for telemedicine by getting patient, provider, and political/financial buy-in.
- Develop appropriate contracts for vendors, providers, and financial/reimbursement institutions.
- Design the workflow, integrating digital technology into the clinical workflow, taking into consideration

patient privacy acts and laws and health-care data security.
- Prepare the telemedicine "care team" who will take care of "all telemedicine patients."
- Develop patient partnership documents based on information gathered during the need identification and patient buy-in steps.
- Implement the process in pilot mode first before full telemedicine project implementation.
- Monitor and evaluate to improve the process.
- Scale your success measures to position the telemedicine practice for expansion.

LESSONS LEARNED

In the WHO Southeast Asia region, telemedicine supported the strengthening of primary care. Lessons from the COVID-19 pandemic experiences include implementing integrated information systems, stakeholder engagement, capacity building, and carefully managing the transition that could further help in mainstreaming telemedicine as the new normal in comprehensive health services delivery.

Telemedicine has shown potential in salvaging the dwindling health-care system in low- and middle-income countries but faced certain challenges that may create new health inequalities especially based on income.

In the study, "Pulse Oximetry for Monitoring Patients with COVID-19 at Home—A Pragmatic, Randomized Trial," a Philadelphia U.S. randomized trial that assessed a text message–based remote-monitoring program (COVID Watch) supplemented with monitoring of oxygen saturation by means of a home pulse oximeter, remote monitoring was implemented using pulse oximetry. Telemedicine visits were documented visits between a licensed prescriber (advanced practice practitioner or physician) and patient, typically with the use of videoconference technology. Monitored for 30 days, among patients with COVID-19, the addition of home pulse oximetry to remote monitoring, did not show any significant difference in survival, that is, days alive and out of the hospital, when compared to those with subjective assessments of dyspnea alone, with no continuous monitoring at home. Home monitoring (COVID Watch) showed the same outcomes as non-home monitoring (physician videoconference) modalities and did not have a worse outcome.

POTENTIAL LIMITATIONS OF TELEHEALTH

Adaptations to telehealth may need to be considered in certain situations where in-person visits are more appropriate such as:
- due to urgency, a person's underlying health conditions, or the fact that a physical exam or laboratory testing is needed for medical decision-making
- if sensitive topics need to be addressed, especially if there is patient discomfort or concern for privacy
- limited access to technological devices (e.g., phones, tablets, computers) or connectivity, which may be especially true for those living in rural settings
- when health-care workers or patients may be less comfortable using the technology and may prefer an in-person visit
- when virtual visits are not readily accepted in lieu of in-person visits by health-care workers or patients[3]

---

[3] "Telehealth and Telemedicine during COVID-19 in Low Resource Non-U.S. Settings," Centers for Disease Control and Prevention (CDC), May 19, 2022. Available online. URL: www.cdc.gov/coronavirus/2019-ncov/global-covid-19/telehealth-covid19-nonUS.html. Accessed January 3, 2023.

Part 4 | Coronavirus Vaccines and Immunizations

Chapter 30 | Getting Your COVID-19 Vaccine

Chapter Contents
Section 30.1—How Do You Find a COVID-19
            Vaccine or Booster? 349
Section 30.2—Types of COVID-19 Vaccines 350
Section 30.3—Stay Up-to-Date with COVID-19
            Vaccines Including Boosters 359
Section 30.4—COVID-19 Vaccines for Specific
            Groups of People 368

Section 30.1 | How Do You Find a COVID-19 Vaccine or Booster?

FIND COVID-19 VACCINES OR BOOSTERS NEAR YOU

There are other ways you can look for vaccine providers near you in the United States.

- Ask your doctor, pharmacist, or community health center, or visit their website (www.vaccines.gov).
- Contact your state health department.
- Check your local pharmacy's website to see if vaccination appointments are available. Some pharmacies may offer vaccines to those who walk in without making an appointment ahead of time.

If You Are Homebound

- Contact your health-care provider or your state or local health department for information about getting a COVID-19 vaccine.
- In many states, you may also dial 211 to connect to essential community services.
- Contact groups that are advocates for people who are homebound or that provide home health services.
  - Call The Aging Network (https://eldercare.acl.gov/Public/About/Aging_Network/Index.aspx) at 800-677-1116.
  - Search for services by the ZIP code with the Eldercare Locator (https://eldercare.acl.gov/Public/Index.aspx).
  - Contact the Disability Information and Access Line (DIAL; https://acl.gov/DIAL) at 888-677-1199.
  - Call the hotline for Medicare recipients at 800-633-4227 (TTY: 877-486-2048).

SCHEDULING VACCINATION APPOINTMENTS

To schedule your COVID-19 vaccine appointment, visit a vaccine provider's online scheduling services. If you have a question about

scheduling your appointment, contact the vaccination provider directly.
- To verify, reschedule, or cancel a COVID-19 vaccination appointment, contact the location that set up your appointment.
- You can get your vaccines at different locations.

The Centers for Disease Control and Prevention (CDC) cannot schedule, verify, reschedule, or cancel a vaccination appointment.[1]

Section 30.2 | Types of COVID-19 Vaccines

TYPES OF COVID-19 VACCINES AVAILABLE
There are four approved or authorized vaccines in the United States:
- Pfizer-BioNTech and Moderna COVID-19 vaccines are messenger ribonucleic acid (mRNA) vaccines.
- The Novavax COVID-19 vaccine is a protein subunit vaccine.
- Johnson & Johnson's Janssen (J&J/Janssen) COVID-19 vaccine is a viral vector vaccine and can be given in some situations.

These vaccines are given as a shot in the muscle of the upper arm or in the thigh of a young child. COVID-19 vaccine ingredients are considered safe for most people. Nearly all of the ingredients in COVID-19 vaccines are ingredients found in many foods—fats, sugar, and salts. None of the COVID-19 vaccines affect or interact with your deoxyribonucleic acid (DNA), and the following are not included in the vaccines:
- No preservatives such as thimerosal or mercury or any other preservatives.
- No antibiotics such as sulfonamide or any other antibiotics.

---
[1] "How Do I Find a COVID-19 Vaccine or Booster?" Centers for Disease Control and Prevention (CDC), September 15, 2022. Available online. URL: www.cdc.gov/coronavirus/2019-ncov/vaccines/How-Do-I-Get-a-COVID-19-Vaccine.html. Accessed December 16, 2022.

Getting Your COVID-19 Vaccine

- No medicines or therapeutics such as ivermectin or any other medications.
- No tissues such as aborted fetal cells, gelatin, or any materials from any animal.
- No food proteins such as eggs or egg products, gluten, peanuts, tree nuts, nut products, or any nut by-products. COVID-19 vaccines are not manufactured in facilities that produce food products.
- No metals such as iron, nickel, cobalt, titanium, or rare earth alloys. They also do not have any manufactured products such as microelectronics, electrodes, carbon nanotubes or other nanostructures, or nanowire semiconductors.
- No latex. The vial stoppers used to hold the vaccine also do not contain latex.

After the body produces an immune response, it discards all of the vaccine ingredients, just as it would discard any substance that cells no longer need. This process is a part of normal body functioning.

PFIZER-BIONTECH AND MODERNA mRNA COVID-19 VACCINES

mRNA vaccines use mRNA created in a laboratory to teach your cells how to make a protein—or even just a piece of a protein—that triggers an immune response inside your bodies. The mRNA from the vaccines is broken down within a few days after vaccination and discarded from the body.

Pfizer-BioNTech
COMIRNATY NAME CHANGE

After receiving U.S. Food and Drug Administration (FDA) approval on August 23, 2021, the Pfizer-BioNTech COVID-19 vaccine for people aged 16 years and older began to be marketed under the COMIRNATY brand name. The vaccine was also FDA-approved for preteens and teens aged 12–15 on July 8, 2022. No change was made to the vaccine's formula with the name change.

The Pfizer-BioNTech vaccine label remains for people aged six months to 11 years since the vaccine is FDA authorized but not yet approved for these age groups.

INGREDIENTS IN VACCINE FORMULA FOR CHILDREN

Table 30.1 shows the Pfizer-BioNTech COVID-19 vaccine for children aged six months to 11 years contains only the following ingredients.

Table 30.1. A List of Ingredients in the Vaccine Formulation for Children

Type of Ingredient	Ingredient	Purpose
mRNA	• nucleoside-modified mRNA encoding the viral spike (S) glycoprotein of severe acute respiratory syndrome coronavirus 2 (SARS-CoV-2)	Provides instructions the body uses to build a harmless piece of a protein from the virus that causes COVID-19. This protein causes an immune response that helps protect the body from getting sick with COVID-19 in the future.
Lipids (fats)	• 2((polyethylene glycol (PEG))-2000)-N,N-ditetradecylacetamide • 1,2-distearoyl-sn-glycero-3-phosphocholine • cholesterol (plant-derived) • ((4-hydroxybutyl)azanediyl) bis(hexane-6,1-diyl)bis(2-hexyldecanoate)	Work together to help the mRNA enter cells.
Sugar and acid stabilizers	• sucrose (table sugar) • tromethamine • tromethamine hydrochloride	Work together to help keep the vaccine molecules stable while the vaccine is manufactured, frozen, shipped, and stored until it is ready to be given to a vaccine recipient.

INGREDIENTS IN THE VACCINE FORMULA FOR TEENS AND ADULTS

Table 30.2 shows the Pfizer-BioNTech COVID-19 vaccine for teens and adults aged 12 years and older contains only the following ingredients.

Getting Your COVID-19 Vaccine

Table 30.2. Ingredients in the Teens and Adult Vaccine Formula

Type of Ingredient	Ingredient	Purpose
mRNA	• nucleoside-modified mRNA encoding the viral spike (S) glycoprotein of SARS-CoV-2	Provides instructions the body uses to build a harmless piece of a protein from the virus that causes COVID-19. This protein causes an immune response that helps protect the body from getting sick with COVID-19 in the future.
Lipids (fats)	• 2[(polyethylene glycol (PEG))-2000]-N,N-ditetradecylacetamide • 1,2-distearoyl-sn-glycero-3-phosphocholine • cholesterol (plant-derived) • ((4-hydroxybutyl)azanediyl)bis(hexane-6,1-diyl)bis(2-hexyldecanoate)	Work together to help the mRNA enter cells.
Sugar and acid stabilizers	• sucrose (table sugar) • tromethamine • tromethamine hydrochloride	Work together to help keep the vaccine in good condition (molecules remain stable) while the vaccine is manufactured, frozen, shipped, and stored until it is ready to be given to a vaccine recipient.

Moderna
SPIKEVAX NAME CHANGE

After receiving FDA approval on January 31, 2022, the Moderna COVID-19 vaccine for people aged 18 years and older began to be marketed under the Spikevax brand name. No change was made to the vaccine's formula with the name change.

The Moderna vaccine name remains for people aged six months to 17 years since the vaccine is authorized by the FDA but not yet approved for these age groups.

INGREDIENTS

Table 30.3 shows the Moderna COVID-19 vaccine for everyone aged six months and older contains only the following ingredients.

Table 30.3. Ingredients That Make Up the Moderna COVID-19 Vaccine

Type of Ingredient	Ingredient	Purpose
mRNA	• nucleoside-modified mRNA encoding the viral spike (S) glycoprotein of SARS-CoV-2	Provides instructions the body uses to build a harmless piece of a protein from the virus that causes COVID-19. This protein causes an immune response that helps protect the body from getting sick with COVID-19 in the future.
Lipids (fats)	• PEG2000-DMG: 1,2-dimyristoyl-rac-glycerol, methoxypolyethylene glycol • 1,2-distearoyl-sn-glycero-3-phosphocholine • BotaniChol® (nonanimal origin cholesterol) • SM-102: heptadecane-9-yl 8-((2-hydroxyethyl) (6-oxo-6-(undecyloxy) hexyl) amino) octanoate	Work together to help the mRNA enter cells.
Salt, sugar, acid stabilizers, and acid	• sodium acetate • sucrose (basic table sugar) • tromethamine • tromethamine hydrochloride • acetic acid (the main ingredient in White household vinegar)	Work together to help keep the vaccine in good condition (molecules remain stable) while the vaccine is manufactured, frozen, shipped, and stored until it is ready to be given to a vaccine recipient.

NOVAVAX PROTEIN SUBUNIT COVID-19 VACCINE

Protein subunit vaccines contain pieces (proteins) of the virus that causes COVID-19. The virus pieces are the spike protein. The Novavax COVID-19 vaccine contains another ingredient called an "adjuvant." It helps the immune system respond to that spike protein. After learning how to respond to the spike protein, the immune system will be able to respond quickly to the actual virus spike protein and protect you against COVID-19.

When to Consider Getting a Monovalent Novavax Booster

You may get a monovalent Novavax booster if you are unable or unwilling to receive a Pfizer or Moderna updated (bivalent) COVID-19 booster and you meet the following requirements:
- You are 18 years of age or older.
- You completed a COVID-19 vaccine primary series at least six months ago.
- You have not gotten any other booster dose.

INGREDIENTS

Table 30.4 shows the ingredients that the Novavax COVID-19 vaccine contains.

JOHNSON AND JOHNSON'S JANSSEN (J&J/JANSSEN) VIRAL VECTOR COVID-19 VACCINE

Viral vector vaccines use a harmless, modified version of a different virus (a vector virus) and not the virus that causes COVID-19. The vector virus delivers important instructions to your cells on how to recognize and fight the virus that causes COVID-19.

Table 30.4. Ingredients That Make Up the Novavax COVID-19 Vaccine

Type of Ingredient	Ingredient	Purpose
Protein	• SARS-CoV-2 recombinant spike protein	Causes an immune response that helps protect the body from getting sick with COVID-19 in the future.
Lipids (fats)	• cholesterol • phosphatidylcholine	Work together to help the recombinant spike protein enter cells.
Adjuvant	Fraction-A and fraction-C of Quillaja saponaria Molina extract	Facilitates activation of the cells of the innate immune system.

Table 30.4. Continued

Type of Ingredient	Ingredient	Purpose
Salts, sugar, and acid	• disodium hydrogen phosphate heptahydrate • disodium hydrogen phosphate dihydrate • polysorbate-80 • potassium chloride (common food salt) • potassium dihydrogen phosphate (common food salt) • sodium chloride (basic table salt) • sodium dihydrogen phosphate monohydrate • sodium hydroxide or hydrochloric acid • water	Work together to help keep the vaccine molecules stable while the vaccine is manufactured, shipped, and stored until it is ready to be given to a vaccine recipient. The vaccine may also contain very small amounts of ingredients from the manufacturing stage, which can be found in the Emergency Use Authorization (EUA) fact sheet.

When to Consider Getting the J&J/Janssen COVID-19 Vaccine

In most situations, Pfizer-BioNTech, Moderna, or Novavax COVID-19 vaccines are recommended over the J&J/Janssen COVID-19 vaccine for primary and booster vaccination due to the risk of serious adverse events. Vaccine recipients should talk to their health-care provider about which vaccine is right for them. They must be informed of the risks and benefits of J&J/Janssen COVID-19 vaccination. The J&J/Janssen COVID-19 vaccine may be considered in some situations, including for persons who:

- had a severe reaction after an mRNA vaccine dose or who have a severe allergy to an ingredient of Pfizer-BioNTech or Moderna (mRNA COVID-19 vaccines)
- would otherwise remain unvaccinated for COVID-19 due to limited access to Pfizer-BioNTech or Moderna (mRNA COVID-19 vaccines) or to Novavax
- want to get the J&J/Janssen COVID-19 vaccine despite the safety concerns
- are 18 years and older

Getting Your COVID-19 Vaccine

INGREDIENTS

Table 30.5 shows the J&J/Janssen COVID-19 vaccine contains only the following ingredients.

Table 30.5. Ingredients That Make Up the J&J/Janssen COVID-19 Vaccine

Type of Ingredient	Ingredient	Purpose
A harmless version of a virus unrelated to the COVID-19 virus	• recombinant, replication-incompetent Ad26 vector, encoding a stabilized variant of the SARS-CoV-2 Spike (S) protein	Provides instructions the body uses to build a harmless piece of a protein from the virus that causes COVID-19. This protein causes an immune response that helps protect the body from getting sick with COVID-19 in the future.
Sugars, salts, acid, and acid stabilizer	• polysorbate-80 • 2-hydroxypropyl-β-cyclodextrin • trisodium citrate dihydrate • sodium chloride (basic table salt) • citric acid monohydrate (closely related to lemon juice) • ethanol (a type of alcohol)	Work together to help keep the vaccine molecules stable while the vaccine is manufactured, shipped, and stored until it is ready to be given to a vaccine recipient.

HOW WELL DO COVID-19 VACCINES WORK?

- People who are up-to-date have a lower risk of severe illness, hospitalization, and death from COVID-19 than people who are unvaccinated or who have only received the primary series.
- Updated COVID-19 boosters can help restore protection that has decreased since the previous vaccination. The updated boosters provide added protection against the Omicron subvariants that are more contagious than the previous ones. The recent subvariants, BA.4 and BA.5, are very closely related to the original variant, Omicron, with very small differences between itself and the original variant.

SAFETY OF COVID-19 VACCINES

COVID-19 vaccines have undergone—and will continue to undergo—the most intensive safety monitoring in U.S. history. Evidence from the hundreds of millions of COVID-19 vaccines already administered in the United States, as well as the billions of vaccines administered globally, demonstrates that they are safe and effective.

Side Effects
- Side effects that happen within seven days of getting vaccinated are common but are mostly mild. Sometimes, they may affect a person's ability to do daily activities.
- Side effects throughout the body (such as fever, chills, tiredness, and headache) are more common after the second dose of a Pfizer-BioNTech, Moderna, or Novavax COVID-19 vaccine.

Adverse Events
- Severe allergic reactions to vaccines are rare but can happen.
- There is a rare risk of myocarditis and pericarditis associated with mRNA COVID-19 vaccination, mostly among males aged 12–39 years. The rare risk may be further reduced with a longer interval between the first and second dose.
- Cases of myocarditis and pericarditis have also been reported in people who received the Novavax COVID-19 vaccine.
- There is a potential cause-and-effect relationship between the J&J/Janssen COVID-19 vaccine and a rare and serious adverse event. It is blood clots with low platelets (thrombosis with thrombocytopenia syndrome or TTS). TTS occurs at a rate of about four cases per million Janssen's Johnson and Johnson doses and has resulted in deaths. Because of this risk, vaccination with COVID-19 vaccines other than the J&J/Janssen vaccine is preferred.

Getting Your COVID-19 Vaccine

IF YOU ARE ALLERGIC TO AN INGREDIENT IN A COVID-19 VACCINE OR HAD A PREVIOUS SEVERE ALLERGIC REACTION

- If in the past you have had a severe allergic reaction to an ingredient in a COVID-19 vaccine or if you have a known allergy to an ingredient in a COVID-19 vaccine, you should not get that COVID-19 vaccine. Examples are as follows:
  - If you are allergic to polyethylene glycol (PEG), you should not get Pfizer-BioNTech or Moderna COVID-19 vaccines.
  - If you are allergic to polysorbate, you should not get Novavax or J&J/Janssen COVID-19 vaccines.
- If you are not able to get one type of COVID-19 vaccine, talk to your doctor about your options for getting a different type of COVID-19 vaccine.[2]

Section 30.3 | Stay Up-to-Date with COVID-19 Vaccines Including Boosters

ABOUT COVID-19 VACCINES

COVID-19 vaccines available in the United States are effective at protecting people from getting seriously ill, being hospitalized, and dying. As with other vaccine-preventable diseases, you are protected best from COVID-19 when you stay up-to-date with the recommended vaccinations, including recommended boosters.
- Updated (bivalent) boosters became available on:
  - September 2, 2022, for people 12 years of age and older
  - October 12, 2022, for people aged 5–11

---

[2] "Overview of COVID-19 Vaccines," Centers for Disease Control and Prevention (CDC), November 1, 2022. Available online. URL: www.cdc.gov/coronavirus/2019-ncov/vaccines/different-vaccines/overview-COVID-19-vaccines.html. Accessed December 19, 2022.

- The Centers for Disease Control and Prevention (CDC) recommends everyone stay up-to-date with COVID-19 vaccines for their age group:
  - children and teens aged six months to 17 years
  - adults aged 18 years and older
- Getting a COVID-19 vaccine after you recover from COVID-19 infection provides added protection against COVID-19.
- If you recently had COVID-19, you may consider delaying your next vaccine dose (primary dose or booster) by three months from when your symptoms started or, if you had no symptoms, when you first received a positive test.
- People who are moderately or severely immunocompromised have different recommendations for COVID-19 vaccines.
- COVID-19 vaccine and booster recommendations may be updated as the CDC continues to monitor the latest COVID-19 data.

Four COVID-19 vaccines are approved or authorized in the United States:
- Pfizer-BioNTech
- Moderna
- Novavax
- Johnson & Johnson's Janssen (J&J/Janssen; however, the CDC recommends that the J&J/Janssen COVID-19 vaccine should only be considered in certain situations due to safety concerns)

Updated (Bivalent) Boosters

The updated (bivalent) boosters are called "bivalent" because they protect against both the original virus that causes COVID-19 and the Omicron variants BA.4 and BA.5. Previous boosters are called "monovalent" because they were designed to protect against the original virus that causes COVID-19. They also provide some protection against Omicron but not as much as the updated (bivalent) boosters.

Getting Your COVID-19 Vaccine

The virus that causes COVID-19 has changed over time. The different versions of the virus that have developed over time are called "variants." Two COVID-19 vaccine manufacturers, Pfizer and Moderna, have developed updated (bivalent) COVID-19 boosters.

WHEN ARE YOU UP-TO-DATE?

You are up-to-date with your COVID-19 vaccines if you have completed a COVID-19 vaccine primary series and received the most recent booster dose recommended for you by the CDC.

- If you have completed your primary series—but are not yet eligible for a booster—you are also considered up-to-date.
- If you become ill with COVID-19 after you received all COVID-19 vaccine doses recommended for you, you are also considered up-to-date. You do not need to be revaccinated or receive an additional booster.

COVID-19 vaccine recommendations are based on three things:
- your age
- the vaccine you first received
- the length of time since your last dose

People who are moderately or severely immunocompromised have different recommendations for COVID-19 vaccines.

GETTING VACCINES IF YOU HAD OR CURRENTLY HAVE COVID-19

If you recently had COVID-19, you may consider delaying your next vaccine dose (whether a primary dose or booster) by three months from when your symptoms started or, if you had no symptoms, when you first received a positive test.

Reinfection is less likely in the weeks to months after infection. However, certain factors, such as personal risk of severe disease or risk of disease in a loved one or close contact, local COVID-19 community level, and the most common COVID-19 variant currently causing illness, could be reasons to get a vaccine sooner rather than later.

Children and Teens Aged Six Months to 17 Years
PFIZER-BIONTECH
Age group six months to four years:
- first dose Pfizer-BioNTech primary series
- second dose Pfizer-BioNTech primary series 3–8 weeks after the first dose
- third dose Pfizer-BioNTech primary series at least eight weeks after the second dose

Age group 5–11 years:
- first dose Pfizer-BioNTech primary series
- second dose Pfizer-BioNTech primary series 3–8 weeks after the first dose
- third dose Pfizer-BioNTech updated (bivalent) booster at least two months after the second dose or last booster (children aged five years can only get a Pfizer-BioNTech booster, and children aged 6–11 years can get a Pfizer-BioNTech or Moderna booster)

Age group 12–17 years:
- first dose Pfizer-BioNTech primary series
- second dose Pfizer-BioNTech primary series 3–8 weeks after the first dose
- third dose Pfizer-BioNTech or Moderna updated (bivalent) booster at least two months after the second dose or last booster

MODERNA
Age group six months to five years:
- first dose Moderna primary series
- second dose Moderna primary series 4–8 weeks after the first dose
- third dose Pfizer-BioNTech updated (bivalent) booster (children five years of age can get a Pfizer-BioNTech booster at least two months after their second dose; children six months to four years are not recommended for a booster)

Age group 6–17 years:
- first dose Moderna primary series
- second dose Moderna primary series 4–8 weeks after the first dose
- third dose Pfizer-BioNTech or Moderna updated (bivalent) booster at least two months after the second primary series dose

NOVAVAX

Age group 12–17 years: Novavax is not authorized as a booster dose at this time.
- first dose Novavax primary series
- second dose Novavax primary series 3–8 weeks after the first dose
- third dose Pfizer-BioNTech or Moderna updated (bivalent) booster at least two months after the second primary series dose

Adults Aged 18 Years and Older
PFIZER-BIONTECH
- first dose Pfizer-BioNTech primary series
- second dose Pfizer-BioNTech primary series 3–8 weeks after the first dose
- third dose Pfizer-BioNTech or Moderna updated (bivalent) booster at least two months after the second primary series dose or last booster

MODERNA
- first dose Moderna primary series
- second dose Moderna primary series 4–8 weeks after the first dose
- third dose Pfizer-BioNTech or Moderna updated (bivalent) booster at least two months after the second primary series dose or last booster

NOVAVAX
- first dose Novavax primary series
- second dose Novavax primary series 3–8 weeks after the first dose
- third dose Pfizer-BioNTech or Moderna updated (bivalent) booster at least two months after the second primary series dose (a monovalent Novavax booster is available in limited situations)

JOHNSON AND JOHNSON'S JANSSEN
Age group 18 years and older:
- first dose Johnson and Johnson's Janssen primary series
- second dose Pfizer-BioNTech or Moderna updated (bivalent) booster at least two months after the second primary series dose (a monovalent J&J/Janssen booster is available in limited situations)

GETTING YOUR SECOND DOSE
Talk to your health-care or vaccine provider about the timing for the second dose in your primary series.
- People aged six months through 64 years, especially males aged 12 through 39 years, may consider getting the second primary Pfizer-BioNTech, Moderna, or Novavax eight weeks after the first dose.
  - A longer time between the first and second primary doses may increase how much protection the vaccines offer and further minimize the rare risk of myocarditis and pericarditis.
- Anyone wanting protection due to high levels of community transmission, people aged 65 years and older, or people who are likely to get very sick from COVID-19 should get the second dose of the following:
  - the Pfizer-BioNTech COVID-19 vaccine three weeks (or 21 days) after the first dose

Getting Your COVID-19 Vaccine

- the Moderna COVID-19 vaccine four weeks (or 28 days) after the first dose
- the Novavax COVID-19 vaccine three weeks (or 21 days) after the first dose

STAYING UP-TO-DATE
- If you have completed your primary series but are not yet eligible for a booster, you are also considered up-to-date.

NOVAVAX BOOSTER
- You may get a monovalent Novavax booster if you are unable or unwilling to receive a Pfizer or Moderna updated (bivalent) COVID-19 booster and you meet the following requirements:
  - You are 18 years of age or older.
  - You completed a COVID-19 vaccine primary series at least six months ago.
  - You have not gotten any other booster dose.

MIXING COVID-19 VACCINE PRODUCTS
Do Not Mix Primary Series
The CDC does not recommend mixing products for your primary series doses. If you received Pfizer-BioNTech, Moderna, or Novavax for the first dose of your primary series, you should get the same product for all the following primary series doses.

Mixing Boosters
The following information applies to people who want to get different products for their booster vaccine.

CHILDREN AGED SIX MONTHS TO FOUR YEARS
Children aged six months to four years should get the same product for all their primary series and booster, if eligible. However, children who only completed two doses of Pfizer-BioNTech COVID-19

vaccines should get the Pfizer-BioNTech updated (bivalent) vaccine as the third dose in their primary series.

Children aged six months to four years who completed the two-dose Moderna primary series should get an updated (bivalent) Moderna booster.

PEOPLE AGED FIVE YEARS AND OLDER

Children aged five years who completed the Pfizer-BioNTech primary series should only get the updated (bivalent) Pfizer-BioNTech booster. Children aged five years who completed the Moderna primary series can get a different product for their updated (bivalent) booster compared with what they got for their primary series.

People aged six years and older can get a different product for their updated (bivalent) booster compared with what they got for their primary series or last booster.

VACCINATION RECEIVED OUTSIDE THE UNITED STATES

Specific recommendations for people vaccinated outside the United States depend on whether:
- the vaccine(s) received are accepted in the United States as valid vaccinations
- the primary series was completed, and if eligible, a booster dose was received

These recommendations apply only to people who are not moderately or severely immunocompromised.

COVID-19 Vaccines Available Abroad That Are Accepted in the United States as Valid Vaccinations

Vaccines listed for emergency use by the World Health Organization (WHO) currently include those that are listed above and the following:
- AstraZeneca/Oxford vaccine
- Sinopharm
- Sinovac
- COVAXIN

Getting Your COVID-19 Vaccine

- Covovax
- CanSino

If You Receive a Vaccine That Is Not in the U.S. Accepted List Above
- Wait at least 28 days after the last dose you received of that vaccine and then start COVID-19 vaccination over with a COVID-19 vaccine that has been approved or authorized by the U.S. Food and Drug Administration (FDA).
- If the FDA has not approved or authorized a vaccine, there may be limited data available or reviewed on the safety or effectiveness of the COVID-19 vaccine.

How to Complete a Primary Series
- Receive one dose of a single-dose accepted COVID-19 vaccine.
- Receive two doses of a two-dose accepted COVID-19 vaccine.

The CDC does not recommend mixing different COVID-19 vaccines for the primary series, but the CDC is aware that mixing COVID-19 vaccines for the primary series is increasingly common in many countries outside the United States. Therefore, people who receive a mixed primary series, meaning two different COVID-19 vaccines, have completed the series.

If You Started but Did Not Complete a Primary Series
You will need to complete the primary series. If you got the first dose of Moderna, Novavax, or Pfizer-BioNTech, it is best to get the same vaccine again to complete the primary series.

After Completing a Primary Series
If you are not yet eligible for a booster, you are considered up-to-date. Otherwise, stay up-to-date by getting the booster recommended for you as soon as a booster is recommended for you

based on your age and the appropriate time that has passed since completing the primary series.

The Vaccination Card in the United States

The white CDC COVID-19 vaccination cards are issued only to people vaccinated in the United States. The CDC recommends that people vaccinated outside of the United States keep their documentation of being vaccinated in another country as proof of vaccination. The CDC does not keep vaccination records nor determine how vaccination records are used. People can update their records with vaccines they received while outside of the United States by:

- contacting the immunization information system (IIS) in their state
- contacting their health-care provider or local or state immunization program through their state's health department[3]

Section 30.4 | COVID-19 Vaccines for Specific Groups of People

COVID-19 VACCINATION FOR CHILDREN AND TEENS WITH DISABILITIES

Children and youth with special health-care needs require more care for their physical, developmental, behavioral, or emotional differences than their typically developing peers. A special health-care need can include physical, intellectual, and developmental disabilities, as well as long-standing medical conditions, such as asthma, diabetes, a blood disorder, or muscular dystrophy (MD).

---

[3] "Stay Up-to-Date with COVID-19 Vaccines including Boosters," Centers for Disease Control and Prevention (CDC), November 1, 2022. Available online. URL: www.cdc.gov/coronavirus/2019-ncov/vaccines/stay-up-to-date.html. Accessed December 19, 2022.

Getting Your COVID-19 Vaccine

Children and Teens with Disabilities Are at an Increased Risk for Severe Illness from COVID-19

Many children and teens with disabilities have underlying medical conditions such as lung, heart, or kidney disease, a weakened immune system, cancer, obesity, diabetes, some blood diseases, or conditions of the muscular or central nervous system. Children and teens with one or more underlying medical conditions are likely to get severely ill from COVID-19.

Similarly, children and teens with developmental disabilities, such as cerebral palsy, an intellectual disability, or autism, may be likely to experience mental health conditions from social isolation. They can also experience barriers to getting needed health care and other support and can have other characteristics that increase their risk of COVID-19, including the following:
- limited mobility
- need for important support services
- challenges practicing preventive measures, such as wearing a mask
- challenges communicating symptoms of illness or being sick

Getting Children and Teens with Disabilities Vaccinated against COVID-19
THE BENEFITS OF COVID-19 VACCINATION OUTWEIGH THE KNOWN AND POTENTIAL RISKS
- COVID-19 vaccines have been shown to be safe and effective at protecting against COVID-19 and preventing severe illness if infected.
  - In clinical trials, about 20 percent of children and teens who participated had an underlying medical condition.
- Some children and teens with a weakened immune system should get an additional dose of vaccine as part of their primary COVID-19 vaccination series.

Prepare all children and teens for the vaccination visit and use resources such as picture stories for support during and after vaccination.

After vaccination, parents and caregivers should continue following all current prevention measures recommended by the Centers for Disease Control and Prevention (CDC).

REQUESTING ACCOMMODATIONS AT COVID-19 VACCINATION SITES
When making an appointment or arriving for vaccination, parents and caregivers can let staff and/or volunteers know their child might need some accommodations.

COVID-19 VACCINE DISABILITY INFORMATION AND ACCESS LINE (DIAL)
Call 888-677-1199 Monday–Friday from 9 a.m. to 8 p.m. (EST), email DIAL@usaginganddisability.org, or visit their website, https://wecandothis.hhs.gov/resource/covid-19-vaccine-disability-information-and-access-line-dial, to help:
- find local vaccination locations
- make appointments
- connect to local services such as accessible transportation

HOME VISITS
If a child under your care is unable to leave the home, contact your state, territorial, local, or tribal health department to request an in-home vaccination.

COVID-19 VACCINES FOR PEOPLE WHO WOULD LIKE TO HAVE A BABY/ARE PLANNING PREGNANCY
The Centers for Disease Control and Prevention and Medical Professionals Recommend COVID-19 Vaccination for People Who Want to Have Children
Professional medical organizations serving people of reproductive age, including adolescents, emphasize that there is no evidence that COVID-19 vaccination causes problems with fertility.

PREGNANCY AFTER VACCINATION
Many people have become pregnant after receiving a COVID-19 vaccine, including some who got vaccinated during COVID-19

Getting Your COVID-19 Vaccine

vaccine clinical trials. In addition, a recent report using the V-safe COVID-19 vaccine pregnancy safety monitoring system data showed that 4,800 people had a positive pregnancy test after receiving the first dose of a messenger ribonucleic acid (mRNA) COVID-19 vaccine. Another report using data from eight U.S. health-care systems documented more than 1,000 people who completed COVID-19 vaccination (with any COVID-19 vaccine) before becoming pregnant.

NO EVIDENCE THAT COVID-19 VACCINES AFFECT FERTILITY
There is currently no evidence that vaccine ingredients or antibodies made following COVID-19 vaccination would cause any problems with becoming pregnant now or in the future:
- Recent studies have found no differences in pregnancy success rates among women who had antibodies from COVID-19 vaccines or from a recent COVID-19 infection and women who had no antibodies, including for patients undergoing assisted reproductive technology procedures (e.g., in vitro fertilization).
- A study of more than 2,000 females aged 21–45 years and their partners found that COVID-19 vaccination of either partner did not affect the likelihood of becoming pregnant.

Like with all vaccines, scientists continue to study COVID-19 vaccines carefully and will continue to report findings as they become available.

LIMITED, TEMPORARY IMPACT OF COVID-19 VACCINES ON MENSTRUAL CYCLES
Results from recent research studies show that people who menstruate may observe small, temporary changes in menstruation after COVID-19 vaccination, including the following:
- longer-lasting menstrual periods
- shorter intervals between periods
- heavier bleeding than usual

Despite these temporary changes in menstruation, there is no evidence that COVID-19 vaccines cause fertility problems.

RESEARCH STUDIES OF FERTILITY IN HEALTHY MEN
- Currently, no evidence shows that any vaccines, including COVID-19 vaccines, cause male fertility problems. A recent small study of 45 healthy men who received an mRNA COVID-19 vaccine looked at sperm characteristics, such as quantity and movement, before and after vaccination. Researchers found no significant changes in these sperm characteristics after vaccination.
  - However, one study found that COVID-19 infection may be associated with a decline in fertility for men for up to 60 days after infection.
- Fever from any illness has been associated with a short-term decrease in sperm production in healthy men. Although fever can be a side effect of COVID-19 vaccination, there is no current evidence that fever after COVID vaccination affects sperm production. Fever is also a common symptom of COVID-19 infection.

SAFETY MONITORING
COVID-19 vaccines are undergoing the most intense safety monitoring in U.S. history. Data continue to accumulate and show that COVID-19 vaccines are safe and effective for use before and during pregnancy.

MANAGING SIDE EFFECTS
If you have side effects after COVID-19 vaccination, talk to your health-care provider about taking over-the-counter (OTC) medicine, such as ibuprofen, acetaminophen, or antihistamines, for any pain or discomfort you may experience, including fever. You can take these medications to relieve short-term side effects after getting vaccinated if you have no medical reasons that prevent you from taking these medications.

Fever, for any reason, has been associated with adverse pregnancy outcomes. Fever in pregnancy may be treated with acetaminophen as needed, in moderation and in consultation with a health-care provider. It is not recommended you take these medicines before vaccination to try to prevent side effects.

COVID-19 VACCINES WHILE PREGNANT OR BREASTFEEDING
People Who Are Pregnant

Although the overall risks are low, if you are pregnant or were recently pregnant:

- You are more likely to get very sick from COVID-19 than people who are not pregnant. People who get very sick from COVID-19 may require hospitalization, admission to an intensive care unit (ICU), or use of a ventilator or special equipment to breathe. Severe COVID-19 illness can also lead to death.
- You are at an increased risk of complications that can affect your pregnancy and developing baby. For example, COVID-19 during pregnancy increases the risk of delivering a preterm or stillborn infant.

Getting a COVID-19 vaccine can protect you and others around you from getting very sick from COVID-19, and keeping you as healthy as possible during pregnancy is important for the health of your baby.

The CDC recommends COVID-19 vaccines for everyone aged six months and older, including people who are pregnant, breastfeeding, trying to get pregnant now, or those who might become pregnant in the future. This recommendation includes getting boosters when it is time to get one.

Safety and Effectiveness of COVID-19 Vaccination during Pregnancy

Evidence continues to build showing that COVID-19 vaccination before and during pregnancy is safe, effective, and beneficial to both the pregnant person and the baby. The benefits of receiving a COVID-19 vaccine outweigh any potential risks of vaccination during pregnancy. Below is a brief summary of the growing evidence:

- COVID-19 vaccines do not cause COVID-19, including in people who are pregnant or their babies. None of the COVID-19 vaccines contain the live virus. They cannot make anyone sick with COVID-19, including people who are pregnant or their babies.
- Data on the safety of receiving an mRNA COVID-19 vaccine (Moderna or Pfizer-BioNTech) before and during pregnancy are reassuring.
  - Data from vaccine safety monitoring systems have not found any safety concerns for people who received an mRNA COVID-19 vaccine late in pregnancy or for their babies.
  - Scientists have not found an increased risk for miscarriage among pregnant people who received an mRNA COVID-19 vaccine just before or during early pregnancy (before 20 weeks of pregnancy).
  - Data from American, European, and Canadian studies showed that vaccination with an mRNA COVID-19 vaccine during pregnancy was not associated with an increased risk for pregnancy complications, including preterm birth, stillbirth, bacterial infection of the placenta, and excessive maternal blood loss after birth.
  - A Chicago study has shown that vaccination of pregnant people with a COVID-19 vaccine prior to and during the first trimester was not associated with an increased risk of birth defects detectable on prenatal ultrasound.
  - The monitoring of the effect of COVID-19 vaccination during pregnancy is ongoing. The CDC will continue to follow people vaccinated during all trimesters of pregnancy to better understand any effects of the vaccine on pregnancies and babies.

Getting Your COVID-19 Vaccine

- Data show that receiving an mRNA COVID-19 vaccine during pregnancy reduces the risk of severe illness and other health effects from COVID-19 for people who are pregnant. Recent studies compared people who were pregnant and received an mRNA COVID-19 vaccine with pregnant people who did not. Scientists found that COVID-19 vaccination was effective at reducing the risk of getting very sick from COVID-19. One study that looked at people who were hospitalized during pregnancy found that most were not vaccinated. Other studies have shown that by reducing the risk of severe illness in pregnant people, COVID-19 vaccination might also help prevent stillbirths.
- Vaccination during pregnancy builds antibodies that can help protect the baby. Much like people who are not pregnant, when people who are pregnant receive an mRNA COVID-19 vaccine, their bodies build antibodies against COVID-19. Antibodies made after pregnant people received an mRNA COVID-19 vaccine have been found in their baby's umbilical cord blood. This means COVID-19 vaccination during pregnancy can help protect babies against COVID-19 by passing antibodies from the mother to her baby. More data are needed to determine how these antibodies may provide protection to the baby.
  - A recent small study found that at six months old, the majority (57%) of infants born to pregnant people who were vaccinated during pregnancy had detectable antibodies against COVID-19, compared with eight percent of infants born to pregnant people who had COVID-19 illness during pregnancy.
  - Recent data show that completing a two-dose primary mRNA COVID-19 vaccine series during pregnancy can help protect babies younger than aged six months from hospitalization due to COVID-19. In these reports, the majority of babies

hospitalized with COVID-19 were born to pregnant people who were not vaccinated during pregnancy.
- Another study found that receiving a booster dose with an mRNA COVID-19 vaccine during pregnancy significantly increased the levels of antibodies found in umbilical cord blood. This means that getting a COVID-19 booster during pregnancy can help further protect babies against COVID-19.
- No safety concerns were found in animal studies. Studies in animals receiving a COVID-19 vaccine before or during pregnancy found no safety concerns in pregnant animals or their babies.

More clinical trials on the safety of COVID-19 vaccines and how well they work in people who are pregnant are underway or planned. Vaccine manufacturers are also collecting and reviewing data from people in the completed clinical trials who received a vaccine and became pregnant during the trial.

TALK TO YOUR HEALTH-CARE PROVIDER

If you are pregnant, talk to your health-care provider about COVID-19 vaccination. While such a conversation might be helpful, it is not required before vaccination. You can receive a COVID-19 vaccine, including a booster shot, without any additional documentation from your health-care provider.

Common Questions about Vaccination during Pregnancy
WHAT ARE THE LONG-TERM EFFECTS ON THE BODY WHEN A PERSON GETS THE COVID-19 VACCINE DURING PREGNANCY?

Scientific studies to date have shown no safety concerns for babies born to people who were vaccinated against COVID-19 during pregnancy. Based on how these vaccines work in the body, experts believe they are unlikely to pose a risk for long-term health effects. The CDC continues to monitor, analyze, and disseminate information from people vaccinated during all trimesters of pregnancy to better understand effects on pregnancy and babies.

WHEN DURING PREGNANCY SHOULD A PERSON GET A COVID-19 VACCINE?

The CDC and professional medical organizations, including the American College of Obstetricians and Gynecologists and the Society for Maternal-Fetal Medicine, recommend COVID-19 vaccination at any point in pregnancy, as well as booster doses when it is time to get one. COVID-19 vaccination can protect you from getting very sick from COVID-19. Keeping yourself as healthy as possible during pregnancy is important for the health of your baby.

WHICH COVID-19 VACCINE SHOULD PREGNANT PEOPLE RECEIVE?

You can choose to get either an mRNA COVID-19 vaccine (Moderna or Pfizer-BioNTech) or Novavax COVID-19 vaccine. The J&J/Janssen COVID-19 vaccine is authorized for use only in certain limited situations.

CAN PREGNANT PEOPLE GET A COVID-19 VACCINE AT THE SAME TIME AS OTHER VACCINES?

Children, teens, and adults, including pregnant people, may get a COVID-19 vaccine and other vaccines, including a flu vaccine, at the same time.

People Who Are Breastfeeding

The CDC recommends that people who are breastfeeding get vaccinated and stay up-to-date with their COVID-19 vaccines, including getting a COVID-19 booster shot when it is time to get one.

Clinical trials for the COVID-19 vaccines currently used in the United States did not include people who were breastfeeding. Therefore, limited data are available on the following:
- safety of COVID-19 vaccines in people who are breastfeeding
- effects of vaccination on the breastfed baby
- effects on milk production or excretion

Available data on the safety of COVID-19 vaccination while breastfeeding indicate no severe reactions after the first or second dose, neither in the breastfeeding person nor in the breastfed child. There has been no evidence to suggest that COVID-19 vaccines are harmful to either people who have received a vaccine and are breastfeeding or to their babies.

COVID-19 vaccines cannot cause COVID-19 in anyone, including pregnant people and their babies. None of the COVID-19 vaccines contain the live virus. Vaccines are effective at preventing COVID-19 in people who are breastfeeding. Recent reports have shown that breastfeeding people who have received mRNA COVID-19 vaccines have antibodies in their breast milk, which could help protect their babies. More data are needed to determine what level of protection these antibodies might provide to the baby.

People Who Would Like to Have a Baby

The CDC recommends that people who are trying to get pregnant now or might become pregnant in the future, as well as their partners, get vaccinated and stay up-to-date with their COVID-19 vaccines, including getting a COVID-19 booster shot when it is time to get one. COVID-19 vaccines are not associated with fertility problems in women or men.

Vaccine Side Effects

Side effects can occur after receiving any of the available COVID-19 vaccines, especially after the second dose for vaccines that require two doses or after a booster.

People who are pregnant have not reported different side effects from people who are not pregnant after vaccination with mRNA COVID-19 vaccines (Moderna and Pfizer-BioNTech vaccines).
- Fever during pregnancy, for any reason, has been associated with adverse pregnancy outcomes.
- Fever in pregnancy may be treated with acetaminophen as needed, in moderation and in consultation with a health-care provider.
- Learn more at Possible Side Effects after Getting a COVID-19 Vaccine (www.cdc.gov/coronavirus/2019-ncov/vaccines/expect/after.html).

Getting Your COVID-19 Vaccine

Although rare, some people have had severe allergic reactions after receiving a COVID-19 vaccine. Talk with your health-care provider if you have a history of allergic reaction to any other vaccine or injectable therapy (intramuscular, intravenous, or subcutaneous).

Key considerations you can discuss with your health-care provider include the following:
- The benefits of vaccination.
- The unknown risks of developing a severe allergic reaction.
- If you have an allergic reaction after receiving a COVID-19 vaccine during pregnancy, you can receive treatment for it.[4]

---

[4] "COVID-19 Vaccines for Specific Groups of People," Centers for Disease Control and Prevention (CDC), June 19, 2022. Available online. URL: www.cdc.gov/coronavirus/2019-ncov/vaccines/recommendations/specific-groups.html. Accessed December 19, 2022.

Chapter 31 | Effectiveness and Benefits of Getting a COVID-19 Vaccine

All currently approved or authorized COVID-19 vaccines are safe and effective and reduce your risk of severe illness. Vaccination can reduce the spread of disease, which helps protect those who get vaccinated and the people around them.

COVID-19 VACCINES PROTECT AGAINST COVID-19 INFECTIONS AND HOSPITALIZATIONS

Vaccines reduce the risk of COVID-19, including the risk of severe illness and death among people who are fully vaccinated. In addition to data from clinical trials, evidence from real-world vaccine effectiveness studies shows that COVID-19 vaccines help protect against COVID-19 infections, with or without symptoms (asymptomatic infections). Vaccine effectiveness against hospitalizations has remained relatively high over time, although it tends to be slightly lower for older adults and for people with weakened immune systems.

MOST PEOPLE NEED BOOSTER SHOTS

COVID-19 vaccines are working well to prevent severe illness, hospitalization, and death. However, public health experts see reduced protection over time against mild and moderate disease, especially among certain populations. For the best protection, everyone six months and older is recommended to stay up-to-date with their COVID-19 vaccines, which includes getting boosters if eligible.

VACCINE BREAKTHROUGH INFECTIONS

COVID-19 vaccines are effective at preventing severe disease, hospitalization, and death. However, since vaccines are not 100 percent effective at preventing infection, some people who are up-to-date with the recommended vaccines will still get COVID-19. This is called "a breakthrough infection." When people who are vaccinated develop symptoms of COVID-19, they tend to experience less severe symptoms than people who are unvaccinated.

COVID-19 VACCINES ARE EFFECTIVE AGAINST MOST VARIANTS

Viruses are constantly changing to create new types of the virus called "variants." COVID-19 vaccines used in the United States continue to protect against severe disease, hospitalization, and death from known circulating variants. They may not be as effective in preventing infection from these variants. The Centers for Disease Control and Prevention (CDC) will continue to monitor vaccine effectiveness to see what impact, if any, variants have on how well COVID-19 vaccines work in real-world conditions.[1]

VACCINE EFFECTIVENESS

Vaccine effectiveness is a measure of how well vaccination protects people against outcomes such as infection, symptomatic illness, hospitalization, and death. Vaccine effectiveness is typically measured through observational studies specifically designed to estimate individual protection from vaccination under "real-world" conditions.[2]

---

[1] "COVID-19 Vaccines Work," Centers for Disease Control and Prevention (CDC), June 28, 2022. Available online. URL: www.cdc.gov/coronavirus/2019-ncov/vaccines/effectiveness/work.html. Accessed November 29, 2022.

[2] "COVID-19 Vaccines Are Effective," Centers for Disease Control and Prevention (CDC), June 29, 2022. Available online. URL: www.cdc.gov/coronavirus/2019-ncov/vaccines/effectiveness/index.html. Accessed November 29, 2022.

Effectiveness and Benefits of Getting a COVID-19 Vaccine

MONITORING COVID-19 VACCINE EFFECTIVENESS

The CDC continuously monitors vaccine effectiveness to understand how COVID-19 vaccines protect people in real-world conditions.

The CDC monitors COVID-19 vaccine effectiveness to understand how well the vaccines:
- protect different age groups, such as children, adolescents, and adults, including adults aged 65 years and older
- protect specific groups, such as people with underlying health conditions or health-care workers
- protect against new variants
- lower the risk of infection, including infection without symptoms
- protect against milder COVID-19 illness
- prevent more serious outcomes, such as hospitalization or death
- prevent complications from COVID-19, such as post-COVID conditions and multisystem inflammatory syndrome (MIS)
- prevent spreading COVID-19 to others
- provide long- and short-term protection
- perform among people who have received one or more booster doses

ASSESSING HOW VACCINES WORK IN THE REAL WORLD HELPS YOU
- Adjust vaccine recommendations, as needed, such as booster doses.
- Guide vaccine policy and vaccine distribution.
- Inform development of vaccine technologies.[3]

---

[3] "Monitoring COVID-19 Vaccine Effectiveness," Centers for Disease Control and Prevention (CDC), June 23, 2022. Available online. URL: www.cdc.gov/coronavirus/2019-ncov/vaccines/effectiveness/how-they-work.html. Accessed November 29, 2022.

COVID-19 AFTER VACCINATION: POSSIBLE BREAKTHROUGH INFECTION

COVID-19 vaccines help protect against severe illness, hospitalization, and death. COVID-19 vaccines also help protect against infection. People who are vaccinated may still get COVID-19. When people who have been vaccinated get COVID-19, they are much less likely to experience severe symptoms than people who are unvaccinated.

When someone who is vaccinated with either a primary series or a primary series plus a booster dose gets infected with the virus that causes COVID-19, it is referred to as a "vaccine breakthrough infection."

People who get vaccine breakthrough infections can spread COVID-19 to other people. When a community reports more COVID-19 infections, that means more viruses are circulating. When more viruses are circulating, more breakthrough infections will occur even when vaccination rates are high. Even if you are vaccinated, if you live in a county with a high COVID-19 community level, you and others in your community, whether vaccinated or not, should take more steps to protect yourself and others, such as wearing a mask in indoor public places.

The CDC monitors reported vaccine breakthrough infections to better understand patterns of COVID-19 among people who are vaccinated and unvaccinated. The latest rates of COVID-19 cases and deaths by vaccination status are available on the CDC COVID Data Tracker (https://covid.cdc.gov/covid-data-tracker/#rates-by-vaccine-status).[4]

BENEFITS OF GETTING A COVID-19 VACCINE

There are many benefits of getting vaccinated against COVID-19:
- **Prevents serious illness.** COVID-19 vaccines available in the United States are safe and effective at protecting people from getting seriously ill, being hospitalized, and dying.

---

[4] "COVID-19 after Vaccination: Possible Breakthrough Infection," Centers for Disease Control and Prevention (CDC), June 23, 2022. Available online. URL: www.cdc.gov/coronavirus/2019-ncov/vaccines/effectiveness/why-measure-effectiveness/breakthrough-cases.html. Accessed November 29, 2022.

Effectiveness and Benefits of Getting a COVID-19 Vaccine

- **A safer way to build protection**. Getting a COVID-19 vaccine is a safer, more reliable way to build protection than getting sick with COVID-19.
- **Offers added protection**. COVID-19 vaccines can offer added protection to people who had COVID-19, including protection against being hospitalized for a new infection.
- **How to be best protected**. As with vaccines for other diseases, people are best protected when they stay up-to-date with the recommended number of doses, including bivalent boosters, when eligible.

COVID-19 VACCINES PROTECT YOUR HEALTH

COVID-19 vaccines are effective at protecting people from getting seriously ill, being hospitalized, and dying. Vaccination remains the safest strategy for avoiding hospitalizations, long-term health outcomes, and death.

PREVENT SEVERE ILLNESS, HOSPITALIZATION, AND DEATH

Use Vaccines.gov—to find a COVID-19 vaccine near you.
- All unvaccinated persons should start their primary series as soon as possible.
- The CDC recommends everyone stay up-to-date with COVID-19 vaccines for their age group:
  - children and teens aged six months to 17 years
  - adults aged 18 years and older

Severe Illness

Messenger ribonucleic acid (mRNA) COVID-19 vaccines are highly effective in preventing the most severe outcomes from a COVID-19 infection.

Myocarditis is a condition where the heart becomes inflamed in response to an infection or some other trigger. Myocarditis after COVID-19 vaccination is rare. This study shows that patients with COVID-19 had nearly 16 times the risk for myocarditis compared with patients who did not have COVID-19.

Hospitalization

COVID-19 vaccines can help prevent you from becoming hospitalized if you do get infected with COVID-19.

Death

COVID-19 vaccines can help prevent you from dying if you do get infected with COVID-19.[5]

---

[5] "Benefits of Getting a COVID-19 Vaccine," Centers for Disease Control and Prevention (CDC), December 22, 2022. Available online. URL: www.cdc.gov/coronavirus/2019-ncov/vaccines/vaccine-benefits.html. Accessed December 29, 2022.

Chapter 32 | Side Effects and COVID-19 Vaccine Safety

Chapter Contents
Section 32.1—Possible Side Effects after Getting a
  COVID-19 Vaccine 389
Section 32.2—COVID-19 Vaccine Safety and
  Monitoring 392
Section 32.3—Vaccine Adverse Event Reporting System 394
Section 32.4—COVID-19 Vaccine Safety in
  Specific Population 399

Section 32.1 | Possible Side Effects after Getting a COVID-19 Vaccine

COMMON SIDE EFFECTS

Side effects after a COVID-19 vaccination tend to be mild, temporary, and such as those experienced after routine vaccinations. They can vary across different age groups.

- Side effects after getting a COVID-19 vaccine can vary from person to person.
- Some people experience a little discomfort and can continue to go about their day. Others have side effects that affect their ability to do daily activities.
- Side effects generally go away in a few days.
- Even if you do not experience any side effects, your body is building protection against the virus that causes COVID-19.
- Adverse events (serious health problems) are rare but can cause long-term health problems. They usually happen within six weeks of getting a vaccine.

CHILDREN AND TEENS AGED SIX MONTHS TO 17 YEARS

The common side effects for the age group six months to three years can include the following:

- pain on the leg or arm where the shot was given
- swollen lymph nodes
- irritability or crying
- sleepiness
- loss of appetite

The side effects for the age group 4–17 years are more common after the second dose and can include the following:

- pain, swelling, and redness on the arm where the shot was given
- tiredness
- headache

- muscle or joint pain
- chills
- swollen lymph nodes

ADULTS 18 YEARS AND OLDER
The following are the side effects on the arm where you got the shot:
- pain
- redness
- swelling

The following are the side effects throughout the rest of your body:
- tiredness
- headache
- muscle pain
- chills
- fever
- nausea

After a Second Shot or Booster
Reactions reported after getting a booster shot are similar to those after the two- or single-dose primary shots. Most side effects were mild-to-moderate. The most commonly reported side effects were as follows:
- fever
- headache
- fatigue (tiredness)
- pain at the injection site

HELPFUL TIPS TO RELIEVE SIDE EFFECTS
Adults
To relieve pain or swelling on the arm where you got the shot, follow the below procedures:
- Apply a clean, cool, wet washcloth over the area.
- Use or keep moving your arm.
- Also, if possible, get some rest.

Side Effects and COVID-19 Vaccine Safety

To reduce discomfort from fever, follow the below procedures:
- Drink plenty of fluids.
- Dress in comfortable clothes.
- Talk to your doctor about taking over-the-counter (OTC) medicine, such as ibuprofen, acetaminophen, aspirin (only for people aged 18 years or older), or antihistamines.
  - It is not recommended to take these medicines before vaccination to try to prevent side effects as it is not known how OTC medicines might affect how well the vaccine works.

Children
Ask your child's health-care provider for advice on using a nonaspirin pain reliever and learn about other steps you can take at home to comfort your child after vaccination. Call a doctor or health-care provider about a side effect if the following conditions occur:
- Redness or tenderness where the shot was given gets worse after 24 hours.
- Side effects are worrying or do not seem to be going away after a few days.

ADVERSE EVENTS AFTER COVID-19 VACCINATION ARE RARE
Adverse events, including severe allergic reactions, after COVID-19 vaccination are rare but can happen. For this reason, everyone who receives a COVID-19 vaccine is monitored by their vaccination provider for at least 15 minutes.

After leaving a vaccination provider site, if you think you or your child might be having a severe allergic reaction, seek immediate medical care by calling 911.

REPORTING SIDE EFFECTS AND ADVERSE EVENTS
Use V-safe or the Vaccine Adverse Event Reporting System (VAERS) to report your side effects:
- V-safe, a smartphone-based tool, provides quick and confidential health check-ins via text messages and web

surveys. It does this, so you can quickly and easily share with the Centers for Disease Control and Prevention (CDC) how you or your child feels after getting a COVID-19 vaccine.
- The VAERS can be used by you or your health-care provider to report a side effect, adverse event, or reaction from the COVID-19 vaccine.[1]

Section 32.2 | COVID-19 Vaccine Safety and Monitoring

Vaccine safety monitoring systems are used to check for potential vaccine safety problems (sometimes called "adverse events") that may not have been seen during clinical trials. The Centers for Disease Control and Prevention (CDC) uses new and established systems to actively monitor for possible adverse events related to COVID-19 vaccination. The CDC and vaccine safety experts quickly assess unexpected adverse events to help guide U.S. vaccine recommendations.
- **Vaccine Adverse Event Reporting System (VAERS).** It is the nation's early warning system, used to monitor adverse events that happen after vaccination. Anyone can report possible health problems after vaccination to the VAERS. The CDC and U.S. Food and Drug Administration (FDA) review the reports for unusual patterns that might indicate a vaccine safety problem needing deeper investigation. The VAERS cannot determine if a vaccine causes an adverse event. The CDC might use the Clinical Immunization Safety Assessment (CISA) project or Vaccine Safety Datalink (VSD) to conduct follow-up studies.
- **V-safe.** People who receive a COVID-19 vaccine can enroll in V-safe, a new smartphone-based tool that

---

[1] "Possible Side Effects after Getting a COVID-19 Vaccine," Centers for Disease Control and Prevention (CDC), September 14, 2022. Available online. URL: www.cdc.gov/coronavirus/2019-ncov/vaccines/expect/after.html. Accessed December 14, 2022.

provides quick health check-ins. People can share if they have side effects. The CDC may call to check on people who report a health problem to get more information and submit a report to the VAERS.
- **Clinical Immunization Safety Assessment (CISA) project.** This is a collaboration between the CDC and seven medical research centers. The CISA consults with U.S. health-care providers and health departments about vaccine safety, conducts clinical research, and helps investigate safety issues. The VSD is a collaboration between the CDC and nine health-care organizations. Participating sites link patient vaccination and electronic health record (EHR) data. The CDC monitors the data for vaccine safety concerns and research opportunities.
- **VSD.** This is a collaboration between the CDC and nine health-care organizations. Participating sites link patient vaccination and EHR data. The CDC monitors the data for vaccine safety concerns and research opportunities.
- **V-safe COVID-19 Pregnancy Registry.** The CDC invites some people enrolled in V-safe who received a COVID-19 vaccine shortly before or during pregnancy to participate in the v-safe COVID-19 Pregnancy Registry. The CDC monitors information collected from participants to ensure the continued safety of COVID-19 vaccinations.[2]

VACCINE SAFETY AND MONITORING
- COVID-19 vaccines were developed using science that has been around for decades.
- COVID-19 vaccines are safe and meet the FDA's rigorous scientific standards for safety, effectiveness, and manufacturing quality.

[2] "CDC Monitors Health Reports Submitted after COVID-19 Vaccination to Ensure Continued Safety," Centers for Disease Control and Prevention (CDC), July 22, 2021. Available online. URL: www.cdc.gov/coronavirus/2019-ncov/downloads/vaccines/323652-A_COVID-19_VaccineSafety_MonitoringSystems_v9.pdf. Accessed December 14, 2022.

- COVID-19 vaccines are effective at preventing severe illness from COVID-19 and limiting the spread of the virus that causes it.
- Millions of people in the United States have received COVID-19 vaccines.
- COVID-19 vaccines are monitored by the most intense safety monitoring efforts in U.S. history.

The CDC recommends COVID-19 vaccines for everyone aged six months and older and boosters for everyone five years and older, if eligible.[3]

Section 32.3 | Vaccine Adverse Event Reporting System

The Vaccine Adverse Event Reporting System (VAERS) is the nation's early warning system that monitors the safety of vaccines after they are authorized or licensed for use by the U.S. Food and Drug Administration (FDA). The VAERS is part of the larger vaccine safety system in the United States that helps make sure vaccines are safe. The system is comanaged by the Centers for Disease Control and Prevention (CDC) and the FDA.

The VAERS accepts and analyzes reports of possible health problems—also called "adverse events"—after vaccination. As an early warning system, the VAERS cannot prove that a vaccine caused a problem. Specifically, a report to the VAERS does not mean that a vaccine caused an adverse event. But the VAERS can give the CDC and the FDA important information. If it looks as though a vaccine might be causing a problem, the FDA and the CDC will investigate further and take action if needed.

Anyone can submit a report to the VAERS—health-care professionals, vaccine manufacturers, and the general public. The VAERS

---

[3] "Ensuring COVID-19 Vaccine Safety in the U.S.," Centers for Disease Control and Prevention (CDC), December 22, 2022. Available online. URL: www.cdc.gov/coronavirus/2019-ncov/vaccines/safety.html. Accessed December 14, 2022.

welcomes all reports, regardless of seriousness and regardless of how likely the vaccine may have been to have caused the adverse event.

TOP SIX THINGS TO KNOW ABOUT THE VACCINE ADVERSE EVENT REPORTING SYSTEM

- It is a national vaccine safety surveillance program that helps detect unusual or unexpected reporting patterns of adverse events for vaccines.
- It accepts reports from anyone, including patients, family members, health-care providers, and vaccine manufacturers.
- It is not designed to determine if a vaccine caused or contributed to an adverse event. A report to the VAERS does not mean the vaccine caused the event.
- It is a passive surveillance system, meaning it relies on people sending in reports of their experiences after vaccination.
- Health-care providers and vaccine manufacturers are required by law to report certain events after vaccination.
- If the VAERS detects a pattern of adverse events following vaccination, other vaccine safety monitoring systems conduct follow-up studies.

HOW DOES THE VACCINE ADVERSE EVENT REPORTING SYSTEM WORK?

The VAERS is part of the larger postlicensure vaccine safety monitoring system in the United States. After vaccines are licensed or authorized for use by the FDA, they are continually monitored for safety by multiple, complementary systems. These systems also conduct safety studies in populations that are larger and more diverse than those typically included in vaccine clinical trials.

As a passive reporting system, the VAERS relies on individuals to send in reports of adverse health events following vaccination. From these reports, VAERS scientists can:
- assess the safety of newly licensed vaccines
- detect new, unusual, or rare adverse events that happen after vaccination

- monitor increases in known side effects, such as arm soreness where a shot was given
- identify potential patient risk factors for particular types of health problems related to vaccines
- identify and address possible reporting clusters
- recognize persistent safe-use problems and administration errors
- watch for unexpected or unusual patterns in adverse event reports
- serve as a monitoring system in public health emergencies

The information collected by the VAERS can quickly provide an early warning of a potential safety problem with a vaccine. Patterns of adverse events, or an unusually high number of adverse events reported after a particular vaccine, are called "signals." If a signal is identified through the VAERS, scientists may conduct further studies to find out if the signal represents an actual risk.

Further studies are done in safety systems such as the CDC's Vaccine Safety Datalink (VSD) or the Clinical Immunization Safety Assessment (CISA) project. These systems can better assess health risks and possible connections between adverse events and a vaccine.

INFORMATION COLLECTED FROM REPORTS

The number of VAERS reports submitted varies each year. In 2019, the VAERS received over 48,000 reports. About 85–90 percent of the reports described mild side effects such as fever, arm soreness, or mild irritability. The remaining reports are classified as serious, which means that the reported adverse event resulted in permanent disability, hospitalization, prolongation of existing hospitalization, life-threatening illness, congenital deformity/birth defect, or death. While these events can happen after vaccination, they are rarely caused by the vaccine.

Adverse event information collected by the VAERS includes the following:
- the type of vaccine received
- the date of vaccination

Side Effects and COVID-19 Vaccine Safety

- when the adverse event began
- current illnesses and medications
- medical history
- past history of adverse events following vaccination
- demographic information

In some cases, multiple reports are submitted for the same adverse event. For example, the person who experienced the adverse event and their health-care provider could submit a report for the same adverse event. VAERS scientists review the reports, identify any duplicates, and attach them to the original submission. This review process ensures the same adverse event is not counted more than once, even in cases where there are multiple reports on the same adverse event. Only the primary reports are shown in the public data system, not additional or follow-up reports for the same event.

STRENGTHS AND LIMITATIONS OF VACCINE ADVERSE EVENT REPORTING SYSTEM DATA

When evaluating VAERS data, it is important to understand the strengths and limitations.

Strengths

- The VAERS accepts reports from anyone. This also allows the VAERS to act as an early warning system to detect rare adverse events.
- It collects information about the vaccine, the person vaccinated, and the adverse event. Scientists obtain follow-up information on serious reports.
- All data (without identifying patient information) are publicly available.

Limitations

- The VAERS is a passive reporting system, meaning that reports about adverse events are not automatically

collected. Instead, someone who had or is aware of an adverse event following vaccination must file a report.
- VAERS reports are submitted by anyone and sometimes lack details or contain errors.
- VAERS data alone cannot determine if the vaccine caused the reported adverse event.
- This specific limitation has caused confusion about the publicly available data, specifically regarding the number of reported deaths. In the past, there have been instances where people misinterpreted reports of death following vaccination as death caused by the vaccines; that is a mistake.
- It accepts all reports of adverse events following vaccination without judging whether the vaccine caused the adverse health event. Some reports to the VAERS might represent true vaccine reactions, and others might be coincidental adverse health events not related to vaccination at all.
- Generally, a causal relationship cannot be established using information from VAERS reports alone.
- The number of reports submitted to the VAERS may increase in response to media attention and increased public awareness.
- It is not possible to use VAERS data to calculate how often an adverse event occurs in a population.[4]

---

[4] "Vaccine Adverse Event Reporting System (VAERS)," Centers for Disease Control and Prevention (CDC), September 8, 2022. Available online. URL: www.cdc.gov/coronavirus/2019-ncov/vaccines/safety/vaers.html. Accessed December 14, 2022.

Section 32.4 | COVID-19 Vaccine Safety in Specific Population

MONITORING COVID-19 VACCINE SAFETY DURING PREGNANCY

The Centers for Disease Control and Prevention (CDC) and the U.S. Food and Drug Administration (FDA) currently have five safety monitoring systems in place to capture information about vaccination during pregnancy and closely monitor that information reported to each system.

- **CDC and FDA**. The Vaccine Adverse Event Reporting System (VAERS) is a national system to which health-care professionals, vaccine manufacturers, and the public can report possible side effects or health problems that happen after vaccination. Scientists investigate reports of events that are unexpected, appear to happen more often than expected, or have unusual patterns. The VAERS reporting (https://vaers.hhs.gov/reportevent.html) form has a question to identify pregnant people. CDC clinicians review all pregnancy reports related to COVID-19 vaccinations.
- **CDC**. V-safe COVID-19 Vaccine Pregnancy Registry—V-safe is a smartphone-based, after-vaccination health checker for people who receive COVID-19 vaccines. The V-safe COVID-19 Vaccine Pregnancy Registry is a registry to collect additional health information from V-safe participants who report being pregnant at the time of vaccination or a positive pregnancy test after vaccination. This information helps the CDC monitor the safety of COVID-19 vaccines in people who are pregnant.
- **CDC**. Vaccine Safety Datalink (VSD)—It is a network of nine integrated health-care organizations across the United States that monitor and evaluate the safety of vaccines. The system is also used to help determine whether possible side effects identified using the

VAERS are actually related to vaccination. Through the VSD, the CDC will study the following:
- weekly counts and rates of COVID-19 vaccination in pregnant people
- miscarriage and stillbirth that occur among people who received the COVID-19 vaccine during pregnancy
- adverse outcomes in pregnancy following COVID-19 vaccination, including the following:
  - pregnancy complications
  - birth outcomes
  - infant outcomes for the first year of life (includes infant death, birth defects, and developmental disorders)
- **CDC**. Clinical Immunization Safety Assessment (CISA) Project—This project is a collaboration between the CDC and seven medical research centers to provide expert consultation on individual cases of adverse events after vaccination and conduct clinical research studies about vaccine safety. It will implement a clinical research study on COVID-19 vaccine safety among pregnant people at three sites. The study will carry out the following:
  - Enroll pregnant people who plan to receive COVID-19 vaccination; COVID-19 vaccines will be given as part of the study.
  - Collect baseline maternal health information, including if they previously had COVID-19.
  - Follow people during pregnancy and for three months after delivery.
    - Follow babies through their first three months of life.
- **CDC**. Birth Defects Study to Evaluate Pregnancy Exposures (BD-STEPS)—This is an ongoing study that collects information, including COVID-19 vaccination information, from people who have recently been

pregnant to understand the potential causes of birth defects and how to prevent them.[5]

COVID-19 VACCINE SAFETY IN CHILDREN AND TEENS

- The CDC recommends COVID-19 vaccines for everyone aged six months and older and COVID-19 boosters for everyone aged five years and older, if eligible.
- Through continued safety monitoring, COVID-19 vaccination has been found to be safe for children and teens.
- Millions of children and teens aged 5–17 years have already received at least one dose of a COVID-19 vaccine.
- The known risks and possible severe complications of COVID-19 outweigh the potential risks of having a rare, adverse reaction to vaccination.
- Use the CDC's COVID-19 booster tool to learn if and when your child or teen can get boosters to stay up-to-date with their COVID-19 vaccines.

CLINICAL TRIALS AND ONGOING SAFETY MONITORING SHOW THAT COVID-19 VACCINATION IS SAFE FOR CHILDREN AND TEENS

Before authorizing or approving COVID-19 vaccines, scientists conducted clinical trials with thousands of children and teens to establish their safety and effectiveness.

COVID-19 vaccines are being monitored under the most comprehensive and intense vaccine safety monitoring program in U.S. history. The CDC monitors all COVID-19 vaccines after they are authorized or approved for use. The CDC and the FDA continue to monitor vaccines, keep people informed of findings, and use data to make COVID-19 vaccination recommendations.

---

[5] "COVID-19 Vaccine Monitoring Systems for Pregnant People," Centers for Disease Control and Prevention (CDC), August 25, 2021. Available online. URL: www.cdc.gov/widgets/micrositeCollectionViewerMed/index.html. Accessed December 14, 2022.

SERIOUS HEALTH EVENTS AFTER COVID-19 VACCINATION ARE RARE

Serious reactions after COVID-19 vaccination in children and teens are rare. When they are reported, serious reactions most frequently occur within a few days after vaccination.

Rare cases of myocarditis (inflammation of the heart muscle) and pericarditis (inflammation of the outer lining of the heart) have been reported after children and teens aged five years and older got the Pfizer-BioNTech COVID-19 vaccine. New studies have shown the rare risk of myocarditis and pericarditis associated with mRNA COVID-19 vaccination (Pfizer-BioNTech and Moderna)—mostly among males between the ages of 12 and 39 years—may be further reduced with a longer time between the first and second dose.

- In children aged 5–11 years, there were 20 confirmed reports of myocarditis out of approximately 18.1 million doses given of the Pfizer-BioNTech COVID-19 vaccine between November 2021 and April 2022.
- In reports of myocarditis following mRNA-based COVID-19 vaccination from December 2020 to August 2021, the risk of myocarditis was the highest following the second dose of the Pfizer-BioNTech vaccine in adolescent and young adult males.
- Reporting rates were around 70 cases per million doses in males aged 12–15 years and 105 cases per million doses in males aged 16–17 years.

Febrile seizures were rare in COVID-19 vaccine clinical trials for young children and occurred at similar rates for both Pfizer and Moderna COVID-19 vaccines.

A severe allergic reaction, such as anaphylaxis, may happen after any vaccination, including COVID-19 vaccination, but this is rare. If your child experiences a severe allergic reaction after getting a COVID-19 vaccine, vaccine providers can rapidly provide care and call for emergency medical services, if needed.[6]

---

[6] "COVID-19 Vaccine Safety in Children and Teens," Centers for Disease Control and Prevention (CDC), July 20, 2022. Available online. URL: www.cdc.gov/coronavirus/2019-ncov/vaccines/vaccine-safety-children-teens.html. Accessed December 14, 2022.

Chapter 33 | Myths and Facts about the COVID-19 Vaccines

Accurate vaccine information is critical and can help stop common myths and rumors. It can be difficult to know which sources of information you can trust.

BUST COMMON MYTHS AND LEARN THE FACTS

Myth. The ingredients in COVID-19 vaccines are dangerous.

Fact. Nearly all the ingredients in COVID-19 vaccines are also ingredients in many foods—fats, sugars, and salts.

Exact vaccine ingredients vary by manufacturer. Pfizer-BioNTech and Moderna COVID-19 vaccines also contain messenger ribonucleic acid (mRNA), and the Johnson & Johnson/Janssen COVID-19 vaccine contains a harmless version of a virus unrelated to the virus that causes COVID-19. The Novavax COVID-19 vaccine includes harmless pieces (proteins) of the virus that causes COVID-19; they are pieces of what is often called the "spike protein." These give instructions to cells in your body to create an immune response. This response helps protect you from getting sick with COVID-19 in the future. After the body produces an immune response, it discards all the vaccine ingredients just as it would discard any information that cells no longer need. This process is a part of normal body functioning.

COVID-19 vaccines do not contain ingredients such as preservatives, tissues (such as aborted fetal cells), antibiotics, food proteins, medicines, latex, or metals.

Myth. The natural immunity you get from being sick with COVID-19 is better than the immunity you get from COVID-19 vaccination.

Fact. Getting a COVID-19 vaccination is a safer and more dependable way to build immunity to COVID-19 than getting sick with COVID-19.

COVID-19 vaccination causes a more predictable immune response than infection with the virus that causes COVID-19. Getting a COVID-19 vaccine gives most people a high level of protection against COVID-19 and can provide added protection for people who already had COVID-19. One study showed that, for people who already had COVID-19, those who do not get vaccinated after their recovery are more than two times as likely to get COVID-19 again than those who get fully vaccinated after their recovery.

All COVID-19 vaccines currently available in the United States are effective at preventing COVID-19. Getting sick with COVID-19 can offer some protection from future illness, sometimes called "natural immunity," but the level of protection people get from having COVID-19 may vary depending on how mild or severe their illness was, the time since their infection, and their age. Getting a COVID-19 vaccination is also a safer way to build protection than getting sick with COVID-19. COVID-19 vaccination helps protect you by creating an antibody response without you having to experience sickness.

Getting vaccinated yourself may also protect people around you, particularly people at an increased risk for severe illness from COVID-19. Getting sick with COVID-19 can cause severe illness or death, and you cannot reliably predict who will have mild or severe illness. If you get sick, you can spread COVID-19 to others. You can also continue to have long-term health issues after COVID-19 infection.

Myth. COVID-19 vaccines cause variants.

Fact. COVID-19 vaccines do not create or cause variants of the virus that causes COVID-19. Instead, COVID-19 vaccines can help prevent new variants from emerging.

Myths and Facts about the COVID-19 Vaccines

New variants of a virus happen because the virus that causes COVID-19 constantly changes through a natural ongoing process of mutation (change). As the virus spreads, it has more opportunities to change. High vaccination coverage in a population reduces the spread of the virus and helps prevent new variants from emerging. The Centers for Disease Control and Prevention (CDC) recommends COVID-19 vaccines for everyone aged six months and older and boosters for everyone five years and older, if eligible.

Myth. All events reported to the Vaccine Adverse Event Reporting System (VAERS) are caused by vaccination.

Fact. Anyone can report events to the VAERS, even if it is not clear whether a vaccine caused the problem. Because of this, VAERS data alone cannot determine if the reported adverse event was caused by a COVID-19 vaccination.

Some VAERS reports may contain information that is incomplete, inaccurate, coincidental, or unverifiable. Vaccine safety experts study these adverse events and look for unusually high numbers of health problems or a pattern of problems after people receive a particular vaccine.

Recently, the number of deaths reported to the VAERS following COVID-19 vaccination has been misinterpreted and misreported as if this number means deaths that were proven to be caused by vaccination. Reports of adverse events to the VAERS following vaccination, including deaths, do not necessarily mean that a vaccine caused a health problem.

Myth. The mRNA vaccine is not considered a vaccine.

Fact. mRNA vaccines, such as Pfizer-BioNTech and Moderna, work differently than other types of vaccines, but they still trigger an immune response inside your body.

This type of vaccine is new, but research and development on it has been underway for decades.

The mRNA vaccines do not contain any live virus. Instead, they work by teaching your cells to make a harmless piece of a "spike protein," which is found on the surface of the virus that causes COVID-19. After making the protein piece, cells display it on their surface. Your immune system then recognizes that it does not belong there and responds to get rid of it. When an immune response begins, antibodies are produced, creating the same response that happens in a natural infection.

In contrast to mRNA vaccines, many other vaccines use a piece of, or a weakened version of, the germ that the vaccine protects against. This is how the measles and flu vaccines work. When a weakened or small part of the virus is introduced to your body, you make antibodies to help protect against future infection.

Myth. COVID-19 vaccines contain microchips.

Fact. COVID-19 vaccines do not contain microchips. Vaccines are developed to fight against disease and are not administered to track your movement.

Vaccines work by stimulating your immune system to produce antibodies, exactly like it would if you were exposed to the disease. After getting vaccinated, you develop immunity to that disease, without having to get the disease first.

Myth. Receiving a COVID-19 vaccine can make you magnetic.

Fact. Receiving a COVID-19 vaccine will not make you magnetic, including at the site of vaccination which is usually your arm.

COVID-19 vaccines do not contain ingredients that can produce an electromagnetic field at the site of your injection. All COVID-19 vaccines are free from metals.

Myth. COVID-19 vaccines authorized for use in the United States shed or release their components.

Fact. Vaccine shedding is the release or discharge of any of the vaccine components in or outside of the body and can only occur when a vaccine contains a live weakened version of the virus.

None of the vaccines authorized for use in the United States contain a live virus. mRNA and viral vector vaccines are the two types of currently authorized COVID-19 vaccines available.

Myth. COVID-19 vaccines can alter your deoxyribonucleic acid (DNA).

Fact. COVID-19 vaccines do not change or interact with your DNA in any way.

Both mRNA and viral vector COVID-19 vaccines work by delivering instructions (genetic material) to your cells to start building protection against the virus that causes COVID-19.

Myths and Facts about the COVID-19 Vaccines

After the body produces an immune response, it discards all the vaccine ingredients just as it would discard any information that cells no longer need. This process is a part of normal body functioning. The genetic material delivered by mRNA vaccines never enters the nucleus of your cells, which is where your DNA is kept. Viral vector COVID-19 vaccines deliver genetic material to the cell nucleus to allow your cells to build protection against COVID-19. However, the vector virus does not have the machinery needed to integrate its genetic material into your DNA, so it cannot alter your DNA.

Myth. A COVID-19 vaccine can make you sick with COVID-19.

Fact. Because none of the authorized COVID-19 vaccines in the United States contain the live virus that causes COVID-19, the vaccine cannot make you sick with COVID-19.

COVID-19 vaccines teach your immune systems how to recognize and fight the virus that causes COVID-19. Sometimes, this process can cause symptoms, such as fever. These symptoms are normal and are signs that the body is building protection against the virus that causes COVID-19.

OTHER MYTHS AND FACTS

Myth. COVID-19 vaccines will affect your fertility.

Fact. Currently, no evidence shows that any vaccines, including COVID-19 vaccines, cause fertility problems (problems trying to get pregnant) in women or men.

COVID-19 vaccination is recommended for people who are pregnant, trying to get pregnant now, or might become pregnant in the future, as well as their partners.

Myth. Being near someone who received a COVID-19 vaccine will affect your menstrual cycle.

Fact. Your menstrual cycle cannot be affected by being near someone who received a COVID-19 vaccine.

Many things can affect menstrual cycles, including stress, changes in your schedule, problems with sleep, and changes in diet or exercise. Infections may also affect menstrual cycles.

Myth. Getting a COVID-19 vaccine will cause you to test positive on a viral test.

Fact. None of the authorized and recommended COVID-19 vaccines can cause you to test positive on viral tests, which are used to see if you have a current infection.

If your body develops an immune response to vaccination, which is the goal, you may test positive on some antibody tests. Antibody tests indicate you had a previous infection and that you may have some level of protection against the virus.[1]

---

[1] "Myths and Facts about COVID-19 Vaccines," Centers for Disease Control and Prevention (CDC), July 20, 2022. Available online. URL: www.cdc.gov/coronavirus/2019-ncov/vaccines/facts.html. Accessed December 14, 2022.

Chapter 34 | Herd Immunity against COVID-19

"Herd immunity" can happen once a large part of a population—say 70–90 percent—develops immunity to a disease. This generally happens by infection (conferring natural immunity) or vaccination. Herd immunity can help slow or stop a disease's spread, but many people may die before it happens.

It is currently unclear how herd immunity could happen for COVID-19. For example, the data are insufficient to show how much immunity infection confers or whether it is enough to prevent reinfection. How long any immunity will last is also unknown. Related viruses confer some immunity after infection, but that immunity does not seem to last longer than a year.

WHY THIS MATTERS

Increasing the immunity of a population to an infectious disease such as COVID-19 can slow the spread of infection and protect those most vulnerable. However, with limited information about important aspects of COVID-19, there are challenges to understanding the implications of herd immunity in the current pandemic.

THE SCIENCE

- What is it? A population can establish herd immunity to an infectious disease once a large enough portion of the population—typically 70–90 percent—develops immunity. Reaching this "herd immunity threshold" limits the likelihood that a nonimmune person will be infected. In general, immunity develops through either infection (resulting in natural immunity) or vaccination (resulting in vaccine-induced immunity). Herd immunity helps protect people not immune to a disease by reducing their chances of interacting with an infected individual. This process slows or stops the spread of the disease.

- How does it work? Once a community has established herd immunity, someone without immunity is less likely to be exposed to an infectious individual during an outbreak. For example, because there are more people with immunity in the population, there are fewer people susceptible to infection, and thus, the number of potential transmissions is limited. Similarly, those who are immune will not be infected and thus will not transmit the disease to others. Both of these situations help limit the size of the outbreak.

If an effective vaccine is available for a virus, achieving herd immunity can require a high rate of vaccination in the community. For diseases that spread more easily, more people must have vaccine-induced immunity or natural immunity to achieve herd immunity. However, if a virus mutates quickly, the community's herd immunity may be relatively short-lived because the immunity from prior infection or vaccination may no longer be effective. Also, the disease can still circulate in segments of the population that are not immune, such as those with weakened immune systems who cannot effectively form immunity.

For diseases where no vaccination is available, it is possible to develop herd immunity through exposure to, and recovery from, the disease. However, if COVID-19 runs its natural course, this approach would entail the risk of severe disease or death. Given the risk associated with COVID-19 infections, achieving herd immunity without a vaccine could result in significant morbidity and mortality rates.

Herd Immunity against COVID-19

- How mature is it? Knowledge of previous infectious disease outbreaks where a vaccine was available has allowed researchers to identify how herd immunity was achieved for those diseases. However, researchers currently have insufficient data on the factors that could contribute to herd immunity for the COVID-19 pandemic. These factors include the herd immunity threshold, the number of secondary cases typically generated by an infected individual, the viral mutation rate, and the length of time immunity lasts.

At this stage in the COVID-19 pandemic, researchers have insufficient data to draw definitive conclusions about the level of immunity conferred by an infection or how long immunity to the disease might last. For example, in order to determine the herd immunity threshold, it is important to know how contagious the disease is—which is affected by factors such as how many susceptible people an infected person can infect. While researchers have developed estimates for how contagious COVID-19 is, uncertainties about case reporting and testing—such as uncertainty in the accuracy of some tests—make this calculation difficult. Some peer-reviewed research on COVID-19 suggests the average number of people infected by a contagious person ranges from about one to seven (refer to Figure 34.1).

While analyses of viruses related to the novel coronavirus have shown that infection can provide some level of immunity, such immunity did not appear to last longer than a year. Studies of other infectious diseases, such as polio, exhibit a range in the threshold for herd immunity, the average number of people infected by an infected person, and how long people remained immune, among other factors.

OPPORTUNITIES

- **Halt disease spread**. Achieving herd immunity will slow or stop the spread of a disease within a population and limit the size of outbreaks.

Disease	Percentage of the population who must be immune to reach herd immunity	The average number of people infected by a contagious person	Estimated duration of immunity
Polio	80-86%	5-7	~18 years
Smallpox	80-85%	5-7	~3-5 years
Measles	91-94%	11-18	Lifelong
Rubella	83-94%	6-14	~15-20 years
COVID-19	Unknown	~1-7	Unknown

Figure 34.1. Immunity Data of Previous Outbreaks and COVID-19

Source: GAO adaptation of Johns Hopkins University School of Hygiene and Public Health, Health Department Catalonia (column 1), Johns Hopkins University School of Hygiene and Public Health, Health Department Catalonia, Umea University (column 2), and University of Auckland, and the Centers for Disease Control and Prevention, (column 3).
Note: *While data on previous disease outbreaks are available, for COVID-19, we do not yet have all of the necessary data for many of the relevant factors.*

- **Support economic recovery**. Established herd immunity could help bolster the economy by allowing people to safely return to work and conduct other activities.
- **Restore medical capacity**. Established herd immunity could help ease the burden on the medical system as fewer patients seek treatment.

CHALLENGES

- **Limited data on immunity**. Currently, there are a number of unknown factors, such as whether a COVID-19 infection leads to immunity and how long immunity might last. It may be necessary for more time to pass to monitor individuals who have been infected and recovered and thus determine how long they show disease immunity. This information is needed to determine the herd immunity threshold.

Herd Immunity against COVID-19

- **Implications of natural herd immunity.** Relying on natural immunity from the disease progression of COVID-19 could allow a population to establish herd immunity. However, such an approach risks exposing people to a debilitating and potentially fatal disease.
- **Testing limitations.** If infection confers immunity, researchers need accurate data on the number of recovered individuals and other disease transmission parameters to determine if or when herd immunity is achieved. Accurate testing data are critical to understanding these parameters. However, there are still challenges associated with the use and availability of antibody tests, as well as with determining their accuracy.
- **Lack of the vaccine.** A vaccine could help a population safely achieve herd immunity. However, developing a vaccine is a complicated process that is costly, typically requiring 10–15 years or more, and many candidates fail during the development process. Efforts are underway, however, to accelerate the process for COVID-19.
- **Inconsistent immunity.** Even if herd immunity is eventually achieved, outbreaks may still occur because immunity may not be uniform across the general population.[1]

---

[1] "Science & Tech Spotlight: Herd Immunity for COVID-19," U.S. Government Accountability Office (GAO), July 7, 2020. Available online. URL: www.gao.gov/products/gao-20-646sp. Accessed December 15, 2022.

Part 5 | Long-Term Effects of COVID-19 Infection

Chapter 35 | Post-COVID Health Conditions

Some people who have been infected with the virus that causes COVID-19 can experience long-term effects from their infection, known as "post-COVID conditions" or "long COVID." People call post-COVID conditions by many names, including post-acute COVID-19, post-acute sequelae of severe acute respiratory syndrome coronavirus 2 (SARS-COV-2) infection (PASC), and chronic COVID.[1]

Post-COVID conditions are associated with a spectrum of physical, social, and psychological consequences, as well as functional limitations that can present substantial challenges to patient wellness and quality of life. Post-COVID conditions are referred to by a wide range of names, including the following:
- long COVID
- post-acute COVID-19
- long-term effects of COVID
- post-acute COVID syndrome
- chronic COVID
- long-haul COVID
- late sequelae
- PASC

Although standardized case definitions are still being developed, in the broadest sense, post-COVID conditions can be considered a

---

[1] "Long COVID or Post-COVID Conditions," Centers for Disease Control and Prevention (CDC), September 1, 2022. Available online. URL: www.cdc.gov/coronavirus/2019-ncov/long-term-effects/index.html. Accessed December 15, 2022.

lack of return to a usual state of health following acute COVID-19 illness. Post-COVID conditions might also include the development of new or recurrent symptoms or the unmasking of a preexisting condition that occurs after the symptoms of acute COVID-19 illness have resolved.

TIME FRAME
The Centers for Disease Control and Prevention (CDC) considers post-COVID conditions to be present if recovery does not occur after the four-week acute phase even though many patients continue to recover between four and 12 weeks.
- While patients may still recover after 12 weeks, persistent illness becomes likely.
- The CDC uses the four-week time frame in describing post-COVID conditions to emphasize the importance of initial clinical evaluation and supportive care during the initial 4–12 weeks after acute COVID-19.

PRESENTATION
Different onset patterns for post-COVID conditions have been identified that further exemplify their heterogeneity, including the following:
- persistent symptoms and conditions that begin at the time of acute COVID-19 illness
- new-onset signs, symptoms, or conditions following asymptomatic disease or a period of acute symptom relief or remission
- an evolution of symptoms and conditions that include some persistent symptoms (e.g., shortness of breath) with the addition of new symptoms or conditions over time (e.g., cognitive difficulties)
- worsening of preexisting symptoms or conditions

Factors that may further complicate the presentation of post-COVID conditions include the following:
- pre-COVID comorbidities (underlying medical conditions)

Post-COVID Health Conditions

- physical deconditioning at baseline or after a prolonged acute disease course that can be nonspecific to COVID-19
- physical and mental health consequences of illness with a long or complicated disease course, including depression and anxiety
- social, environmental, and economic stressors caused by the COVID-19 pandemic

Some presentations may share similarities with other postinfectious syndromes, such as myalgic encephalomyelitis/chronic fatigue syndrome (ME/CFS), postural orthostatic tachycardia syndrome (POTS) and other forms of dysautonomia, or mast cell activation syndrome (MCAS). Some of these types of conditions were also reported in patients following severe acute respiratory syndrome (SARS) and Middle East respiratory syndrome (MERS), two other life-threatening illnesses resulting from coronavirus infections.

NEW OR ONGOING SYMPTOMS

A wide range of other new or ongoing symptoms and clinical findings can occur in people with varying degrees of illness from acute SARS-CoV-2 infection, including patients who have had mild or asymptomatic SARS-CoV-2 infection. These effects can overlap with multiorgan complications or with the effects of treatment or hospitalization. This category is heterogeneous, as it can include patients who have clinically important but poorly understood symptoms (e.g., difficulty thinking or concentrating, postexertional malaise (PEM)) that can be persistent or intermittent after initial acute infection with SARS-CoV-2. Commonly reported symptoms include the following:
- dyspnea or increased respiratory effort
- fatigue
- PEM* and/or poor endurance
- cognitive impairment or "brain fog"
- cough
- chest pain
- headache

- palpitations and tachycardia
- arthralgia
- myalgia
- paresthesia
- abdominal pain
- diarrhea
- insomnia and other sleep difficulties
- fever
- light-headedness
- impaired daily function and mobility
- pain
- rash (e.g., urticaria)
- mood changes
- anosmia or dysgeusia
- menstrual cycle irregularities
- erectile dysfunction

*PEM is the worsening of symptoms following even minor physical or mental exertion, with symptoms typically worsening 12–48 hours after activity and lasting for days or even weeks.

PREVALENCE

The prevalence of post-COVID conditions has been challenging to estimate, with estimates ranging widely (5–30%). Reasons for these wide-ranging estimates include the following:
- differing symptoms or conditions investigated
- the temporal criteria used (three weeks up to many months following SARS-CoV-2 infection)
- the study settings included (outpatient versus inpatient)
- how symptoms and conditions are assessed (e.g., self-report versus electronic health record database)

The CDC posts data on post-COVID conditions and provides analyses, the most recent of which can be found on the U.S. Census Bureau's Household Pulse Survey (www.cdc.gov/nchs/covid19/pulse/long-covid.htm).

POSSIBLE CAUSES

It can be difficult to distinguish symptoms caused by post-COVID conditions from symptoms that occur for other reasons. Alternative reasons for health problems need to be considered, such as other diagnoses, unmasking of preexisting health conditions, or even SARS-CoV-2 reinfection.

It is also possible that some patients with post-COVID conditions will not have had positive test results for SARS-CoV-2 because of a lack of testing or inaccurate testing during the acute period or because of waning antibody levels or false-negative antibody testing during follow-up.

Post-COVID conditions are heterogeneous and may be attributable to different underlying pathophysiologic processes. Researchers are working to characterize and differentiate the multiple possible etiologies, such as the following:

- organ damage resulting from acute phase infection
- complications from a dysregulated inflammatory state
- ongoing viral activity associated with an intrahost viral reservoir
- autoimmunity
- inadequate antibody response
- other potential causes

MULTIORGAN SYSTEM EFFECTS OF COVID-19

Autoimmune conditions can also occur after COVID-19. A wide variety of health effects can persist after the acute COVID-19 illness has resolved (e.g., pulmonary fibrosis, myocarditis). Patients who experienced multisystem inflammatory syndrome (MIS) during or after COVID-19 illness may be at a higher risk for ongoing multiorgan system effects and post-COVID conditions. It is unknown how long multiorgan system effects might last and whether the effects could lead to chronic health conditions.

EFFECTS OF COVID-19 ILLNESS OR HOSPITALIZATION

Some of these effects are similar to those from hospitalization for other respiratory infections or other conditions.

- This category can also encompass post-intensive care syndrome (PICS), which includes a range of health effects that remain after a critical illness.
- These effects can include severe weakness and post-traumatic stress disorder (PTSD).

Though the effects of hospitalization may not be unique to COVID-19 illness, they are considered post-COVID conditions if they occur after a SARS-CoV-2 infection and persist for four or more weeks.[2]

---

[2] "Post-COVID Conditions: Information for Healthcare Providers," Centers for Disease Control and Prevention (CDC), December 16, 2022. Available online. URL: www.cdc.gov/coronavirus/2019-ncov/hcp/clinical-care/post-covid-conditions.html#assessment-and-testing. Accessed December 21, 2022.

Chapter 36 | Assessment and Testing for Post-COVID Conditions

For most patients with possible post-COVID conditions, healthcare professionals should choose a conservative diagnostic approach in the first 4–12 weeks following SARS-CoV-2 infection. Laboratory and imaging studies can often be normal or nondiagnostic in patients experiencing post-COVID conditions, and symptoms may improve or resolve during the first few months after acute infection in some patients, further supporting an initial conservative approach to diagnostic testing. However, workup and testing should not be delayed when there are signs and symptoms of urgent and potentially life-threatening clinical conditions (e.g., pulmonary embolism, myocardial infarction, pericarditis with effusion, stroke, and renal failure). Symptoms that persist beyond three months should prompt further evaluation.

PHYSICAL EXAMINATION AND VITAL SIGNS

For patients who report a previous infection with SARS-CoV-2, in addition to standard vital signs (i.e., blood pressure, heart rate, respiratory rate, pulse oximetry and body temperature) and the body mass index, health-care professionals should evaluate ambulatory pulse oximetry for individuals presenting with respiratory symptoms, fatigue, or malaise. Orthostatic vital signs should be evaluated for individuals reporting postural symptoms, dizziness, fatigue, cognitive impairment, or malaise.

LABORATORY TESTING

A positive SARS-CoV-2 viral test (i.e., nucleic acid amplification test (NAAT) or antigen test) or serologic (antibody) test can help assess for current or previous infection; however, these laboratory tests are not required to establish a diagnosis of post-COVID conditions. SARS-CoV-2 real-time reverse transcription–polymerase chain reaction (RT-PCR) and antigen testing are not 100 percent sensitive. Furthermore, testing capacity was limited early in the pandemic, so some infected and recovered persons had no opportunity to obtain laboratory confirmation of SARS-CoV-2 infection. Finally, some patients who develop post-COVID conditions were asymptomatic with their acute infection and would not have had a reason to be tested.

Before ordering laboratory testing for post-COVID conditions, the goals of testing should be clear to the health-care professional and to the patient. Laboratory testing should be guided by the patient history, physical examination, and clinical findings.

- A basic panel of laboratory tests might be considered for patients with ongoing symptoms (including testing for non-COVID-19-related conditions that may be contributing to illness) to assess for conditions that may respond to treatment (refer to Table 36.1).
- More specialized testing may not be needed in patients who are being initially evaluated for post-COVID conditions; however, expanded testing should be considered if symptoms persist for 12 weeks or longer (refer to Table 36.2).

The absence of laboratory-confirmed abnormalities or the decision to forgo extensive laboratory testing should not lead to dismissing the possible impact of a patient's symptoms on their daily function. Where clinically indicated, symptom management and a comprehensive rehabilitation plan can be initiated simultaneously with laboratory testing for most patients.

Assessment and Testing for Post-COVID Conditions

Table 36.1. Basic Diagnostic Laboratory Testing for Patients with Post-COVID Conditions

Category	Laboratory Tests
Blood count, electrolytes, and renal function	Complete blood count with possible iron studies to follow, basic metabolic panel, urinalysis
Liver function	Liver function tests or complete metabolic panel
Inflammatory markers	C-reactive protein, erythrocyte sedimentation rate, ferritin
Thyroid function	TSH and free T4
Vitamin deficiencies	Vitamin D, vitamin B12

Table 36.2. Specialized Diagnostic Laboratory Testing for Patients with Post-COVID Conditions

Category	Laboratory Tests
Rheumatological conditions	Antinuclear antibody, rheumatoid factor, anticyclic citrullinated peptide, anticardiolipin, and creatine phosphokinase
Coagulation disorders	D-dimer, fibrinogen
Myocardial injury	Troponin
Differentiate symptoms of cardiac versus pulmonary origin	B-type natriuretic peptide

OTHER ASSESSMENT AND TESTING TOOLS

Symptom inventories and assessment tools, such as those embedded within electronic health records (EHRs) at many healthcare organizations, can help evaluate and monitor the status of post-COVID conditions. Functional testing can also be helpful to quantitatively document clinical status over time.

A selection of some available assessment tools is shown in Tables 36.3 and 36.4. These and other measures can also be found in the health measures toolbox (www.healthmeasures.net/index.php) and the American Academy of Physical Medicine & Rehabilitation's functional assessments (www.now.aapmr.org/functional-assessment/), along with assessment tools for other rehabilitation needs (e.g., bowel and bladder function, pain, activities of daily living, cognition, mobility, sleep).

Testing should be tailored to the patient's symptoms and presentation.

Health-care professionals should use caution when conducting exercise capacity testing with some patients, especially those with postexertional malaise (PEM; i.e., the worsening of symptoms following even minor physical or mental exertion, with symptoms

Table 36.3. Selected Assessment Tools for Evaluating People with Post-COVID Conditions

Category	Tools
Functional status or quality of life (QoL)	• Patient-Reported Outcomes Measurement Information System (PROMIS; e.g., Cognitive Function 4a) • Post-Covid-19 Functional Status Scale (PCFS) • EuroQol-5D (EQ-5D)
Respiratory conditions	• Modified Medical Research Council (mMRC) Dyspnea Scale
Neurologic conditions	• Montreal Cognitive Assessment (MoCA) • Mini Mental Status Examination (MMSE) • Compass 31 (for dysautonomia) • Neurobehavioral Symptom Inventory
Psychiatric conditions	• Generalized Anxiety Disorder-7 (GAD-7) • Patient Health Questionnaire-9 (PHQ-9) • PTSD Symptom Scale (PSS) • Screen for Posttraumatic Stress Symptoms (SPTSS) • PTSD Checklist for DSM-5 (PCL-5) • Impact of Event Scale-Revised (IESR) • Hospital Anxiety and Depression Scale (HADS)
Other conditions	• Wood Mental Fatigue Inventory (WMFI) • Fatigue Severity Scale • Insomnia Severity Index (ISI) • Connective Tissue Disease Screening Questionnaire

Assessment and Testing for Post-COVID Conditions

Table 36.4. Selected Functional and Other Testing Tools for Evaluating People with Post-COVID Conditions

Category	Tools
Exercise capacity	• 1-minute sit-to-stand test • 2-minute step test • 10-meter walk test (10MWT) • 6-minute walk test
Balance and fall risk	• BERG Balance Scale • Tinetti Gait and Balance Assessment Tool
Other	• Tilt-table testing (e.g., for POTS) • Orthostatic HR assessment

typically worsening 12–48 hours after activity and lasting for days or even weeks).
- For these patients, and others who may not have the stamina for extended or lengthy assessments, modifications in the testing plan may also be needed.
- Exercise capacity tests should be scheduled for a dedicated follow-up appointment so that patients can prepare additional home supports.
- Ensuring that the testing circumstances best support the patient to perform maximally and then documenting this performance can create an objective reliable record of functional status that may be needed for assessment for other services or disabilities.

Additional diagnostic testing should be guided by findings from the patient history and physical examination and results of previous diagnostic testing and may include a chest x-ray, pulmonary function tests (PFTs), electrocardiogram (ECG), or echocardiogram (Echo) for persistent or new respiratory or cardiac concerns although additional studies and more clinical evidence are needed to support the utility of specific imaging tests for evaluation of post-COVID conditions.

For patients who may require imaging based on clinical findings, symptom management and a rehabilitation plan can often be initiated simultaneously with the imaging workup. In patients with normal chest x-rays and normal oxygen saturation, computed tomography (CT) imaging of the chest might have a lower yield for assessing pulmonary disease. In patients without an elevated D-dimer and compatible symptoms, CT pulmonary angiogram may be a lower yield in the context of a pulmonary embolism workup. In patients with brain fog symptoms, magnetic resonance imaging (MRI) of the brain might not be revealing for pathologic findings in the absence of focal neurological deficits. Further caution may be exercised in ordering imaging in children without a high index of suspicion of pathology. More specialized (e.g., cardiac MRI) imaging studies might merit consultation with specialists.[1]

---

[1] "Post-COVID Conditions: Information for Health-Care Providers," Centers for Disease Control and Prevention (CDC), December 16, 2022. Available online. URL: www.cdc.gov/coronavirus/2019-ncov/hcp/clinical-care/post-covid-conditions.html#assessment-and-testing. Accessed December 21, 2022.

Chapter 37 | Patient Tips: Health-Care Provider Appointments for Post-COVID Conditions

BEFORE YOUR APPOINTMENT
If you think you or a loved one may have a post-COVID condition (new or persistent conditions occurring four or more weeks after initial infection with severe acute respiratory syndrome coronavirus 2 (SARS-CoV-2), the virus that causes COVID-19), taking a few steps to prepare for your meeting with a health-care provider can make all the difference in getting the proper medical evaluation, diagnosis, and treatment. You play a vital role in helping health-care providers understand your or your family member's symptoms and how they affect your daily life.

- Preparing for an appointment can make all the difference in getting the proper evaluation, diagnosis, and treatment.
- To help get the most out of appointments for post-COVID conditions, download the Healthcare Appointment Checklist (www.cdc.gov/coronavirus/2019-ncov/downloads/long-term-effects/Lista_de_verificacion_para_las_citas_de_atencion_medica-ES-508.PDF).

- Try to arrive early or log on a few minutes ahead of the appointment and ensure the paperwork is completed on your appointment day.
- After visiting your health-care provider, review your notes to prepare for your next appointment.

List Your Health-Care Providers
- Prepare a list of your current and past health-care providers and your current and past medical conditions, especially if you are seeing a new health-care provider.

Write Down Your History
- Prepare a brief history that summarizes your experience with COVID-19 and post-COVID conditions. For example, write down a list of the symptoms you think started after your COVID-19 infection:
  - the date of the onset of original COVID-19 illness and/or positive COVID-19 test, if known
  - when your post-COVID condition symptoms started
  - a list of prior treatments and diagnostic tests related to your post-COVID symptoms (blood work, x-rays, etc.)
  - things that make your symptoms worse
  - how the symptoms affect your activities, including challenges that affect daily living, working, attending school, and so on
  - how often symptoms occur
  - how you have been feeling
  - examples of your best and worst days
  - most important issues (sometimes referred to as "chief complaints")

List Your Medications
- Prepare a list of medications and supplements you are taking. Most health-care providers will ask you to provide this information at each appointment. Bringing your list with you will help keep track.

Patient Tips: Health-Care Provider Appointments for Post-COVID Conditions

Talk with a Family Member or Friend

Consider discussing your appointment with a trusted family member or friend immediately before and after you see your health-care provider. This person can help you take notes and remember what was discussed at the appointment while it is still fresh in your mind. If your health-care provider's office policy allows it, consider bringing them to your appointment with you.

What to Expect

The provider you meet with could be a doctor, nurse, nurse practitioner, physician assistant, or different type of health-care professional. It may take more than one appointment to evaluate potential post-COVID symptoms and determine an accurate diagnosis to better manage and treat your symptoms. Your provider may ask questions about your medical history, current symptoms, and quality of life. Depending on your symptoms, they may run tests to determine a diagnosis and plan for treatment.

DURING YOUR APPOINTMENT

On the day of your appointment, try to arrive a little early or, for telemedicine appointments, call in or log on a few minutes ahead of the appointment. If your provider is running late, you can use the time to make sure your paperwork or forms have been filled out and the front desk has your correct information. Everyone likes to be seen on time, but it is important to remember that each patient should receive the same attention from the provider once it is their turn. The list below can help you during your appointment.

Bring Your List of Concerns

- Since appointment time is often limited, it will be helpful if you make a list of why you are coming in for an appointment. Start with your most concerning issues (sometimes called "chief complaints").
- Focus on talking to your provider as this can be the most valuable part of the visit. If your provider still needs any of

your past medical records, ask them to sign the required forms to give your permission to have these records sent.

Ask and Answer Questions

- Ask questions, starting with the most important ones. Do not hesitate to ask your health-care provider to clarify the answers if they are not clear to you.
- Be prepared to discuss your activity levels, what activities make your illness worse, and any medications that seem to improve or worsen the symptoms.
- Answer the provider's questions. Explain how you feel. Be straightforward and do not be embarrassed to talk about anything.
- Let your provider know if there have been any changes to your prescribed medications and supplements.

Know Your Next Steps

- Make sure you understand the next steps. Bring a pencil and paper to write down instructions or use your handheld device for notes. Repeat back what the provider has told you to check for understanding. (e.g., you might ask: "So, you should go to the lab next week with this paperwork to get your blood drawn?"). Additional questions could include the following:
  - Will you need additional tests?
  - When and how will you get the test results?
  - When should you return for another visit?

Ask for a Summary

- Ask for an appointment summary. You can also ask the provider to write down any instructions, medication names, and so on for you. If there are changes to your treatment plan, make sure you understand what to do. For new medication, ask why it is being given and what you should expect by taking this new medication.

Patient Tips: Health-Care Provider Appointments for Post-COVID Conditions

AFTER YOUR APPOINTMENT

If you have been diagnosed with a post-COVID condition or are waiting to hear back from your provider about a post-COVID condition diagnosis, reviewing your appointment notes and preparing for your next one can help you get the most out of your appointments.

Track Your Appointments
- Make appointments for follow-up and any additional testing.
- Record future appointments on your calendar. Ask a friend or family member to put the appointment(s) on their calendars as well. Ask the provider's office if they will call or email you with an appointment reminder.

Work with Your Health-Care Provider
- If you are confused or do not remember something your provider said, call the provider's office for clarification.
- Follow your provider's instructions as closely as you can.

Document Your Experiences
- Continue to record symptoms in a journal, if possible. Some people with post-COVID conditions find it helpful to include the following:
  - whether symptoms have improved
  - which treatments have improved symptoms
  - any side effects
  - any other new symptoms or changes
- Make a note to give your health-care provider feedback about how recommended interventions have worked for you.
- Write down any issues you did not have time to talk about at the last appointment.
- Keep track of medications, vitamins, herbs, supplements, and over-the-counter drugs you take, using a current medications and supplements list.

- Remind your provider to share any test results if the expected window for receiving the results has passed.

Set Goals with Your Health-Care Provider

Your provider may run tests that return normal results. This does not change the existence, severity, or importance of your symptoms or conditions. Health-care providers and patients are encouraged to set achievable goals through shared decision-making and to approach treatment by focusing on specific symptoms or conditions.[1]

---

[1] "Patient Tips: Health-Care Provider Appointments for Post-COVID Conditions," Centers for Disease Control and Prevention (CDC), July 11, 2022. Available online. URL: www.cdc.gov/coronavirus/2019-ncov/long-term-effects/post-covid-appointment/index.html. Accessed December 14, 2022.

Chapter 38 | Supporting People with Post-COVID Conditions

Having a post-COVID condition or supporting someone with a post-COVID condition can be challenging. It can be difficult to care for yourself or loved ones, especially when there are few or no immediate answers or solutions. However, there are ways to help relieve some of the additional burdens of experiencing or caring for someone with a new and unknown condition. If you care for someone, remember to take steps to protect yourself and others from COVID-19.

CHILDREN AND ADOLESCENTS

Although post-COVID conditions appear to be less common in children and adolescents than in adults, long-term effects after COVID-19 do occur in children and adolescents. Young children may have trouble describing the problems they are experiencing.

If your child has a post-COVID condition that impacts their ability to attend school, complete schoolwork, or perform their usual activities, it may be helpful to discuss with your child's healthcare professional and school possible accommodations such as extra time on tests, scheduled rest periods throughout the day, a modified class schedule, and so on. School administrators, school counselors, and school nurses can work with families and healthcare professionals to provide learning accommodations for children with post-COVID conditions, particularly those experiencing thinking, concentrating, or physical difficulties. You may also request similar accommodations for activities outside of school, such as daycare, tutoring, sports, scouting, and so on.

UNDERSTAND YOUR EXPERIENCE

Each person copes differently with a long-term illness, and there are different ways to manage the stress, anxiety, and uncertainty of a new illness. Some people find taking an active role in understanding their condition is a comfort for managing their ongoing illness:

- Read about the experiences of other people with a post-COVID condition. Understanding other people's experiences with post-COVID conditions and reflecting on how these experiences may be similar or different from your own can help confirm you are not alone.
- Contribute to ongoing scientific research. Participating in research studies can build a larger understanding of new and unknown illnesses. Information about enrolling in clinical trials related to COVID-19 can be found at CombatCovid.hhs.gov (https://aspr.hhs.gov/COVID-19/treatments/Pages/default.aspx#all) and includes opportunities for persons with and without COVID-19.
- Participate in specific long COVID research. The National Institutes of Health (NIH) is conducting a research project, called the "RECOVER Initiative," to understand how people recover from a COVID-19 infection and why some people do not fully recover and develop long COVID or post-COVID conditions.

People experiencing post-COVID conditions may find different strategies to be helpful. If you are experiencing a post-COVID condition, you should engage in whatever coping strategies are best for your mental and physical health.

SUPPORT PEOPLE WITH POST-COVID CONDITIONS

Experiencing post-COVID conditions can be confusing and frustrating, and a person who feels sick long-term may feel isolated. Everyone experiences these conditions differently and may want different types of support or even no support at all. To determine the most helpful steps you can take for others, first listen with compassion and ask questions about what they need.

The How Right Now campaign of the Centers for Disease Control and Prevention (CDC; www.cdc.gov/howrightnow/index.html) provides helpful tools for navigating conversations about the type of support someone with post-COVID conditions may need.

Listen with Compassion

The unknown and long-term nature of a post-COVID condition can create stress. Taking steps to understand the person's experiences might make them feel less isolated.

WHAT TO DO

- When listening, give feedback that acknowledges and validates what they are going through.

Start a Conversation to Gain Understanding

Support can look different to different people. To best understand what type of support a person needs, start by asking them to talk and ask questions about their experiences.

WHAT TO DO

- When having these conversations, start with an open-ended question, such as "How is it going for you these days?" Then, work to narrow down what you can do to help.
- After taking time to compassionately listen to their responses, directly ask what they need or what you can do to help.

Determine How You Can Help with What They Need

After you have listened and worked to understand what support looks like for the person, determine your role in that support.
- Some people may want someone to listen to their experiences more frequently.
- Others may need more physical support (help with household chores, running errands).

There will be times when you may not be able to support a person exactly as they need, and it is okay to acknowledge that. Just be direct in saying what you can and cannot do.

EXAMPLE
- You understand that you need help getting groceries because you are not feeling up to grocery shopping. You do not have a car, but you can recommend the delivery service you use.

Employers can support employees experiencing post-COVID conditions by offering flexible leave and work schedule policies and by providing access to employee assistance programs.

If you are a caregiver, remember that maintaining healthy behaviors and seeking additional support are important parts of helping other people.[1]

---

[1] "Caring for People with Post-COVID Conditions," Centers for Disease Control and Prevention (CDC), September 1, 2022. Available online. URL: www.cdc.gov/coronavirus/2019-ncov/long-term-effects/care-post-covid.html. Accessed December 15, 2022.

Chapter 39 | Supporting Employees with Long COVID

Millions of Americans have lingering COVID-19 symptoms, a condition known as "long COVID," also called "post-COVID." This refers to various ongoing health problems that are either recurrent or new, experienced four or more weeks after the initial COVID-19 infection. According to the *Clinical Infectious Diseases* journal (https://academic.oup.com/cid/advance-article/doi/10.1093/cid/ciac961/6948437?login=false), close to 19 million adults in the United States have experienced long COVID.

These symptoms include cognitive impairment (brain fog), mood changes, fatigue, muscle or joint pain, heart palpitations, shortness of breath, and sleep difficulties. The effects can be critical enough to disrupt a person's ability to work and function normally. Long COVID syndrome has long-lasting detrimental effects in several organ systems, including the cardiac, respiratory, musculoskeletal, and neurologic.

CONSEQUENCES OF LONG COVID

It is estimated that one in every five adults with a long COVID condition will experience at least one symptom related to the previous COVID-19 infection, and individuals with long COVID syndrome are twice as likely to develop respiratory illnesses.

Moreover, Brookings Metro estimated that long COVID status could contribute to about 15 percent of the current national labor shortage in the United States. The labor force is declining post-COVID, according to the Minneapolis Fed, Lancet, and Trades Union Congress (TUC) data, and hiring and training new employees incur significant costs for an employer. Thus, organizations must find ways to support and retain current employees and support those with long COVID.

CHALLENGES OF LONG COVID EMPLOYEES

- **Cognitive function and mental health.** Long COVID has taken a significant toll on the mental health of employees. Many struggle with brain fog, memory loss, anxiety, and fear. Approximately one-third of employees diagnosed with COVID-19 have also been diagnosed with psychiatric problems, such as posttraumatic stress disorder (PTSD) and depression, within six months of infection.
- **Physical capacity.** The physical symptoms of long COVID can diminish an employee's physical capacity, with many experiencing fatigue, shortness of breath, muscle pain, and other issues that make it difficult to perform even basic tasks.
- **Medical attitudes of the society.** One of the biggest challenges faced by employees with long COVID is the lack of adequate medical knowledge and understanding from the community and society. Coworkers, friends, and family might imagine the symptoms are not real, leading to a lack of support.
- **Fear of returning to the workplace.** Employees with long COVID may also fear returning to the workplace due to the risk of reinfection or spreading the virus. This is particularly concerning for those in high-risk environments, such as hospitals and care facilities.
- **Decreased work capacity.** Long COVID can reduce an employee's work capacity, making it challenging to keep up with job demands and creating fears regarding job security and decreased income.

SUPPORTING EMPLOYEES WITH LONG COVID

Employers must understand the symptoms and effects of long COVID to facilitate workplace accommodations to meet employees' specific needs. To help fight COVID-19, employers should give priority to their employees' mental health and workplace wellbeing. After familiarizing themselves with long COVID symptoms, employers should determine the measures to take to help employees with long COVID and tailor them to each individual's different symptoms. Workplace flexibility is critical for employees with long COVID, especially those experiencing disability for the first time. Employers may undertake a variety of initiatives to support employees with long COVID with the following:

Telework (Working Remotely)

Telework provides a solution for long COVID employees to manage their symptoms better than working in an office. Working from home allows them to avoid a taxing commute, rest when necessary, and work at their own pace, which aids in their recovery. Working remotely may make employees feel safer about reinfection because individuals with long COVID are typically at a higher risk of a COVID relapse. Telework enables them to remain productive and contribute to their organization without compromising their health.

Reduced Work Hours

Reducing an employee's hours or allowing them additional or longer breaks can help. It might enable them to avoid standing for long periods or doing physically straining activities for hours. This may be beneficial in managing employees suffering from long COVID and result in better output and work efficiency in the long run.

Collaborative Work Systems

Effective workplace teams allow employees to work together and support each other to contribute to general productivity. It can help alleviate stress on long COVID sufferers to know that others share responsibility for their projects.

Unpaid Sick Leave

According to the U.S. Department of Labor (DOL), those who work 1,250 hours in a year may be eligible for unpaid leave for up to 12 weeks for medical or domestic reasons. Unpaid leave can help alleviate the stress associated with long COVID and may aid in recovery, but it can also lead to financial worry due to the absence of income.

Information on Organizational Resources

Educating employees with long COVID about organizational resources such as the employee resource group (ERG) or employee assistance program (EAP) is an effective way to support them. These resources can help employees find mental health, financial, and other types of support during their recovery. Employees should be made aware of the services provided by such organizational resources.

Peer Mentorship

This approach matches long COVID employees with peers who have faced similar experiences to provide mutual guidance, support, and encouragement as they work through their recovery. The goal of peer mentorship is to help employees feel more connected to their workplace, develop a sense of community, and build resilience in the face of a challenging situation. Peer mentoring can also help employees feel more confident in their ability to return to work and make a successful transition back to their roles.

Training Human Resource and Management Teams

It is crucial to understand the lingering nature of long COVID effects and suitably assist employees by creating a safe environment for open communication. To meet this critical challenge, management and HR teams should be trained to effectively handle long COVID employee needs and provide clear instructions on whom to contact for assistance.

It is important for employers to recognize the impact that long COVID can have on an employee's ability to perform their job duties. The role of an employer in this situation is to be supportive and understanding while ensuring that the work environment is safe for everyone. When a long COVID employee returns to work, it is crucial to have a conversation with them to understand any challenges they may be facing and how best to accommodate them. This could involve adjusting their workload with other peers, providing additional training, or arranging for flexible working hours.

Long COVID can have a significant impact on an employee's mental and emotional well-being. It is crucial to offer support in this area. This could involve providing occupational therapy services and access to counseling services or listening and offering support or responding to any particular needs of such employees in a timely manner.

The role of an employer in supporting long COVID employees is to be understanding and supportive in finding solutions that work for everyone, exploring various reasonable workplace adjustments, and regularly checking in with the employee about the effectiveness of those adjustments. By taking these measures, employers can help ensure that their long COVID employees can return to work feeling confident and supported and contribute to a safe and productive workplace for everyone.

References

Bach, Katie. "New Data Shows Long COVID Is Keeping as Many as 4 Million People Out of Work," The Brookings Institution, August 24, 2022. Available online. URL: www.brookings.edu/research/new-data-shows-long-covid-is-keeping-as-many-as-4-million-people-out-of-work. Accessed December 22, 2022.

Cust, Fiona and Runacres, Jessica. "Peer Mentoring to Support Staff Well-Being: Lessons from a Pilot," Times Higher Education (THE), December 7, 2022. Available online. URL: www.timeshighereducation.com/campus/peer-mentoring-support-staff-wellbeing-lessons-pilot. Accessed December 22, 2022.

Davis, Hannah E.; Assaf, Gina S.; McCorkell, Lisa; Wei, Hannah; Low, Ryan J.; Re'em, Yochai; et al. "Characterizing Long COVID in an International Cohort: 7 Months of Symptoms and Their Impact," *The Lancet*, July 15, 2021.

Available online. URL: www.thelancet.com/journals/eclinm/
article/PIIS2589-5370(21)00299-6/fulltext. Accessed
December 22, 2022.

Geddes, Linda. "Long COVID and the Workplace: What
Employers Could Do Better," VaccinesWork, June 16,
2022. Available online. URL: www.gavi.org/vaccineswork/
long-covid-and-workplace-what-employers-could-do-
better. Accessed December 22, 2022.

Ham, Dasom. "Long-Haulers and Labor Market Outcomes,"
Federal Reserve Bank of Minneapolis, July 7, 2022.
Available online. URL: www.minneapolisfed.org/research/
institute-working-papers/long-haulers-and-labor-market-
outcomes. Accessed December 22, 2022.

Ho, Solarina. "Don't Lose the Talent: How to Help Employees
with Long COVID," WebMD LLC., October 24, 2022.
Available online. URL: www.webmd.com/covid/
news/20221024/dont-lose-the-talent-how-to-help-
employees-with-long-covid. Accessed December 22, 2022.

"How Managers Can Support Employees with Long COVID,"
ALA–Allied Professional Association (ALA-APA),
June 2022. Available online. URL: https://ala-apa.org/
newsletter/2022/06/14/how-managers-can-support-
employees-with-long-covid. Accessed December 22, 2022.

"Long COVID—Advice for Employers and Employees," The
Advisory, Conciliation and Arbitration Service (ACAS),
May 1, 2021. Available online. URL: www.acas.org.uk/
long-covid. Accessed December 22, 2022.

Lowenstein, Fiona. "How Managers Can Support
Employees with Long COVID," Massachusetts Institute
of Technology, March 14, 2022. Available online. URL:
https://sloanreview.mit.edu/article/how-managers-can-
support-employees-with-long-covid. Accessed
December 22, 2022.

"Nearly One in Five American Adults Who Have Had
COVID-19 Still Have Long COVID," Centers for
Disease Control and Prevention (CDC), June 22, 2022.
Available online. URL: www.cdc.gov/nchs/pressroom/

nchs_press_releases/2022/20220622.htm. Accessed December 22, 2022.

Schwartz, Bryan and Clark, Cassidy. "Accommodating the Telework Employee Post-COVID," Neubauer & Associates, Inc., May 29, 2021. Available online. URL: www.plaintiffmagazine.com/recent-issues/item/accommodating-the-telework-employee-post-covid. Accessed December 22, 2022.

Sidharthan, Chinta. "An Estimated 19 Million US Adults Living with Long-COVID," News-Medical.Net, December 26, 2022. Available online. URL: www.news-medical.net/news/20221226/An-estimated-19-million-US-adults-living-with-long-COVID.aspx. Accessed January 5, 2023.

"Supporting Employees with Long COVID: A Guide for Employers," Job Accommodation Network (JAN), July 27, 2022. Available online. URL: https://askjan.org/publications/upload/Supporting-Employees-with-Long-COVID-A-Guide-for-Employers.pdf. Accessed December 22, 2022.

"Supporting Employees with Long COVID," System Concepts Ltd., July 23, 2021. Available online. URL: www.system-concepts.com/insights/supporting-employees-with-long-covid. Accessed December 22, 2022.

"Supporting Employees with Long COVID to Return to Work," Diversity Council Australia (DCA), July 11, 2022. Available online. URL: www.dca.org.au/blog/supporting-employees-long-covid-return-work. Accessed December 22, 2022.

"Workers' Experiences of Long COVID: A TUC Report," Trades Union Congress (TUC), June 2021. Available online. URL: www.tuc.org.uk/sites/default/files/2021-06/Formatted%20version%20of%20Long%20Covid%20report%20-%20v1.3.pdf. Accessed December 22, 2022.

Chapter 40 | Long COVID as a Disability

Although many people with COVID-19 get better within weeks, some people continue to experience symptoms that can last months after first being infected or may have new or recurring symptoms at a later time. This can happen to anyone who has had COVID-19, even if the initial illness was mild. People with this condition are sometimes called "long-haulers." This condition is known as "long COVID." In light of the rise of long COVID as a persistent and significant health issue, the Office for Civil Rights of the Department of Health and Human Services and the Civil Rights Division of the Department of Justice have joined together to provide this guidance.

This guidance explains that long COVID can be a disability under Titles II (state and local government) and III (public accommodations) of the Americans with Disabilities Act (ADA), Section 504 of the Rehabilitation Act of 1973 (Section 504), and Section 1557 of the Patient Protection and Affordable Care Act (Section 1557). Each of these federal laws protects people with disabilities from discrimination. This guidance also provides resources for additional information and best practices. This chapter focuses solely on long COVID and does not address when COVID-19 may meet the legal definition of disability.

The civil rights protections and responsibilities of these federal laws apply even during emergencies. They cannot be waived.

CAN LONG COVID BE A DISABILITY UNDER THE ADA, SECTION 504, AND SECTION 1557?

Yes, long COVID can be a disability under the ADA, Section 504, and Section 1557 if it substantially limits one or more major life activities. These laws and their related rules define a person with a disability as an individual with a physical or mental impairment that substantially limits one or more of the major life activities of such individual ("actual disability"), a person with a record of such an impairment ("record of"), or a person who is regarded as having such an impairment ("regarded as"). A person with long COVID has a disability if the person's condition or any of its symptoms is a "physical or mental" impairment that "substantially limits" one or more major life activities.

This chapter addresses the "actual disability" part of the disability definition. The definition also covers individuals with a "record of" a substantially limiting impairment or those "regarded as" having a physical impairment (whether substantially limiting or not). This chapter does not address the "record of" or "regarded as" parts of the disability definition, which may also be relevant to claims regarding long COVID.

Long COVID Is a Physical or Mental Impairment

A physical impairment includes any physiological disorder or condition affecting one or more body systems, including, among others, the neurological, respiratory, cardiovascular, and circulatory systems. A mental impairment includes any mental or psychological disorder, such as an emotional or mental illness.

Long COVID is a physiological condition affecting one or more body systems. For example, some people with long COVID experience the following:
- lung damage
- heart damage, including inflammation of the heart muscle
- kidney damage
- neurological damage

Long COVID as a Disability

- damage to the circulatory system resulting in poor blood flow
- lingering emotional illness and other mental health conditions

Accordingly, long COVID is a physical or mental impairment under the ADA, Section 504, and Section 1557.

Long COVID Can Substantially Limit One or More Major Life Activities

Major life activities include a wide range of activities, such as the following:
- caring for oneself
- performing manual tasks
- seeing
- hearing
- eating
- sleeping
- walking
- standing
- sitting
- reaching
- lifting
- bending
- speaking
- breathing
- learning
- reading
- concentrating
- thinking
- writing
- communicating
- interacting with others
- working

The term also includes the operation of a major bodily function, such as the functions of the immune system, cardiovascular system, neurological system, and circulatory system, or the operation of an organ.

The term "substantially limits" is construed broadly under these laws and should not demand extensive analysis. The impairment does not need to prevent or significantly restrict an individual from performing a major life activity, and the limitations do not need to be severe, permanent, or long-term. Whether an individual with long COVID is substantially limited in a major bodily function or other major life activity is determined without the benefit of any medication, treatment, or other measures used by the individual to lessen or compensate for symptoms. Even if the impairment comes and goes, it is considered a disability if it would substantially limit a major life activity when the impairment is active.

Long COVID can substantially limit a major life activity. The situations in which an individual with long COVID might be substantially limited in a major life activity are diverse. Among possible examples, some are as follows:

- A person with long COVID who has lung damage that causes shortness of breath, fatigue, and related effects is substantially limited in respiratory function, among other major life activities.
- A person with long COVID who has symptoms of intestinal pain, vomiting, and nausea that have lingered for months is substantially limited in gastrointestinal function, among other major life activities.
- A person with long COVID who experiences memory lapses and "brain fog" is substantially limited in brain function, concentrating, and/or thinking.

IS LONG COVID ALWAYS A DISABILITY?

No. An individualized assessment is necessary to determine whether a person's long COVID condition or any of its symptoms substantially limits a major life activity. The Centers for Disease Control and Prevention (CDC) and health experts are working to better understand long COVID.

Long COVID as a Disability

WHAT RIGHTS DO PEOPLE WHOSE LONG COVID QUALIFIES AS A DISABILITY HAVE UNDER THE ADA, SECTION 504, AND SECTION 1557?

People whose long COVID qualifies as a disability are entitled to the same protections from discrimination as any other person with a disability under the ADA, Section 504, and Section 1557. Put simply, they are entitled to full and equal opportunities to participate in and enjoy all aspects of civic and commercial life.

For example, this may mean that businesses or state or local governments will sometimes need to make changes to the way that they operate to accommodate a person's long-COVID-related limitations. For people whose long COVID qualifies as a disability, these changes, or "reasonable modifications," may include the following:

- providing additional time on a test for a student who has difficulty concentrating
- modifying procedures so a customer who finds it too tiring to stand in line can announce their presence and sit down without losing their place in line
- providing refueling assistance at a gas station for a customer whose joint or muscle pain prevents them from pumping their own gas
- modifying a policy to allow a person who experiences dizziness when standing to be accompanied by their service animal that is trained to stabilize them.

WHAT FEDERAL RESOURCES ARE THERE FOR PEOPLE WITH SYMPTOMS OF LONG COVID?

- The Office for Civil Rights of the Department of Health and Human Services (HHS) has the following web page on civil rights and COVID-19 (www.hhs.gov/civil-rights/for-providers/civil-rights-covid19/index.html).
  - If you believe that an entity covered by HHS civil rights laws has violated your rights protected under these authorities, you may file a complaint at www.hhs.gov/ocr/complaints/index.html.

- The Civil Rights Division of the Department of Justice has the following web page on its ADA.gov website that discusses topics related to COVID-19 and the ADA (www.ada.gov/emerg_prep.html).
  - If you believe that you or another person has been discriminated against by an entity covered by the ADA, you may file a complaint with the Disability Rights Section (DRS) in the Department of Justice. Information about how to file a complaint is available at www.ada.gov/fact_on_complaint.htm.
- The CDC's website has the following web page on post-COVID conditions, which discusses long COVID (www.cdc.gov/coronavirus/2019-ncov/long-term-effects/index.html).
- The Administration for Community Living's document, "How ACL's Disability and Aging Networks Can Help People with Long COVID," provides information on resources and programs to assist people with long COVID. This document is available at https://acl.gov/sites/default/files/COVID19/ACL_LongCOVID.pdf.
- Individuals who wish to learn more about COVID-19 and employment can visit the following Equal Employment Opportunity Commission (EEOC) web page, which provides COVID-19 information and resources (www.eeoc.gov/coronavirus).
  - The EEOC's main COVID-19 publication, What You Should Know about COVID-19 and the ADA, the Rehabilitation Act, and Other EEO Laws, is available at www.eeoc.gov/wysk/what-you-should-know-about-covid-19-and-ada-rehabilitation-act-and-other-eeo-laws.[1]

---

[1] "Guidance on 'Long COVID' as a Disability under the ADA, Section 504, and Section 1557," U.S. Department of Health and Human Services (HHS), July 26, 2021. Available online. URL: www.hhs.gov/civil-rights/for-providers/civil-rights-covid19/guidance-long-covid-disability/index.html#footnote10_0ac8mdc. Accessed December 21, 2022.

Part 6 | COVID-19 Pandemic and Its Social Impact

Chapter 41 | Pandemics in History

Chapter Contents
Section 41.1—Endemics, Epidemics, and Pandemics:
            An Overview..457
Section 41.2—Pandemics of the Past..461

Section 41.1 | Endemics, Epidemics, and Pandemics: An Overview

LEVELS OF DISEASE

The amount of a particular disease that is usually present in a community is referred to as the baseline or endemic level of the disease. This level is not necessarily the desired level, which may in fact be zero, but rather is the observed level. In the absence of intervention and assuming that the level is not high enough to deplete the pool of susceptible persons, the disease may continue to occur at this level indefinitely. Thus, the baseline level is often regarded as the expected level of the disease.

ENDEMICS

While some diseases are so rare in a given population that a single case warrants an epidemiologic investigation (e.g., rabies, plague, polio), other diseases occur more commonly so that only deviations from the norm warrant investigation. Sporadic refers to a disease that occurs infrequently and irregularly. Endemic refers to the constant presence and/or usual prevalence of a disease or infectious agent in a population within a geographic area. Hyperendemic refers to persistent, high levels of disease occurrence.

EPIDEMICS

Occasionally, the amount of disease in a community rises above the expected level. Epidemic refers to an increase, often sudden, in the number of cases of a disease above what is normally expected in that population in that area. Outbreak carries the same definition of epidemic but is often used for a more limited geographic area. Cluster refers to an aggregation of cases grouped in place and time that are suspected to be greater than the number expected even though the expected number may not be known. Pandemic refers to an epidemic that has spread over several countries or continents, usually affecting a large number of people.

Epidemics occur when an agent and susceptible hosts are present in adequate numbers and the agent can be effectively conveyed

from a source to the susceptible hosts. More specifically, an epidemic may result from:
- a recent increase in the amount or virulence of the agent
- the recent introduction of the agent into a setting where it has not been before
- an enhanced mode of transmission so that more susceptible persons are exposed
- a change in the susceptibility of the host response to the agent
- factors that increase host exposure or involve introduction through new portals of entry

The previous description of epidemics presumes only infectious agents, but noninfectious diseases such as diabetes and obesity exist in epidemic proportions in the United States.

Epidemic Patterns

Epidemics can be classified according to their manner of spread through a population:
- common-source
  - point
  - continuous
  - intermittent
- propagated
- mixed
- other

A common-source outbreak is one in which a group of persons are all exposed to an infectious agent or a toxin from the same source.

If the group is exposed over a relatively brief period so that everyone who becomes ill does so within one incubation period, then the common-source outbreak is further classified as a point-source outbreak. The epidemic of leukemia cases in Hiroshima following the atomic bomb blast and the epidemic of hepatitis A among patrons of the Pennsylvania restaurant who ate green onions each had a point source of exposure. If the number of cases during an epidemic were plotted over time, the resulting graph, called an "epidemic curve," would typically have a steep upslope and a more gradual downslope (a so-called log-normal distribution).

In some common-source outbreaks, case patients may have been exposed over a period of days, weeks, or longer. In a continuous common-source outbreak, the range of exposures and range of incubation periods tend to flatten and widen the peaks of the epidemic curve. The epidemic curve of an intermittent common-source outbreak often has a pattern reflecting the intermittent nature of the exposure.

A propagated outbreak results from transmission from one person to another. Usually, transmission is by direct person-to-person contact, as with syphilis. Transmission may also be vehicle-borne (e.g., transmission of hepatitis B or human immunodeficiency virus (HIV) by sharing needles) or vector-borne (e.g., transmission of yellow fever by mosquitoes). In propagated outbreaks, cases occur over more than one incubation period. The epidemic usually wanes after a few generations, either because the number of susceptible persons falls below some critical level required to sustain transmission or because intervention measures become effective.

Some epidemics have features of both common-source epidemics and propagated epidemics. The pattern of a common-source outbreak followed by secondary person-to-person spread is not uncommon. These are called "mixed epidemics." For example, a common-source epidemic of shigellosis occurred among a group of 3,000 women attending a national music festival. Many developed symptoms after returning home. Over the next few weeks, several state health departments detected subsequent generations of shigella cases propagated by person-to-person transmission from festival attendees.

Finally, some epidemics are neither common-source in their usual sense nor propagated from person to person. Outbreaks of the zoonotic or vectorborne disease may result from sufficient prevalence of infection in host species, sufficient presence of vectors, and sufficient human-vector interaction.[1]

PANDEMICS

A pandemic is a disease outbreak that spans several countries and affects a large number of people. Pandemics are most often caused by viruses, such as COVID-19, which can easily spread from person to person.

A new virus, such as COVID-19, can emerge from anywhere and quickly spread around the world. It is hard to predict when or where the next new pandemic will emerge.

If a pandemic is declared:
- wash your hands often with soap and water for at least 20 seconds and try not to touch your eyes, nose, or mouth
- keep a distance of at least six feet between yourself and people who are not part of your household
- cover your mouth and nose with a mask when in public
- clean and disinfect high-touch objects and surfaces
- stay at home as much as possible to prevent the spread of disease
- follow the guidance of the Centers for Disease Control and Prevention (CDC)

HOW TO PREPARE YOURSELF FOR A PANDEMIC

- Learn how diseases spread to help protect yourself and others. Viruses can be spread from person to person, from a nonliving object to a person, and by people who are infected but do not have any symptoms.
- Prepare for the possibility of schools, workplaces, and community centers being closed. Investigate and prepare for virtual coordination for school, work (telework), and social activities.

---

[1] "Introduction to Epidemiology," Centers for Disease Control and Prevention (CDC), May 18, 2012. Available online. URL: www.cdc.gov/csels/dsepd/ss1978/lesson1/section11.html#:~:text=Epidemic%20refers%20to%20an%20increase,that%20population%20in%20that%20area. Accessed December 9, 2022.

Pandemics in History

- Gather supplies in case you need to stay home for several days or weeks. Supplies may include cleaning supplies, nonperishable foods, prescriptions, and bottled water. Buy supplies slowly to ensure that everyone has the opportunity to buy what they need.
- Create an emergency plan so that you and your family know what to do and what you will need in case an outbreak happens. Consider how a pandemic may affect your plans for other emergencies.
- Review your health insurance policies to understand what they cover, including telemedicine options.
- Create password-protected digital copies of important documents and store them in a safe place. Watch out for scams and fraud.[2]

Section 41.2 | Pandemics of the Past

An influenza pandemic is a global outbreak of a new influenza A virus that is very different from current and recently circulating human seasonal influenza A viruses. Influenza A viruses are constantly changing, making it possible on very rare occasions for nonhuman influenza viruses to change in such a way that they can infect people easily and spread efficiently from person to person.

1918 PANDEMIC (H1N1 VIRUS)

The 1918 influenza pandemic was the most severe pandemic in recent history. It was caused by a hemagglutinin type 1 and neuraminidase type 1 (H1N1) virus with genes of avian origin. Although there is no universal consensus regarding where the virus originated, it spread worldwide during 1918–1919. In the United States, it was first identified in military personnel in the spring of

---

[2] Ready.gov, "Pandemics," U.S. Department of Homeland Security (DHS), November 17, 2022. Available online. URL: www.ready.gov/pandemic. Accessed December 9, 2022.

1918. It is estimated that about 500 million people or one-third of the world's population became infected with this virus. The number of deaths was estimated to be at least 50 million worldwide with about 675,000 occurring in the United States.

History of the 1918 Flu Pandemic

The 1918 influenza pandemic was the most severe pandemic in recent history. It was caused by an H1N1 virus with genes of avian origin. Although there is no universal consensus regarding where the virus originated, it spread worldwide during 1918–1919. In the United States, it was first identified in military personnel in the spring of 1918.

It is estimated that about 500 million people or one-third of the world's population became infected with this virus. The number of deaths was estimated to be at least 50 million worldwide with about 675,000 occurring in the United States. Mortality was high in people younger than five years old, 20–40 years old, and 65 years and older. The high mortality in healthy people, including those in the 20–40 year age group, was a unique feature of this pandemic.

While the 1918 H1N1 virus has been synthesized and evaluated, the properties that made it so devastating are not well understood. With no vaccine to protect against influenza infection and no antibiotics to treat secondary bacterial infections that can be associated with influenza infections, control efforts worldwide were limited to nonpharmaceutical interventions such as isolation, quarantine, good personal hygiene, use of disinfectants, and limitations of public gatherings, which were applied unevenly.

1918 Pandemic Influenza Historic Timeline

In 1918, a new influenza virus emerged. During this same time period, World War I (WWI) was taking place. The conditions of WWI (overcrowding and global troop movement) helped the 1918 flu spread. The vulnerability of healthy young adults and the lack of vaccines and treatments created a major public health crisis, causing at least 50 million deaths worldwide, including approximately

Pandemics in History

675,000 in the United States. Below is a historical timeline of major events that took place during this time period.

April 1917
- The United States enters WWI with 378,000 in the armed services.

June 1917
- A draft is established to increase the number of soldiers; Army begins training recruits at 32 large camps, each housing 25,000–55,000 soldiers.

March 1918
- Outbreaks of flu-like illness are first detected in the United States.
- More than 100 soldiers at Camp Funston in Fort Riley, Kansas, become ill with flu. Within a week, the number of flu cases quintuples.
- Sporadic flu activity spreads unevenly through the United States, Europe, and possibly Asia over the next six months.

April 1918
- First mention of influenza appears in an April 5 weekly public health report. The report informs officials of 18 severe cases and three deaths in Haskell, Kansas.

May 1918
- By May, hundreds of thousands of soldiers travel across the Atlantic each month as they are deployed for WWI.

September 1918
- The second wave of flu emerges at Camp Devens, a U.S. Army training camp just outside of Boston, and at a naval facility in Boston.
- Between September and November, a second wave of flu peaks in the United States. This second wave is highly fatal and responsible for most of the deaths attributed to the pandemic.

- New York City's Board of Health adds flu to the list of reportable diseases and requires all flu cases to be isolated at home or in a city hospital.
- By the end of September, more than 14,000 flu cases are reported at Camp Devens—equaling about one-quarter of the total camp, resulting in 757 deaths.

October 1918
- The 1918 flu pandemic virus kills an estimated 195,000 Americans during October alone.
- In the fall of 1918, the United States experiences a severe shortage of professional nurses because of the deployment of large numbers of nurses to military camps in the United States and abroad and the failure to use trained African American nurses.
- Chicago chapter of the American Red Cross issues urgent calls for volunteers to help nurse the ill.
- Philadelphia is hit hard with the pandemic flu viruses— more than 500 corpses await burial, some for more than a week. Cold-storage plants are used as temporary morgues, and a manufacturer of trolley cars donates 200 packing crates for use as coffins.
- Chicago, along with many other cities across the United States, closes theaters, movie houses, and night schools and prohibits public gatherings.
- San Francisco's Board of Health requires any person serving the public to wear masks and issues a strong recommendation to all residents to wear masks in public.
- New York City reports a 40 percent decline in shipyard productivity due to flu illnesses in the midst of WWI.

November 1918
- The end of WWI enables a resurgence of influenza as people celebrate Armistice Day and soldiers begin to demobilize.

Pandemics in History

- Salt Lake City officials place quarantine signs on the front and rear doors of 2,000 homes where occupants have been struck with flu.
- By the end of WWI, the U.S. military grew in size from 378,000 soldiers in April 1918 to 4.7 million soldiers.

December 1918
- Public health officials begin education programs and publicity about the dangers of coughing and sneezing and careless disposal of "nasal discharges."
- Committee of the American Public Health Association encourages stores and factories to stagger opening and closing hours and for people to walk to work when possible instead of using public transport to prevent overcrowding.

January 1919
- A third wave of influenza occurs in the winter and spring of 1919, killing many more. The third wave subsides in the summer.
- In San Francisco, 1,800 flu cases and 101 deaths are reported in the first five days of January.
- Many San Antonio citizens begin complaining that new flu cases are not being reported and that this is fueling another influenza surge.
- Seven-hundred and six cases of influenza and 67 deaths are reported in New York City, triggering fear of a recurrence of severe flu activity.
- Trustees of the Boston City Hospital ask the mayor for a special appropriation of $3,000 to study the treatment of influenza.

February 1919
- Influenza appears to be nearly eradicated in New Orleans as the number of reported cases drops.

- Illinois passes a bill to create a one-year course to become a "practical nurse," an effort to address the nursing shortage the pandemic had exposed.

April 1919
- At Versailles Peace Conference, while negotiating the end of WWI with other world leaders, U.S. President Woodrow Wilson collapses. Some historians speculate he was weak from influenza, which was still rampant in Paris.

1957–1958 PANDEMIC (H2N2 VIRUS)

In February 1957, a new influenza A (H2N2) virus emerged in East Asia, triggering a pandemic ("Asian Flu"). This H2N2 virus comprised three different genes from an H2N2 virus that originated from an avian influenza A virus, including the H2 hemagglutinin and the N2 neuraminidase genes. It was first reported in Singapore in February 1957, Hong Kong in April 1957, and in coastal cities in the United States in the summer of 1957. The estimated number of deaths was 1.1 million worldwide and 116,000 in the United States.

Influenza Historic Timeline

Below is a historical timeline of major scientific and public health events and milestones in influenza prevention.

1930s
- Influenza viruses are isolated from people, proving that influenza is caused by a virus not a bacterium.
  - Smith, Andrewes, and Laidlaw isolate influenza A virus in ferrets in 1933.
  - Francis isolates influenza B virus in 1936.
  - In 1936, Burnet discovers that influenza virus can be grown in embryonated hens' eggs.

1940s
- 1940s: Thomas Francis, Jr., MD, and Jonas Salk, MD, serve as lead researchers at the University of Michigan to develop the first inactivated flu vaccine with support

from the U.S. Army. Their vaccine uses fertilized chicken eggs in a method that is still used to produce most flu vaccines today. The Army is involved with this research because of their experience with troop loss from flu illness and deaths during WWI. This original vaccine only includes an inactivated influenza A virus.
- 1940s: First-generation mechanical ventilators become available. These machines support breathing in patients suffering respiratory complications.
- 1940: Influenza B viruses are discovered.
- 1942: A bivalent (two-component) vaccine that offers protection against influenza A and influenza B viruses is produced after the discovery of influenza B viruses.
- 1944: Use of cell cultures for virus growth is discovered. This allows viruses to be cultured outside the body for the first time. The ability to culture influenza from respiratory secretions allows the diagnosis of influenza.
- 1945: Inactivated influenza vaccine is licensed for use in civilians.
- 1946: The Communicable Disease Center (CDC) opens in the old offices of the Malaria Control in War Areas, located on Peachtree Street in Atlanta, Georgia, with a satellite campus in Chamblee. Launched with fewer than 400 employees, the organization—today the Centers for Disease Control and Prevention–moves to its current main campus on Clifton Road in Atlanta in 1947 after paying $10 to Emory University for 15 acres of land.
- 1947: During the seasonal flu epidemic of 1947, investigators determine that changes in the antigenic composition of circulating influenza viruses have rendered existing vaccines ineffective, highlighting the need for continuous surveillance and characterization of circulating flu viruses.
- 1948: The World Health Organization (WHO) Influenza Centre is established at the National Institute for Medical Research in London. The primary tasks of the organization are to collect and characterize

influenza viruses, develop methods for the laboratory diagnosis of influenza virus infections, establish a network of laboratories, and disseminate data accumulated from their investigations.

1950s
- 1952: The Global Influenza Surveillance and Response System (GISRS) is created by WHO to monitor the evolution of influenza viruses. The GISRS network originally includes 26 laboratories.
- 1956: The CDC's Influenza Branch in Atlanta is designated a WHO Collaborating Centre for Surveillance, Epidemiology and Control of Influenza.
- 1957: A new H2N2 flu virus emerges to trigger a pandemic. There are about 1.1 million deaths globally, with about 116,000 in the United States.

1960s
- 1960: In 1960, the U.S. Surgeon General, in response to substantial morbidity and mortality during the 1957–1958 pandemic, recommends annual influenza vaccination for people with chronic debilitating disease, people aged 65 years or older, and pregnant women.
- 1961: An outbreak in South Africa raises the possibility of wild birds as a possible reservoir for influenza A viruses.
- 1962: the CDC launches the 122 Cities Mortality Reporting System. Each week, the vital statistics office of 122 cities across the United States report the total number of death certificates processed and the number of those for which pneumonia or influenza is listed as an underlying or contributing cause of death by age group. The system is retired in October 2016.
- 1966: The U.S. Food and Drug Administration (FDA) licenses amantadine, a new antiviral medication, as a prophylactic (preventive medicine) against influenza A. It is not effective against influenza B.
- 1967: Dr. H.G. Pereira and colleagues propose a relationship between human and avian flu viruses

Pandemics in History

after a study shows an antigenic relationship between the 1957 human pandemic A virus and an influenza A virus isolated from a turkey. The study raises the question and triggers the body of work on whether human influenza viruses are of avian origin.
- 1968: A new influenza A virus subtype H3N2 (H3N2) emerges to trigger another pandemic, resulting in roughly 100,000 deaths in the United States and one million worldwide. Most of those deaths are in age group 65 and older. H3N2 viruses circulating today are descendants of the H3N2 virus that emerges in 1968.

1970s
- An H1N1 (swine flu) outbreak among recruits at Fort Dix leads to a vaccination program to prevent a pandemic. Within 10 months, roughly 25 percent of the U.S. population is vaccinated (48 million people), about twice the level needed to provide coverage for the at-risk population. Cases of Guillain-Barre syndrome, a neurologic condition that in rare instances has been associated with vaccination, among vaccine recipients appeared to be in excess of what was expected, so officials determine the vaccination program should be halted.

1980s
- 1981: CDC begins collecting reports of influenza outbreaks from state and territorial epidemiologists.

1990s
- 1993: The Vaccines for Children (VFC) Program is established as a result of a measles outbreak to provide vaccines at no cost to children whose parents or guardians might not be able to afford them. The program increases the likelihood of children getting recommended vaccinations on schedule.
- 1993: The costs of the influenza vaccine become a covered benefit under Medicare Part B.

- 1994: Rimantadine, derived from amantadine, is approved by the FDA to treat influenza A.
- 1996: An avian influenza H5N1 virus is first isolated from a farmed goose in China.
- 1997: The first human infection with an avian influenza A H5N1 virus is identified in Hong Kong.
- 1997: FluNet, a web-based flu surveillance tool, is launched by the WHO. It is a critical tool for tracking the movement of flu viruses globally. Country data is updated weekly and is publically available.
- 1998: Influenza virus surveillance in swine, conducted by the the U.S. Department of Agriculture, begins in the United States. A virus that is a hybrid of human, bird, and swine flu viruses is detected in pigs. This virus becomes the dominant flu virus in U.S. pigs by 1999.
- 1999: A pandemic planning framework is published by the WHO emphasizing the need to enhance influenza surveillance, vaccine production and distribution, antiviral drugs, influenza research, and emergency preparedness.
- 1999: The neuraminidase inhibitors oseltamivir (Tamiflu®) and zanamivir (Relenza®) are licensed to treat influenza infection.

2000s
- April 2002: The Advisory Committee on Immunization Practices (ACIP) encourages that children aged 6–23 months be vaccinated annually against influenza.
- 2003: Public health officials are concerned about a reemergence of H5N1 avian influenza reported in China and Vietnam.
- June 2003: The first nasal spray flu vaccine is licensed.
- 2004: The National Incident Management System (NIMS) is established to coordinate responses for public health incidents that require actions by all levels of government, as well as public, private, and nongovernmental organizations.

Pandemics in History

- 2005: The U.S. Government National Strategy for Pandemic Influenza is published.
- 2005: The entire genome of the 1918 H1N1 pandemic influenza virus is sequenced.
- 2006: The CDC stops recommending adamantanes during the 2005–2006 season after high levels of resistance among influenza A viruses. In the United States, resistance increased from 1.9 percent during the 2003–2004 season to 11 percent in the 2004–2005 season.
- 2006: The National Strategy for Pandemic Influenza Implementation Plan is published. The section outlines U.S. preparedness and response to prevent the spread of a pandemic.
- 2007: The American Veterinary Medical Association (AVMA) establishes the One Health initiative Task Force, an effort to attain optimal health for people, animals, and the environment.
- 2007: The American Medical Association unanimously approves a resolution calling for increased collaboration between human and veterinary medical communities. The term "one health," which looks at the interactions between animal and human health, enters the medical and scientific lexicon.
- 2007: The One Health approach is recommended for pandemic preparedness during the International Ministerial Conference on Avian and Pandemic Influenza.
- 2007: The FDA approves the first U.S. vaccine for people against an avian influenza A (H5N1) virus.
- 2007: Human infection with a novel influenza virus is added to the nationally notifiable disease list.
- 2008: The ACIP expands its influenza vaccination recommendation to include vaccination of children aged 5–18 years.
- 2008: The HHS Pandemic Influenza Operational Plan is published.

- 2008: The CDC receives the FDA approval for a highly sensitive influenza polymerase chain reaction (PCR) assay. These tests can detect influenza with high specificity that enhances diagnosis and treatment options.
- 2008: The Influenza Reagent Resource (IRR) is established by the CDC to provide registered users with reagents, tools, and information to study and detect influenza viruses.
- April 17, 2009: A new H1N1 virus is detected in the United States. The CDC begins working to develop a virus (called a "candidate vaccine virus") that could be used to make a vaccine to protect against this new virus.
- April 25, 2009: The World Health Organization (WHO) declares a public health emergency of international concern.
- June 11, 2009: The WHO officially declares the new 2009 H1N1 outbreak a pandemic.
- 2009: The CDC begins a complex and multifaceted response to the H1N1 pandemic that lasts more than a year.
- 2009: Physicians use point-of-care rapid immunoassay tests to provide influenza results within 15 minutes during the H1N1 pandemic.
- October 5, 2009: The first doses of the monovalent H1N1 pandemic vaccine are administered.

2010s
- August 10, 2010: WHO declares an end to the 2009 H1N1 influenza pandemic.
- 2010: The ACIP recommends annual influenza vaccination for those six months of age and older.
- 2012: Vaccines containing cell-cultured viruses become available. Even though eggs continue to be the primary means of production, cell culture emerges as an alternative method for producing influenza vaccines.

- 2012: The WHO makes first vaccine composition recommendation for a quadrivalent vaccine.
- 2012: The CDC partners with the Association of Public Health laboratories to define the optimal right size for influenza virologic surveillance. The project produces right-size calculators and statistical tools that help states determine the optimal amount of influenza testing needed for desired confidence levels of surveillance.
- 2014: The FDA approves peramivir (Rapivab) to treat influenza in adults. It is the first IV flu medication.
- 2017: The CDC updates guidelines for use of nonpharmaceutical measures to help prevent the spread of pandemic influenza based on the latest scientific evidence. These are actions that individuals and communities can take to help slow the spread of the flu such as staying home when sick, covering a cough or sneeze, and frequently washing hands.

1968 PANDEMIC (H3N2 VIRUS)

The 1968 pandemic was caused by an influenza A (H3N2) virus that comprised two genes from an avian influenza A virus, including a new H3 hemagglutinin, but also contained the N2 neuraminidase from the 1957 H2N2 virus. It was first noted in the United States in September 1968. The estimated number of deaths was one million worldwide and about 100,000 in the United States. Most excess deaths were in people 65 years and older. The H3N2 virus continues to circulate worldwide as a seasonal influenza A virus. Seasonal H3N2 viruses, which are associated with severe illness in older people, undergo regular antigenic drift.

2009 H1N1 PANDEMIC (H1N1PDM09 VIRUS)

In the spring of 2009, a novel influenza A (H1N1) virus emerged. It was detected first in the United States and spread quickly across the United States and the world. This new H1N1 virus contained a unique combination of influenza genes not previously identified in animals or people. This virus was designated as influenza A

Pandemic Disease Mexico 2009 ((H1N1)pdm09) virus. Ten years later, work continues to better understand influenza, prevent disease, and prepare for the next pandemic.

The 2009 H1N1 Pandemic: A New Flu Virus Emerges

The (H1N1)pdm09 virus was very different from the H1N1 viruses that were circulating at the time of the pandemic. Few young people had any existing immunity (as detected by antibody response) to the (H1N1)pdm09 virus, but nearly one-third of people over 60 years old had antibodies against this virus, likely from exposure to an older H1N1 virus earlier in their lives. Since the (H1N1)pdm09 virus was very different from circulating H1N1 viruses, vaccination with seasonal flu vaccines offered little cross-protection against (H1N1)pdm09 virus infection. While a monovalent (H1N1)pdm09 vaccine was produced, it was not available in large quantities until late November—after the peak of illness during the second wave had come and gone in the United States. From April 12, 2009, to April 10, 2010, the CDC estimated there were 60.8 million cases (range: 43.3–89.3 million), 274,304 hospitalizations (range: 195,086–402,719), and 12,469 deaths (range: 8,868–18,306) in the United States due to the (H1N1)pdm09 virus.

Additionally, the CDC estimated that 151,700–575,400 people worldwide died from (H1N1)pdm09 virus infection during the first year the virus circulated. **Globally, 80 percent of (H1N1)pdm09 virus-related deaths were estimated to have occurred in people younger than 65 years of age. This differs greatly from typical seasonal influenza epidemics, during which about 70–90 percent of deaths are estimated to occur in people 65 years and older.

**Estimated global mortality associated with the first 12 months of 2009 pandemic influenza A H1N1 virus circulation: a modeling study.

Though the 2009 flu pandemic primarily affected children and young and middle-aged adults, the impact of the (H1N1)pdm09 virus on the global population during the first year was less severe than that of previous pandemics. Estimates of pandemic influenza

Pandemics in History

mortality ranged from 0.03 percent of the world's population during the 1968 H3N2 pandemic to 1–3 percent of the world's population during the 1918 H1N1 pandemic. It is estimated that 0.001–0.007 percent of the world's population died of respiratory complications associated with (H1N1)pdm09 virus infection during the first 12 months the virus circulated.

The United States mounted a complex, multifaceted, and long-term response to the pandemic, summarized in the 2009 H1N1 Pandemic: Summary Highlights, April 2009–April 2010. On August 10, 2010, the WHO declared an end to the global 2009 H1N1 influenza pandemic. However, H1N1pdm09 virus continues to circulate as a seasonal flu virus and cause illness, hospitalization, and deaths worldwide every year.

In 2009, a new H1N1 influenza virus emerged, causing the first global flu pandemic in 40 years. Below is a timeline of major events that took place during the 2009 H1N1 pandemic.

April 15, 2009
- First human infection with new influenza A H1N1 virus detected in California.

April 17, 2009
- Second human infection with the new influenza A H1N1 virus detected in California about 130 miles away from first infection, with no known connection to previous patient.

April 18, 2009
- First novel 2009 H1N1 flu infections were reported by the CDC to the World Health Organization (WHO) through the U.S. International Health Regulations Program.

April 21, 2009
- The CDC publicly reported the first two U.S. infections with the new H1N1 virus.
- The CDC began working to develop a candidate vaccine virus.

April 22, 2009
- The CDC activated its Emergency Operations Center (EOC).

April 23, 2009
- Two additional human infections with 2009 H1N1 were detected in Texas, transforming the investigation into a multistate outbreak and response.

April 24, 2009
- The CDC uploaded complete gene sequences of the new H1N1 2009 virus to a pubically accessible international influenza database.

April 25, 2009
- The WHO declared a public health emergency of international concern.

April 26, 2009
- The U.S. government declared 2009 H1N1 a Public Health Emergency of International Concern, and the CDC began releasing 25 percent of antiviral drugs needed to treat this new influenza virus from the federal stockpile.

April 27, 2009
- The WHO Director-General raised the level of influenza pandemic alert from phase 3 to phase 4, based on data showing person-to-person spread and the ability of the virus to cause community-level outbreaks.

April 28, 2009
- The Food and Drug Administration (FDA) approved a new CDC test to detect 2009 H1N1 infections.
- CDC issued the first CDC Interim Guidance on Closing Schools and Childcare Facilities, recommending a seven-day dismissal in affected

schools and childcare facilities with laboratory-confirmed cases of influenza A H1N1 virus.

April 29, 2009
- The WHO raised the level of influenza pandemic alert from phase 4 to phase 5, signaling that a pandemic was imminent, and requested all countries to immediately activate their pandemic preparedness plans and be on high alert for unusual outbreaks of influenza—such as illness and severe pneumonia.

May 2009
- H1N1 influenza summer activity peaked in the United States during May and June.

May 1, 2009
- Domestic and global shipments of new CDC test to detect 2009 H1N1 began.
- The CDC updated the CDC Interim Guidance on Closing Schools and Childcare Facilities, recommending affected communities with lab-confirmed cases of influenza A H1N1 consider adopting school dismissal and childcare closing measures, including closing for up to 14 days depending on the extent and severity of influenza illness.

May 4, 2009
- The CDC shifted from reporting confirmed cases of 2009 H1N1 to reporting both confirmed and probable cases of 2009 H1N1.

May 5, 2009
- It is the peak school dismissal day in the spring phase of the pandemic. Nine hundred and eighty schools were dismissed, affecting 607,778 students.

May 6, 2009
- The CDC distributed updated recommendations for the use of influenza antiviral medicines to

provide guidance for clinicians in prescribing antiviral medicines for treatment and prevention (chemoprophylaxis) of 2009 H1N1 influenza.

May 8, 2009
- The CDC issued a Morbidity and Mortality Weekly Report (MMWR) updating the 2009 H1N1 influenza situations in Mexico, the United States, and worldwide.

May 12, 2009
- The CDC reported early data on 2009 H1N1 illness among pregnant women in an MMWR.

June 11, 2009
- The World Health Organization (WHO) declared a pandemic and raised the worldwide pandemic alert level to phase 6, which means the virus was spreading to other parts of the world.
- The CDC held its first press conference with former CDC Director Thomas Frieden, MD, MPH. The press conference had 2,355 participants.

June 19, 2009
- All 50 states, the District of Colombia, Puerto Rico and the U.S. Virgin Islands reported cases of 2009 H1N1 infection.
- By late June, more than 30 summer camps in the United States had reported outbreaks of 2009 H1N1 influenza illness. The CDC released guidance for day and residential camps to reduce spread of influenza.

June 25, 2009
- The CDC estimated at least one million cases of 2009 H1N1 influenza had occurred in the United States.

Early July
- Reported cases of 2009 H1N1 nearly doubled since mid-June 2009.

Pandemics in History

- Three 2009 H1N1 influenza viruses that were resistant to the antiviral drug, oseltamivir, were detected in three countries.

July 10, 2009
- The CDC reported findings in an MMWR that indicated a large prevalence of obesity in intensive care patients with confirmed 2009 H1N1 influenza infection.
- After mid-July, 2009 H1N1 influenza activity declined in most countries.

July 22, 2009
- Clinical trials testing the 2009 H1N1 flu vaccine began.

August 2009
- Additional oseltamivir-resistant 2009 H1N1 viruses were detected by the CDC.

August 3, 2009
- The CDC School Dismissal Monitoring System (SDMS) activated.

August 19, 2009
- The CDC Guidance for Businesses and accompanying toolkit posted to CDC.gov.

August 20, 2009
- The CDC Guidance for Institutions of Higher Education (IHE) and accompanying toolkit posted to CDC.gov. Calls were conducted with Secretary Duncan and Sebelius to explain guidance.
- Second wave of 2009 H1N1 influenza activity began in the United States.

August 30, 2009
- New reporting season for the 2009–2010 influenza season began.

September 1, 2009
- More than 1,000 test kits shipped to 120 domestic and 250 international laboratories in 140 countries since May 1, 2009.

September 3, 2009
- The CDC published a study that analyzed data related to H1N1 influenza pediatric deaths reported to the CDC from April to August 2009 in MMWR. Data showed 477 deaths with lab-confirmed 2009 H1N1 flu in the United States had been reported to the CDC as of August 8, 2009.

September 10, 2009
- The HHS secretary and the CDC director joined the National Foundation for Infectious Diseases (NFID) in a news conference to stress the importance of getting vaccinated for the upcoming influenza season.

September 15, 2009
- The FDA announced its approval of four 2009 H1N1 influenza vaccines.

September 30, 2009
- U.S. placed first orders of 2009 H1N1 vaccine.

October 2009
- National influenza 2009 H1N1 vaccination campaign initiated.

October 5, 2009
- First doses of H1N1 vaccine were given in the United States.

October 24, 2009
- Influenza activity reached its highest level in the reporting week ending October 24, 2009, with 48 of 50 states reported widespread activity.

Late October
- Second wave of H1N1 flu activity peaked in the United States.

November 16, 2009
- The FDA announced its approval of a fifth 2009 H1N1 vaccine.

November 23, 2009
- No school closures throughout the United States, first time since August 25, 2009.

December 2009
- Results of trials conducted among adults were published in December, and the data indicated that the immune response among vaccinated adults was excellent.

December 4, 2009
- The CDC published preliminary safety results for the 2009 H1N1 vaccines for the first months of reports received through the U.S. Vaccine Adverse Event Reporting System (VAERS).

December 18, 2009
- First 100 million doses of 2009 H1N1 vaccine were available for ordering.

Late December 2009
- H1N1 vaccination was opened up to anyone who wanted it.

January 2010
- Activity declined to levels below baseline but persisted for several more months at lower levels.

January 10–16, 2010
- The president of the United States proclaimed National Influenza Vaccination Week (NIVW) and encouraged

all Americans to observe the week by getting vaccinated with the 2009 H1N1 flu vaccine.

February 2010
- The FDA's Vaccines and Related Biological Products Advisory Committee (VRBPAC) selected the 2009 H1N1 virus for inclusion in the 2010–2011 seasonal flu vaccine.

February 18, 2010
- The WHO published recommendations for the composition of influenza virus vaccines for the upcoming Northern Hemisphere influenza season. Components included a 2009 H1N1-like virus.

April 2010
- Between April 2009 and April 2010, the CDC held 61 related media events—39 press briefings and 22 telebriefings—reaching more than 35,000 participants.

August 11, 2010
- The WHO announced the end of the 2009 H1N1 influenza pandemic.[3]

---

[3] "Past Pandemics," Centers for Disease Control and Prevention (CDC), August 10, 2018. Available online. URL: www.cdc.gov/flu/pandemic-resources/basics/past-pandemics.html. Accessed December 21, 2022.

Chapter 42 | COVID-19 Impact on the Global Economy

Chapter Contents

Section 42.1—Pandemic Impact on Mortality and Economy Varies across Age Groups and Geographies 485
Section 42.2—The U.S. Economy and the Global Pandemic 490
Section 42.3—Pandemic Effect on the Global Economy across Various Sectors 506
Section 42.4—COVID-19 Economic Relief 519

Section 42.1 | Pandemic Impact on Mortality and Economy Varies across Age Groups and Geographies

The initial impact of the COVID-19 pandemic on the U.S. economy was widespread and affected people across all age groups and all states while the initial mortality impact targeted mostly older people in just a few states according to independent research by the U.S. Census Bureau.

During April 2020, the first full month of the pandemic, the United States experienced an additional 2.4 deaths per 10,000 individuals beyond predictions based on historical mortality trends. This was a 33 percent increase in all-cause national mortality—deaths caused directly or indirectly by the coronavirus.

There was a weak correlation between increased mortality rates and negative economic impact across states. There were states that experienced significant employment displacement but no additional mortality, for example. On the other hand, there were states that experienced large mortality impacts but modest economic impacts.

These additional deaths during the early days of the pandemic were highly concentrated in older age groups and in a few states.

Recent research examined the relationship between the pandemic's mortality and economic impacts across different age groups and geography.

ECONOMIC IMPACT OF THE COVID-19 PANDEMIC

The COVID-19 pandemic has caused a devastating loss of life, but it has also devastated the nation's economy. Similar to the excess mortality concept, the pandemic's economic impact is calculated by taking the difference between what is expected (based on historical trends) and what actually happens during a given period.

The ratio of employment to population is one measure of economic activity that shows the share of the population 16 years and older working full- or part-time. This measure closely tracks other possible measures of economic activity such as unemployment rate, percent of the population with unemployment insurance claims, consumer spending, and small business employment.

Declines in the employment-to-population ratio that exceeded predictions indicate there was additional employment loss in the country due to the pandemic. The decline in the employment-to-population ratio in the United States in April 2020 was significant. Historical trends predicted a 61.3 percent ratio, but it turned out to be 51.5 percent. This additional national decline was 9.9 per 100 individuals in April 2020 refer to Figure 42.1. That means there were fewer people employed than was expected before the pandemic.

IMPACTS VARIED BY GEOGRAPHY

Deaths caused directly or indirectly by COVID-19 during the first full month of the pandemic were highly geographically concentrated. About half of all national excess deaths were in just two states: New York and New Jersey. But the economic impact pattern was completely different because it was more geographically widespread.

Every state, except for Wyoming, experienced a statistically significant decline in the employment-to-population ratio during that

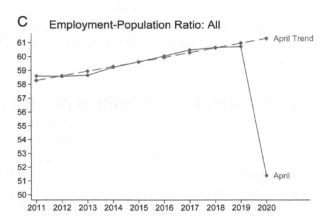

Figure 42.1. U.S Share of Population Working Full- or Part-Time: April 2011–2020

Note: Working population 16 and up. April trend was predicted and observed in the graph.

COVID-19 Impact on the Global Economy

time (refer to Figure 42.2). The two states with the largest initial declines in employment—Nevada and Michigan—only accounted for about seven percent of the national employment displacement.

There was a weak correlation between increased mortality rates and negative economic impact across states. There were states that experienced significant employment displacement but no additional mortality, for example. On the other hand, there were states that experienced large mortality impacts but modest economic impacts (refer to Figure 42.3).

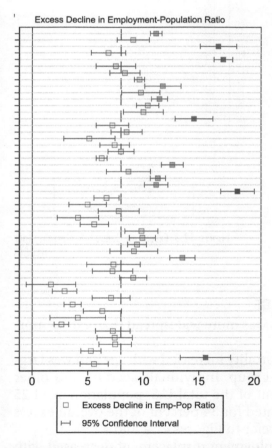

Figure 42.2. Excess Decline in Employment-to-Population Ratio by State: April 2022

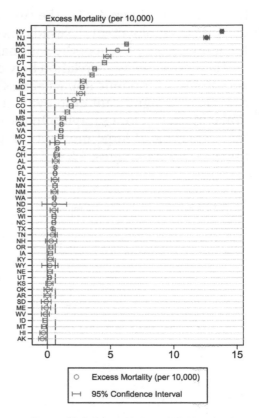

Figure 42.3. Excess All-Cause U.S. Mortality (per 10,000)

DIFFERENT PATTERNS BY AGE

As with geography, job loss was more widespread than excess mortality across age groups.

In April 2020, excess mortality increased with age and was largest among the oldest age group. Individuals aged 85 and older represent only three percent of the total U.S. population aged 25 years and older but accounted for 34 percent of the overall excess mortality in the country (refer to Figures 42.4 and 42.5).

On the other hand, employment displacement decreased with age. It was the largest among the younger age group (aged 25–44).

COVID-19 Impact on the Global Economy

These individuals make up only 39 percent of the U.S. population aged 25 and older but accounted for about half of the people aged 25 and older who lost their jobs nationwide.

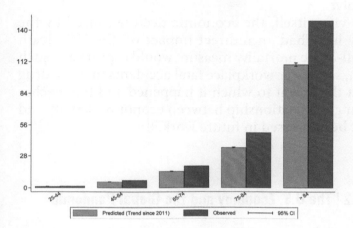

Figure 42.4. All-Cause U.S. Mortality (per 10,000)

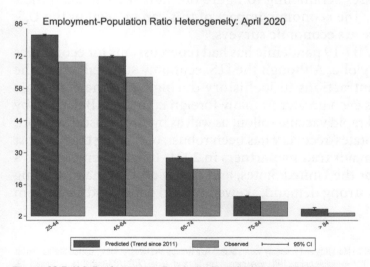

Figure 42.5. U.S. Employment-to-Population Ratio by Age: April 2020

BEYOND THE FIRST MONTH OF THE PANDEMIC

The findings presented here document the pandemic's impacts during April 2020. As the policy response and individuals' behaviors change over time, the mortality and economic impacts will continue to evolve.

Beyond the virus itself, the economic decline caused by the pandemic may have had an indirect impact on the U.S. death count. Excess all-cause mortality measure would capture any such changes—from, say, fewer workplace fatal accidents to more drug overdoses—but the extent to which it happened and the mechanisms underlying the relationship between economic activity and mortality must be addressed in future work.[1]

Section 42.2 | The U.S. Economy and the Global Pandemic

In March 2020, the United States was hit with a global pandemic caused by the coronavirus. The coronavirus pandemic ushered in quarantines, mask mandates, product shortages, business closures, and businesses scrambling to figure out new ways to keep their doors open. The economic impact of this can be seen in the U.S. Census Bureau's economic surveys.

The COVID-19 pandemic has had repercussions for economies around the globe. Although the U.S. economy suffered one of the sharpest contractions in its history during 2020, the economic damage was even greater in many foreign countries. Bolstered by an early and rapid vaccine rollout as well as by strong fiscal support, the United States' recovery has been robust, outpacing that of most of the U.S. major trading partners in 2021. Inflation emerged as a challenge for the United States, and nearly all U.S. major trading partners, as strong demand, skewed toward goods and away from services.

---

[1] "Pandemic Impact on Mortality and Economy Varies across Age Groups and Geographies," United States Census Bureau, March 25, 2022. Available online. URL: www.census.gov/library/stories/2021/03/initial-impact-covid-19-on-united-states-economy-more-widespread-than-on-mortality.html. Accessed December 30, 2022.

COVID-19 Impact on the Global Economy

As a result of the rapid U.S. recovery relative to the rest of the world, the U.S. trade deficit has widened. The strength of the U.S. recovery has led to increased imports, as goods have flowed in from abroad to satisfy resurgent demand from firms and consumers. Although exports have hit record highs, they have increased at a slower pace than imports because many of the countries that buy U.S. goods have not recovered as fast. At the same time, new waves of infection depressed international travel and weighed on the recovery of some services that are important for U.S. exports, such as tourism.

The pandemic highlighted the need to tackle long-standing economic issues, including those resulting from global economic integration. Due to a lack of supportive public policy in the past, many American workers and communities have borne the costs of shifting production around the world but have not fully shared in its benefits, contributing to widening inequality.

Addressing these inadequacies requires policies that broaden the gains from trade while leveling the international economic playing field by countering unfair trade practices and putting in place a more equitable global tax system. Implementing such policy changes in a way that reduces uncertainty and engages with the United States' trade and commercial partners can ensure that American consumers, workers, businesses, and investors benefit from global trade.

This chapter first places America's economic experience during the pandemic in the global context by comparing it with that of the U.S. largest trading partners: the euro area, the United Kingdom, China, Canada, and Mexico. The next section examines how international trade has recovered from its sharp pandemic decline, discussing the causes of the widening U.S. trade deficit and the effects of supply chain bottlenecks internationally on traded inputs such as auto parts and capital goods. The last section discusses how the Biden–Harris Administration is reorienting U.S. international economic policy to mitigate rather than exacerbate economic inequality and to level the international economic playing field.

RECOVERY AMID GLOBAL ECONOMIC CHALLENGES

Placing the U.S. recovery from the COVID-19 pandemic in the global context highlights how U.S. robust fiscal support resulted in a faster return to a strong economy. The backdrop to this demand-driven recovery, however, was a tragic loss of human lives and higher inflation.

The Global Pandemic

The path of the global economy over the past year is best understood in the context of the coronavirus pandemic. The starkest measure of the pandemic's effect is the number of deaths attributed to COVID-19. By the end of 2021, reported deaths due to the virus had exceeded five million people globally, including more than 827,000 in the United States. The true global toll is probably much higher because data collection challenges outside the United States suggest that many other countries may have substantially under-reported deaths. For example, some estimates put the true death toll in India alone in excess of four million. With deaths measured as a share of the population, many of the hardest-hit countries have been middle-income countries in Latin America and Eastern Europe.

Looking at total deaths can obscure the fact that different countries have been hit by waves of differing severity at different times. Which country is faring worst at any point in time has varied significantly. Official data show that the United States, the United Kingdom, and the euro area have all had the highest recorded cases per capita at some point in time. Early in the pandemic, the United States led in per capita cases while the United Kingdom led in deaths. In the second half of 2021, the reverse was true. And the euro area reported the highest per capita cases in the spring of 2021. This variation demonstrates how nearly all major economies have been severely affected at some point during the pandemic.

Progress and timeliness in vaccinating populations have also varied across countries. Both the United States and the United Kingdom managed rapid vaccine rollouts that made them early leaders in the share of the population vaccinated. Rollouts in Canada and the euro area accelerated dramatically in the summer of 2021, and vaccination rates in both places have since reached higher levels than in other major U.S. trading partners. During the second half of 2021, vaccination rates in many middle-income countries, such as Mexico, approached that of the United States, while rates in low-income developing countries remain substantially lower.

The United States' Economic Recovery in the Global Context

The path of real gross domestic product (GDP) since the onset of the COVID-19 pandemic provides the most basic measure of the virus's economic impact. The pandemic was accompanied by historic drops in output in almost all major economies. The U.S. GDP fell by 8.9 percent in the second quarter of 2020, the largest single-quarter contraction in more than 70 years. Most other major economies fared even worse. The GDP of the United Kingdom in 2020 is as follows: Quarter 2 (Q2) was 21.4 percent below its average in 2019. In the euro area, output fell by more than 12.4 percent. Closer to home, Canada's GDP was down 12.4 percent, while Mexico's GDP fell by 19 percent.

The U.S. recovery has outpaced that of all its major trading partners except China. By the second quarter of 2021, the U.S. real GDP exceeded its prepandemic level, ahead of most other major economies. Output growth picked up in the euro area and Canada in the third quarter of 2021 but, at the end of 2021, output in most major U.S. trading partners had only just reached its prepandemic level, while U.S output was three percent higher than before the pandemic. Though many effects of the pandemic are not captured by the GDP, measured by this most basic indicator, the United States' recovery remained farther along than those of nearly all its peers.

The initial drop in real output in China was of a very similar magnitude to that of the United States, but the initial recovery was even faster. By the third quarter of 2020, China's real GDP had not only exceeded its prepandemic level but was also above what would have been expected based on its prepandemic trend. The Chinese government did extend substantial support, primarily through infrastructure spending. However, exports have been a key driver of China's recovery, climbing to more than 40 percent above their prepandemic level by the fourth quarter of 2021. As a result, the contribution of net exports to China's real GDP growth reached nearly 30 percent in 2020, its highest level in more than 20 years.

In this way, China has benefited from the pandemic-induced pivot of global consumption away from services and toward goods, many of which are manufactured in China. Despite continuing support from strong demand for its exports, output growth in China slowed in the second half of 2021 as government support for the economy was withdrawn.

Future research by economists will fully assess what enabled some economies to weather the pandemic shock better or to bounce back more quickly. Based on what is known now, there are two areas of policy where the U.S. response stands out. The first is the speed of the vaccine rollout, discussed above. The fact that more than 40 percent of the U.S. population was fully vaccinated by May 2021, when vaccination rates in most European countries were still less than half that, gave U.S. economic rebound an important head start.

The other area where the United States stands apart is fiscal policy, suggesting that this also played a role in accelerating the recovery beyond those of most of the trading partners. U.S. federal government spending to directly support firms and workers, as well as state and local governments, was substantially larger than comparable efforts in other major economies refer to Figure 42.6. As of the third quarter of 2021, the cumulative U.S. discretionary fiscal response (including not only additional spending but also revenue forgone due to discretionary tax cuts) exceeded 25 percent of GDP. By comparison, the U.K. response was under 20 percent of GDP, and average spending in the euro area was 12 percent of GDP. The scale here helped ensure that by the end of 2021, U.S. consumption had returned to its precrisis trend, while in the euro area, for example, consumption remained below its precrisis level.

THE CHALLENGE OF INFLATION

Inflation has proved a serious challenge for many countries during the recovery. In the 12-month period ending December 2021, headline consumer price inflation in the euro area was 5.0 percent, well above its average of about one percent in the five years before the pandemic. Canada and the United Kingdom have also seen substantially higher inflation than was the case before 2020.

COVID-19 Impact on the Global Economy

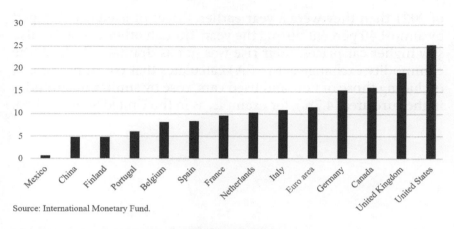

Source: International Monetary Fund.

Figure 42.6. Discretionary Fiscal Response, 2020:Q1–2021:Q3
Percentage of 2020 GDP

Inflation has also risen here; indeed, U.S. inflation has run higher than that of most of its major trading partners although the gap narrowed in the second half of 2021.

The fact that inflation has accelerated in so many countries underscores its common drivers. Pandemic-induced changes in behavior led to relatively more demand for goods than services. In many countries, the balance of consumption remained unusually tilted toward goods throughout 2021, so demand for goods grew substantially faster than would have been the case in a normal recovery. As a result, the world's economic recovery put stress on the already-vulnerable global supply chains for consumer goods. This phenomenon of recovering demand for goods interacting with supply constraints can help explain the relatively higher inflation in the United States, where the recovery was relatively stronger. Looking across countries, inflation was higher where the gap between the real GDP and its prepandemic level—a main measure of progress toward economic recovery—was smaller (refer to Figure 42.7).

Rising prices for motor vehicles were a key driver of U.S. inflation, with prices of new cars nearly 12 percent higher at the end of 2021 than they were a year earlier. Prices of used cars jumped by almost 40 percent during the year. Though other countries also saw higher car prices, their rise was not as dramatic. Indeed, the commodity exchange act (CEA) calculates that consumer prices, excluding those of new and used cars, rose by similar magnitudes in the euro area (4.7%), for example, as in the United States (5.1%).

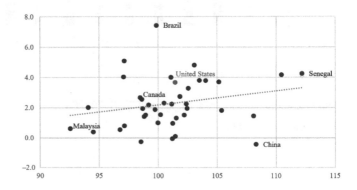

Figure 42.7. Recovery in Output and Inflation
National data organizations
Annualized CPI growth, February 2020–September 2021

Globally, factors pushing up car prices included rebounding demand and a shortage of semiconductors. Car manufacturers both in the United States and abroad have faced production challenges due to the semiconductor shortage, but during 2021, U.S. auto production outpaced that of many peers. At the end of 2021, U.S. auto production stood at just under five percent below its prepandemic level, ahead of the recovery of German, French, and Japanese production. Thus, the greater rise in U.S. prices came in spite of a faster recovery in production. The fact that the rise in car prices has been larger here than abroad stems partly from the particularly resilient demand created by the U.S. recovery passing through to the auto sector—real consumer spending on new motor vehicles rose 16 percent in 2021, a level reaching 18 percent above its prepandemic level. Though higher vehicle prices do pose challenges for American households and businesses, the strength of the recovery in the U.S. auto sector relative to other major auto-producing countries highlights the important benefits of the U.S. demand-driven recovery for workers and businesses.

INTERNATIONAL TRADE, THE ECONOMIC RECOVERY, AND LINGERING COVID-19 CHALLENGES

In 2021, international trade broadly recovered from the sharp decline that followed the onset of the COVID-19 pandemic, with U.S. exports and imports of goods exceeding prepandemic records. Import growth outpaced export growth, widening the U.S. trade deficit. Though trade in goods broadly recovered in 2021, supply bottlenecks slowed the recovery of both imports and exports of such products as automotive and capital goods that are at the heart of the global value chains that were disrupted by pandemic-related challenges.

In contrast, waves of COVID-19 infections have weighed down the recovery of cross-border trade in services. Although trade in services that are less reliant on personal contact followed a recovery pattern similar to goods, others—particularly travel and transportation services—continue to be impaired by the persistence of the virus. The sharp contraction of trade in travel services was a notable drag on the U.S. trade balance in 2021. Exports of these services in the form of foreign tourists, students, and business travelers are typically a significant contributor to the surplus in the U.S. trade balance in services.

The U.S. Trade Balance

The strong domestic demand for goods that has characterized the economic recovery in 2021 is reflected in the deepening deficit of the U.S. trade balance—defined as the difference between the total value of goods and services that U.S. residents buy from abroad and the value of all the U.S. goods and services sold abroad. At four percent of GDP, the 2021 trade deficit is the largest since 2008 (measured as a share of GDP; refer to Figure 42.8). Deeper trade deficits in the United States over the past two decades have been correlated with economic growth because they reflect strong demand; 2021 was no exception.

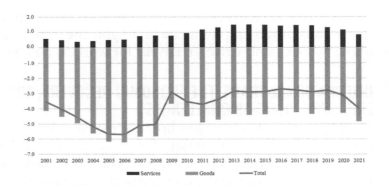

Figure 42.8. U.S. Trade Balance, 2001–2021
Bureau of Economic Analysis (BEA)
Percentage of GDP

Over the past 20 years, the United States has typically maintained a deficit in goods trade that is partially offset by a surplus in services trade. The higher overall trade deficit in 2021 reflected a larger goods trade deficit and a smaller services trade surplus relative to recent years. In particular, the increase in the goods and services trade deficit from 2.8 percent of GDP in 2019 to 4.0 percent in 2021 reflects a 0.5 percentage point reduction in the services surplus and a 0.7 percentage point increase in the goods trade deficit (refer to Figure 42.8). Although both developments can be traced to challenges stemming from COVID-19, the reasons for these outcomes are distinct.

The increases in consumption and investment expenditures that drove strong economic growth in 2021 entailed greater expenditures on both domestically produced and imported goods and services. American producers of goods, challenged by pandemic-induced labor and input supply obstacles, strained to keep pace with the surging domestic demand for goods, which reduced the available supply for exports. The dampening of growth in exports of U.S. goods was amplified by the fact that America's fiscal policy response was larger than most other major economies (refer to Figure 42.6). Though demand here exceeded its prepandemic trend, demand abroad lagged. As a result, American firms and consumers stepped up purchases of imported goods to a greater degree than their foreign counterparts, widening the U.S. trade deficit in goods. Also, contributing to the widening goods trade deficit was the shift in the balance of trade in oil and petroleum products from surplus to deficit. Furthermore, restrictions on foreign nationals entering the United States and rising costs of maritime freight transportation, a service that is primarily provided by foreign-owned firms, brought down the surplus in services trade.

Macroeconomic developments here and abroad have contributed to the widening trade deficit through another channel: exchange rate movements. As the COVID-19 virus spread in early 2020, the U.S. dollar appreciated 9.7 percent from January to late March, reflecting the dollar's status as a safe asset (refer to Figure 42.9). In times of heightened economic uncertainty, investors around the world purchase dollar assets, which they view as a reliable store of value. From the end of March 2020 through the end of 2020, the dollar depreciated as global financial conditions began to normalize and the earlier flight to safety was reversed. That depreciation also reflected the very aggressive action of the Federal Reserve to support the U.S. economy by keeping interest rates low. This benefits American businesses and households that borrow to purchase equipment or homes, but it makes U.S. financial assets less attractive to global investors. Lower foreign demand for U.S. assets, in turn, resulted in dollar depreciation from April through December 2020, as seen in Figure 42.9.

In 2021, the dollar resumed appreciating and ended the year up 3.6 percent against the currencies of its major trading partners, as measured by a Federal Reserve Board index (refer to Figure 42.9). Expectations were that the Federal Reserve would begin to tighten policy earlier than other central banks and that contributed to the rise in the dollar's value. Such expectations reflected two aspects of America's macroeconomic performance relative to the trading partners: the more rapid recovery in U.S. output and the relatively larger rise in inflation. A strengthening dollar tends to widen the trade deficit by making imported goods cheaper for American consumers, which boosts imports, and U.S. exports become more expensive for foreign buyers, depressing exports.

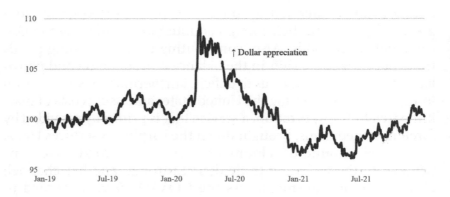

Figure 42.9. Nominal Broad Dollar Index
Federal Reserve Board
Index level: January 2, 2020 = 100

International Trade in Goods

U.S. trade in goods rebounded relatively quickly after the sharp drop at the onset of the COVID-19 pandemic in 2020 and continued to rise through 2021. Both exports and imports of goods broke nominal records set in 2018. Goods imports breached record levels in real terms as well. This swift and robust rebound stands in sharp contrast to the stagnation in trade that followed the Great Recession, beginning in 2008 (refer to Figure 42.10). From the start of the Great Recession, goods exports did not recover from their precrisis peak for more than two years, and goods imports did not systematically rise above their precrisis peak for nearly 10 years.

As discussed in the previous section, 2021 growth in imports generally outpaced that of exports. This has been true throughout the economic recovery. Even though goods imports had fully recovered in real terms to prepandemic levels by November 2020, U.S. exports did not achieve that feat until more than a year later, in October 2021. The faster recovery of imports relative to exports is a direct consequence of the broader macroeconomic context discussed earlier in this chapter. However, the effects of

COVID-19 Impact on the Global Economy

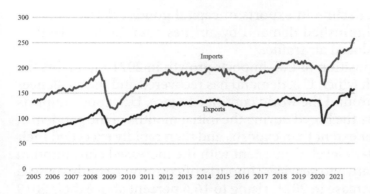

Figure 42.10. U.S. Trade in Goods
Census Bureau
Dollars (in billions)

pandemic-related disruptions inhibited export recovery for some products more than others.

In real terms, U.S. exports of food, feed, and beverages were little affected and exceeded their February 2020 levels for most of the second half of that year. U.S. exports of consumer goods surpassed their prepandemic level in November 2020. By contrast, exports of capital goods did not exceed their prepandemic value until April 2021 and remained at about that level for the rest of the year. Exports of autos and parts were more than 10 percent below their prepandemic level for most of the year.

The relatively swift rebound in exports of consumer goods highlights the global nature of the pandemic-induced switch from services to goods consumption. The softer performance of capital goods and auto exports reflects the flip side of the strong demand unleashed by the economic recovery. Supply challenges for critical inputs disrupted the global value chains that characterize production in the automotive and other capital goods industries, inhibiting their ability to meet surging domestic and foreign demand. The final goods produced and exported by American businesses in these industries are complex. Automotive exports often rely on semiconductors, the global supply of which was notably stressed in 2021. Civilian aircraft, engines, and parts represented the largest share of the decline in exports of capital goods relative to 2019, reflecting diminished demand by airlines after COVID-19 dramatically reduced air traffic.

The composition of U.S. imports growth in 2021 highlights the strength with which U.S. demand has recovered and the challenges economies around the world continue to face. U.S. goods imports dipped across the board during the initial months of the pandemic, but to a lesser extent than exports, and then rapidly exceeded their pre-COVID-19 level. Consistent with the increased consumption of goods relative to services, imports of consumer goods showed a striking increase in 2021, rising to 16.6 percent above their 2019 level. Imports of capital goods, such as machinery used in factories, also rose notably in 2021 to 11.3 percent in real terms above their 2019 level, as domestic American firms expanded to satisfy booming U.S. demand.

The trajectory of automotive imports illustrates the global nature of the supply chain stresses that emerged during 2021. Though automotive imports initially rebounded, they subsequently declined as global supply chains were disrupted. Imports in this category were 9.6 percent below their 2019 level in 2021. This category includes both motor vehicles and parts, but the decline was entirely due to falling imports of finished vehicles, while parts were slightly above their 2019 level. As discussed previously in this chapter, the recovery of the U.S. automotive sector outpaced that of other major auto-manufacturing countries in 2021.

International Trade in Services

In contrast to the relatively swift recovery of trade in goods, the exigencies of containing the spread of COVID-19 continue to suppress global demand for services. The overall decline in both exports and imports of services at the onset of the pandemic (refer to Figure 42.11) is primarily due to a steep drop in trade in travel services (refer to Figure 42.12). Total exports and imports of services other than travel and transportation services—which covers finance, insurance, maintenance, construction, information, personal and government services, intellectual property, and other services—exceeded their 2019 value in 2021.

COVID-19 Impact on the Global Economy

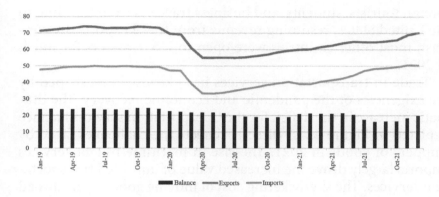

Figure 42.11. Trade in Services

Bureau of Economic Analysis
Dollars (billions)

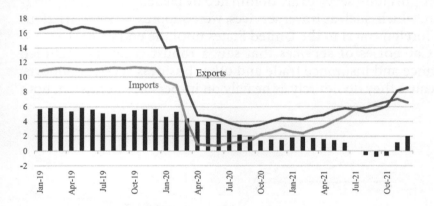

Figure 42.12. Trade in Travel Services

Bureau of Economic Analysis
Dollars (in billions)

Figure 42.12 illustrates that neither imports nor exports of travel services have approached their prepandemic levels. However, while imports of travel services have increased relatively steadily since the pandemic first hit the United States, exports saw only a minimal increase until November 2021 when the Biden-Harris Administration eased travel restrictions that had prevented many foreign tourists, students, and business travelers from traveling to the United States, resuming revenue from travel exports. By contrast, most other countries were open to U.S. travelers for much of 2021.

Trade in transportation services has likewise been shaped by the exigencies of the pandemic and economic recovery. The dramatic increase in the deficit for the transportation services balance depicted in Figure 42.13 directly reflects the challenges faced by shippers of goods in 2021. The rise in maritime freight services imports largely drove the increased value of imported transportation services. The skyrocketing cost of moving goods from abroad to the United States meant that U.S. importers paid dramatically more to shipping companies.

Because nearly all major shipping firms are foreign-owned, these costs register as U.S. service imports. In contrast, U.S. exports of transportation services are dominated by passenger air transportation, which, such as travel services, were suppressed by restrictions on foreign travel to the United States until the end of 2021.

Categories of services that saw a robust recovery included finance and insurance trade and other business services imports. Because they do not rely as heavily on in-person interaction, both

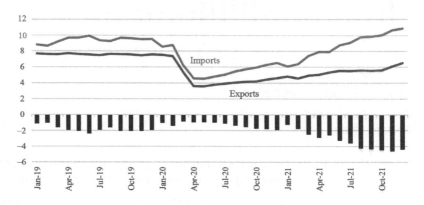

Figure 42.13. Trade in Transportation Services
Bureau of Economic Analysis
Dollars (in billions)

imports and exports increased year-on-year relative to their 2019 levels throughout the pandemic and recovery. Similarly, trade in intellectual property, telecommunications, and other business services recovered quickly and is now above 2019 levels.

CONCLUSION

Comparing the performance of the United States' economy during 2021 with that of the trading partners demonstrates this country's resilience at a time of daunting challenges. Supported by a strong fiscal response and a rapid vaccine rollout, the GDP of the United States exceeded its prepandemic level before those of other major advanced economies. However, as the recovery got under way, demand continued to tilt toward goods and away from services. This shift in global consumption patterns interacted with stressed supply chains to generate inflation in the United States and most of the major trading partners although this effect was particularly pronounced here due to the relative strength of the recovery. The faster pace of the U.S. economic recovery has also resulted in a widening trade deficit.

Openness to international commerce provides substantial benefits to the U.S. economy. However, these benefits have at times come at the cost of wider domestic inequality. You must engage with your partners and allies to make international economic engagement work for all Americans, by ensuring that the global rules are aligned with domestic objectives and values and that these rules are rigorously enforced.[2]

---

[2] "The U.S. Economy and the Global Pandemic," Whitehouse.gov. April 23, 2022. Available online. URL: www.whitehouse.gov/wp-content/uploads/2022/04/Chapter-3-new.pdf. Accessed November 29, 2022.

COVID-19 and the Coronavirus Sourcebook, First Edition

Section 42.3 | **Pandemic Effect on the Global Economy across Various Sectors**

ECONOMIC INDICATORS: SALES, REVENUE, AND VALUE OF SHIPMENTS

The Census Bureau's economic indicator surveys captured the initial shock of the coronavirus pandemic, as well as economic trends since the national emergency was declared on March 13, 2020. Figures 42.14–42.17 show the impact across key sectors of the

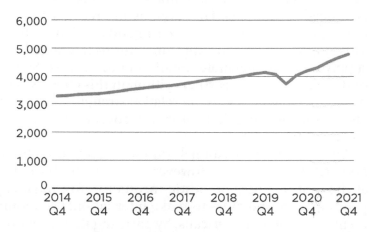

Figure 42.14. Economic Indicator Surveys—Sales, Revenues, and Value of Shipments: 2014–2021—Selected Services Total Quarterly Revenue (Estimates Are Seasonally Adjusted and Presented in Billions of Dollars)

Source: U.S. Census Bureau, Quarterly Services Survey, March 11, 2022 (www.census.gov/services).
Note: Estimates are based on data for employer firms. Data are adjusted for seasonal variation but not for price changes. Differences between estimates may be attributed to sampling or nonsampling error, rather than underlying economic conditions. Caution should be used in drawing conclusions from the estimates and comparisons shown. Information on the survey methodology, including sampling error (e.g., standard errors and relative standard errors) and nonsampling error, is available at www..census.gov/services/qss/how_the_data_are_collected.html. The Census Bureau has reviewed this data product for unauthorized disclosure of confidential information and has approved the disclosure avoidance practices applied.

COVID-19 Impact on the Global Economy

nation's economy, including services, retail trade, wholesale trade, and manufacturing. The data from all four graphs show a dip in estimated sales, revenue, and value of shipments in 2020 followed by a recovery through the fourth quarter of 2021.

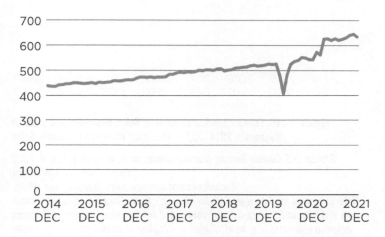

Figure 42.15. Economic Indicator Surveys—Sales, Revenues, and Value of Shipments: 2014–2021—Retail and Food Service Monthly Sales (Estimates Are Seasonally Adjusted and Presented in Billions of Dollars)

Source: U.S. Census Bureau, Advance Monthly Retail Trade Survey, May 17, 2022 (www.census.gov/retail).
Note: Estimates are based on a sample of employer firms. Firms without paid employees, or nonemployers, are represented in the published estimates through the estimation procedure. Data are adjusted for seasonal variation and holiday and trading-day differences but not for price changes. Differences between estimates may be attributed to sampling or nonsampling error, rather than underlying economic conditions. Caution should be used in drawing conclusions from the estimates and comparisons shown. Information on the survey methodology, including sampling error (e.g., standard errors and relative standard errors) and nonsampling error, is available at www.census.gov/retail/how_surveys_are_collected.html. The Census Bureau has reviewed this data product for unauthorized disclosure of confidential information and has approved the disclosure avoidance practices applied.

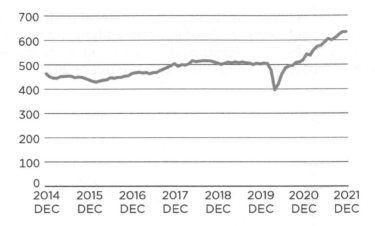

Figure 42.16. Economic Indicator Surveys: Sales, Revenues, and Value of Shipments: 2014–2021—Merchant Wholesaler[1] Monthly Sales

Source: U.S. Census Bureau, Monthly Wholesale Trade Survey, May 9, 2022 (www.census.gov/wholesale).
[1] Excludes manufacturers' sales branches and offices.
Note: Estimates are based on data for employer firms. Data are adjusted for seasonal variation and trading-day differences but not for price changes. Differences between estimates may be attributed to sampling or nonsampling error, rather than underlying economic conditions. Caution should be used in drawing conclusions from the estimates and comparisons shown. Information on the survey methodology, including sampling error (e.g., standard errors and relative standard errors) and nonsampling error, is available at www.census.gov/wholesale/www/how_surveys_are_collected/monthly_methodology.html.
The Census Bureau has reviewed this data product for unauthorized disclosure of confidential information and has approved the disclosure avoidance practices applied.

Manufacturing: Days Closed

As a result of the pandemic, some plants within the manufacturing sector stopped production throughout the year. Manufacturing plants were faced with new safety protocols, falling demand, supply shortages, and reduced worker availability. The average number of days closed varied by subsector as seen in Figure 42.18. Among all subsectors in the manufacturing sector, the Apparel Manufacturing subsector had an average number of days closed of 38.2 days. The Leather and Allied Product Manufacturing subsector had an average number of days closed of 22.6 days.

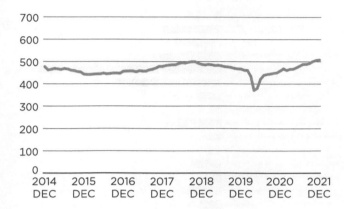

Figure 42.17. Economic Indicator Surveys: Sales, Revenues, and Value of Shipments: 2014–2021—Monthly Value of Shipments of Manufactured Goods (Estimates Are Seasonally Adjusted and Presented in Billions of Dollars)

Source: U.S. Census Bureau, Manufacturers's Shipments, Inventories, and Orders Survey, May 13, 2022 (www.census.gov/manufacturing/m3).
Note: Data are adjusted for seasonality but not price changes. Statistical significance is not measurable for this survey. The Manufacturers' Shipments, Inventories, and Orders estimates are not based on a probability sample, so the sampling error of these estimates cannot be measured nor can the confidence intervals be computed.
The Census Bureau has reviewed this data product for unauthorized disclosure of confidential information and has approved the disclosure avoidance practices applied.

Health Care and Social Assistance: Telemedicine

The COVID-19 pandemic resulted in businesses in the health-care and social assistance sector relying more on telemedicine. Figure 42.19 shows that for most health-care industries offering telemedicine services in 2020, revenue from telemedicine accounted for less than five percent of their total revenue. The three industries with the largest percentage of total revenue from telemedicine services all provided mental health services.

Retail: Changes in Sales and E-commerce Sales

With the pandemic causing store closures, businesses had to adjust and rely on e-commerce. The retail data collected show

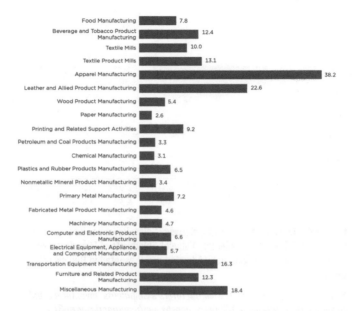

Figure 42.18. Average Number of Days Closed by Manufacturing Subsector: 2020

Source: U.S. Census Bureau, 2020 Annual Survey of Manufactures (https://data.census.gov/cedsci/table?q=AM1831BASIC06&g=0100000US, %240400000&tid=ASMAREA2017.AM1831BASIC06).
Note: Estimates are based on data for employer firms. Differences in estimates may be attributed to sampling or nonsampling error, rather than underlying economic conditions. Caution should be used in drawing conclusions from the estimates and comparisons shown. Information on the survey methodology, including sampling error (e.g., standard errors and relative standard errors) and nonsampling error, is available at www.census.gov/programs-surveys/asm/technical-documentation/methodology.html.

an increase in e-commerce in the industries as shown in Figure 42.20. Non-e-commerce sales were calculated as total sales minus e-commerce sales. The Food and Beverage Store industry experienced the highest growth in e-commerce sales for 2020 with a year-to-year increase of 172.7 percent. Motor Vehicle and Parts Dealers, Health and Personal Care Stores, Gasoline Stations, and General Merchandise Stores are not shown due to confidentiality issues in either or both years.

COVID-19 Impact on the Global Economy

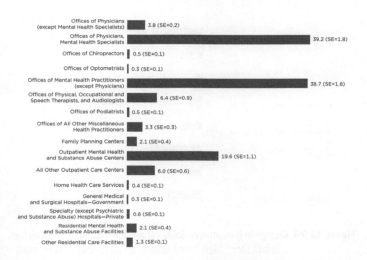

Figure 42.19. Telemedicine as a Percentage of Total Revenue for Select Service Industries: 2020

Source: U.S. Census Bureau, 2020 Service Annual Survey (www.census.gov/data/tables/2020/econ/services/sas-naics.html).
Note: Estimates are based on data for employer firms. Differences in estimates may be attributed to sampling or nonsampling error, rather than underlying economic conditions. Caution should be used in drawing conclusions from the estimates and comparisons shown. Estimates of sampling variability are measured using standard errors (SE). SEs are expressed as percents. Information on the survey methodology, including sampling error (e.g., standard errors and relative standard errors) and nonsampling error, is available at www.census.gov/programs-surveys/sas/technical-documentation/methodology.html. The Census Bureau has reviewed this data product for unauthorized disclosure of confidential information and has approved the disclosure avoidance practices applied.

Generally, e-commerce divisions of brick-and-mortar companies would be included in the Nonstore Retailers subsector as part of the Electronic Shopping and Mail-Order Houses industry as long as they do not fulfill e-commerce orders from their stores.

Wholesale: E-commerce Sales as a Percentage of Total Sales

U.S. merchant wholesalers had sales of $8,037.4 billion in 2020, a 6.6 percent decrease from $8,607.1 billion in 2019. E-commerce

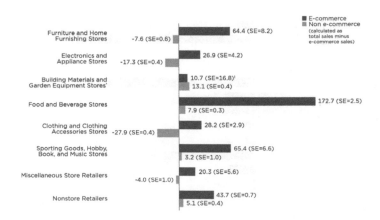

Figure 42.20. Change in E-commerce Sales versus Non-e-commerce Sales by Select Three-Digit Retail Subsector: 2019–2020 (in Percent)

Source: U.S. Census Bureau, 2020 Annual Retail Trade Survey (www.census.gov/data/tables/2020/econ/arts/annual-report.html).
*Percent change estimates for e-commerce and non-e-commerce sales are not significantly different from each other at the 90 percent confidence level.
[1]Percent change estimate is not significantly different from zero at the 90 percent confidence level.
Note: Estimates are based on a sample of employer firms. Firms without paid employees, or nonemployers, are included in the estimates through imputation or administrative data provided by other federal agencies. Estimates are not adjusted for price changes. Differences between estimates may be attributed to sampling or nonsampling error, rather than underlying economic conditions. Caution should be used in drawing conclusions from the estimates and comparisons shown. Estimates of sampling variability are measured using standard errors (SE). SEs are expressed as percents. Information on confidentiality protection, sampling error, nonsampling error, sample design, and definitions is available at www.census.gov/programs-surveys/arts/technical-documentation/methodology.html. The Census Bureau has reviewed this data product for unauthorized disclosure of confidential information and has approved the disclosure avoidance practices applied.

sales of U.S. merchant wholesalers were $2,860.0 billion in 2020, a 1.0 percent decrease from $2,887.9 billion in 2019.

E-commerce as a percentage of total sales, though, increased to 35.6 percent in 2020 from 33.6 percent in 2019. Figure 42.21 shows that Household Appliances and Electrical and Electronic Goods Merchant Wholesalers e-commerce as a percentage of sales was 36.7 percent in 2020 and Grocery and Related Products

COVID-19 Impact on the Global Economy

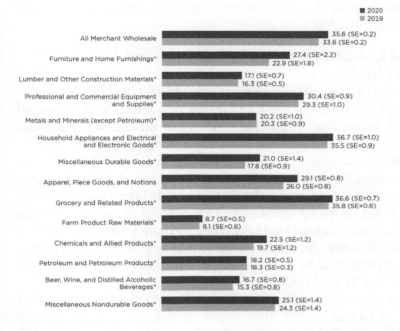

Figure 42.21. E-commerce Sales as a Percentage of Total Sales for U.S. Merchant Wholesalers for Select Industries: 2019 and 2020

Source: U.S. Census Bureau, 2020 Annual Wholesale Trade Survey (www.census.gov/data/tables/2020/econ/awts/annual-reports.html).
*Estimates for 2020 and 2019 are not significantly different from each other at the 90 percent confidence level. [1] Includes manufacturers' sales branches and offices.
Note: Estimates are based on data for employer firms. Differences in estimates may be attributed to sampling or nonsampling error, rather than underlying economic conditions. Caution should be used in drawing conclusions from the estimates and comparisons shown. Estimates of sampling variability are measured using standard errors (SE). SEs are expressed as percents. Additional information on the survey methodology, including sampling error (e.g., standard errors and relative standard errors) and nonsampling error, may be found at www.census.gov/programs-surveys/awts/technical-documentation/methodology.html. The Census Bureau has reviewed this data product for unauthorized disclosure of confidential information and has approved the disclosure avoidance practices applied.

Merchant Wholesalers e-commerce as a percentage of sales was 36.6 percent in 2020.

Financial Assistance Received by Companies and How They Used It

The sources of financial assistance requested/received by companies with employees during the COVID-19 pandemic were collected across 19 sectors in 2020. The majority of businesses requested assistance from the Paycheck Protection Program (PPP).

Financial assistance from the PPP was requested by 61.7 percent of companies with employees and received by 58.3 percent. Financial assistance from the Economic Injury Disaster Loan (EIDL) program was requested by 21.6 percent of companies with employees and received by 18.5 percent. Financial assistance from the Small Business Administration (SBA) Forgiveness Loan program was requested by 21.0 percent of companies with employees and received by 16.2 percent.

Figure 42.22 shows the percentage of companies in six selected sectors of the economy that received financial assistance by source. The selected sectors receiving financial assistance from the PPP include Mining (68.7%), Educational Services (67.9%), and Accommodation and Food Services (67.7%). The selected sectors receiving financial assistance from the EIDL program include Educational Services (23.9%); Health Care and Social Assistance (23.3%); Arts, Entertainment, and Recreational Services (23.8%); and Accommodation and Food Services (33.5%). The selected sectors receiving financial assistance from the SBA Forgiveness Loan program include Manufacturing (19.5%), Health Care and Social Assistance (22.7%), and Accommodation and Food Services (23.1%).

In 2020, 61.0 percent of companies with employees received financial assistance from one or more sources and used the funds to rehire or maintain employees on their payroll; 20.1 percent used the funds to pay the rent/mortgage, 15.3 percent for utilities, 2.2 percent for capital expenditures, and 5.6 percent for all other expenses. Companies may have reported the use of the funds received in more than one category.

Figure 42.23 shows the use of financial assistance for seven selected sectors of the economy. The selected sectors using

COVID-19 Impact on the Global Economy

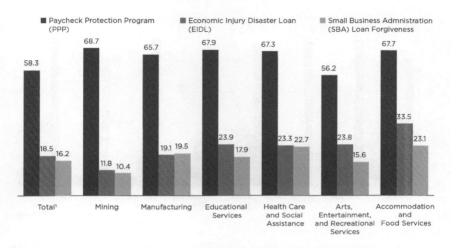

Figure 42.22. Percentage of Companies Receiving Financial Assistance during the Coronavirus Pandemic: 2020 (Companies with Employees)

Source: U.S. Census Bureau, 2020 Annual Capital Expenditures Survey (www.census.gov/library/publications/2022/econ/2020-aces-covid-impact.html).
[1]Percentage of companies for all published sectors.
Note: Estimates are based on data for employer firms. Differences in estimates may be attributed to sampling or nonsampling error, rather than underlying economic conditions. Caution should be used in drawing conclusions from the estimates and comparisons shown. Information on the survey methodology, including sampling error (e.g., standard errors and relative standard errors) and nonsampling error, is available at www.census.gov/programs-surveys/aces/technical-documentation/methodology.html. The Census Bureau has reviewed this data product for unauthorized disclosure of confidential information and has approved the disclosure avoidance practices applied.

financial assistance for payroll include Mining (70.0%), Retail Trade (67.4%), Educational Services (71.3%), Health Care and Social Assistance (70.2%), and Accommodation and Food Services (72.0%). The selected sectors using financial assistance for rent/mortgage include Retail Trade (24.8%); Educational Services (26.0%); Health Care and Social Assistance (27.1%); Arts, Entertainment, and Recreational Services (26.2%); and Accommodation and Food Services (35.6%). The selected sectors using financial assistance for utilities include Manufacturing (20.3%), Retail Trade (19.3%), Health Care and Social Assistance (19.2%), and Accommodation and Food Services (28.4%). The selected sectors using financial assistance for capital

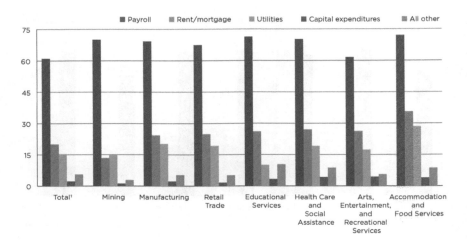

Figure 42.23. Percentage of Companies Using Financial Assistance during the Coronavirus Pandemic: 2020

Source: U.S. Census Bureau, 2020 Annual Capital Expenditures Survey.
Note: Estimates are based on data for employer firms. Differences in estimates may be attributed to sampling or nonsampling error, rather than underlying economic conditions. Caution should be used in drawing conclusions from the estimates and comparisons shown. Information on the survey methodology, including sampling error (e.g., standard errors and relative standard errors) and nonsampling error, is available at www.census.gov/programs-surveys/aces/technical-documentation/methodology.html. The Census Bureau has reviewed this data product for unauthorized disclosure of confidential information and has approved the disclosure avoidance practices applied.

expenditures include Health Care and Social Assistance (4.2%); Arts, Entertainment, and Recreational Services (4.4%); and Accommodation and Food Services (3.9%). Among those selected sectors using financial assistance for all other expenses are Educational Services (10.3%), Health Care and Social Assistance (8.7%), and Accommodation and Food Services (8.6%).

QUARTERLY STATE AND LOCAL TAX REVENUES

The impact of the pandemic is evident in state and local government quarterly tax revenue data, as states followed the federal government's lead in extending tax payment deadlines and delaying tax collections in the spring of 2020. This change disrupted the historical trend of state and local tax collections, especially for individual and corporate income tax payments, which normally peak in the second quarter.

Total state and local tax collections during the second quarter of 2020 were 19 percent lower than in the same quarter of 2019 not only because of the pandemic-related shutdowns and loss of income but also because of the shift in the income tax deadline. By the second quarter of 2021, state and local tax revenue collections rebounded by 46 percent, aided in part by stimulus funding provided by the Coronavirus Aid, Relief, and Economic Security (CARES) Act to assist individuals and businesses.

State Expenditures on Hospital and Health Services

State spending on hospitals and health care is small relative to spending on transportation, education, and public welfare. However, in 2020, spending on hospitals increased by 7.6 percent to $103.5 billion, from $96.1 billion in 2019. During the same time frame, public health care spending rose by 11.4 percent from $69.1 billion to $77.0 billion. Spending on hospitals and health grew by only 6.2 and 6.0 percent, respectively, in 2018 and 2019.

Intergovernmental Revenue

An increase in intergovernmental revenue is a signal of increased movement of funds because of the pandemic. State intergovernmental revenue from federal and local governments increased from $708.5 billion in 2019 to $845.6 billion in 2020, an increase of 19.3 percent compared with an increase of only 3.4 percent from 2018. The dramatic increase in intergovernmental revenue from the federal government specifically for hospitals and health services reflects the eceipt of funding by states for pandemic-related spending. Intergovernmental revenues for hospitals and health from the federal government increased from $25.5 billion in 2019 to $108.6 billion in 2020, a more than fourfold increase.

State and Local Government Pensions

Pensions managers reacted to the uncertainty generated by the pandemic by initially holding more assets in cash and short-term investments. Cash and short-term investments as a proportion of total cash and security holdings increased sharply from 2.9 percent in the fourth quarter of 2019 to 3.8 percent in the first quarter of 2020, then declined slightly to 3.3 percent in the second quarter of 2020. The relative proportion of cash and short-term assets has remained below the peak in the first quarter of 2020, possibly indicating a shift to more risky, high-yielding assets. As the stock market recovered from the pandemic-induced decline in the first quarter of 2020, the value of the public pensions portfolios has increased steadily from the low of $3.7 trillion in the first quarter of 2020 to $5.3 trillion by the fourth quarter of 2021.[3]

---

[3] "The Coronavirus Pandemic's Economic Impact," United States Census Bureau, July 1, 2022. Available online. URL: www2.census.gov/library/publications/2022/economics/coronavirus-pandemics-economic-impact.pdf. Accessed December 30, 2022.

Section 42.4 | COVID-19 Economic Relief

ASSISTANCE FOR AMERICAN FAMILIES AND WORKERS

The COVID-19 public health crisis and resulting economic crisis have created a variety of challenges for families across the country and changed the way you all live and work. The Treasury Department is providing critical assistance to individuals and their families, ensuring people have the opportunity to keep their families safe and thriving, at work and at home.

Economic Impact Payments

The Treasury Department, the Bureau of the Fiscal Service, and the Internal Revenue Service (IRS) rapidly sent out three rounds of direct relief payments during the COVID-19 crisis, and payments from the third round continue to be disbursed to Americans.

Starting in March 2020, the Coronavirus Aid, Relief, and Economic Security Act (CARES Act) provided Economic Impact Payments (EIPs) of up to $1,200 per adult for eligible individuals and $500 per qualifying child under age 17. The payments were reduced for individuals with adjusted gross income (AGI) greater than $75,000 ($150,000 for married couples filing a joint return). For a family of four, these EIPs provided up to $3,400 of direct financial relief.

The COVID-related Tax Relief Act of 2020, enacted in late December 2020, authorized additional payments of up to $600 per adult for eligible individuals and up to $600 for each qualifying child under age 17. The AGI thresholds at which the payments began to be reduced were identical to those under the CARES Act.

The American Rescue Plan Act of 2021 (American Rescue Plan), enacted in early March 2021, provided EIPs of up to $1,400 for eligible individuals or $2,800 for married couples filing jointly, plus $1,400 for each qualifying dependent, including adult dependents.

For this third round of EIPs, the American Rescue Plan requires an additional "plus-up" payment, which is based on information (such as a recently filed 2020 tax return) that the IRS receives after making the initial payment to the eligible individual. In addition, the American Rescue Plan increases direct financial relief to American families by providing $1,400 payments for all qualifying dependents of a family, rather than just qualifying children under age 17.

Normally, a taxpayer will qualify for the full amount of EIP if they have AGI of up to $75,000 for singles and married persons filing a separate return, up to $112,500 for heads of household, and up to $150,000 for married couples filing joint returns and surviving spouses. Payment amounts are reduced for eligible individuals with AGI above those levels.

The Treasury Department and the IRS continue to expand outreach to millions of homeless, rural poor, and other disadvantaged Americans to ensure that they receive EIPs. This includes new and continued relationships with homeless shelters, legal aid clinics, and providing EIP information in more than 35 languages.

Unemployment Compensation

The American Rescue Plan extended employment assistance, starting in March 2021, and waived some federal taxes on unemployment benefits to assist those who lost work due to the COVID-19 crisis.

Across the nation, millions of Americans lost their jobs in the wake of the COVID-19 pandemic and, as a result, claimed unemployment benefits. The American Rescue Plan extended employment assistance, starting in March 2021.

In addition, the American Rescue Plan waives federal income taxes on the first $10,200 of unemployment benefits received in 2020 by individuals with adjusted gross incomes less than $150,000. The tax relief extends to both workers who received benefits through federal unemployment programs as well as those who received traditional benefits through their state unemployment insurance fund. This law will provide tax relief for Americans who lost their jobs and utilized unemployment benefits last year—allowing millions of workers to focus their benefits on covering essentials during the COVID-19 pandemic.

Child Tax Credit

The American Rescue Plan increased the Child Tax Credit and expanded its coverage to better assist families who care for children.

The American Rescue Plan's expansion of the Child Tax Credit will reduce child poverty by:
- supplementing the earnings of families receiving the tax credit
- making the credit available to a significant number of new families

Specifically, the Child Tax Credit was revised in the following ways for 2021:
- The credit amount was increased for 2021. The American Rescue Plan increased the amount of the Child Tax Credit from $2,000 to $3,600 for qualifying children under age six and $3,000 for other qualifying children under age 18.
- The credit was made fully refundable. By making the Child Tax Credit fully refundable, low-income households will be entitled to receive the full credit benefit, as significantly expanded and increased by the American Rescue Plan.
- The credit's scope has been expanded. The American Rescue Plan allowed 17-year-olds to qualify for the Child Tax Credit. Previously, only children 16 and younger qualified.
- Many eligible taxpayers received monthly advance payments of half of their estimated 2021 Child Tax Credit amounts during 2021 from July to December. Families caring for children were able to receive financial assistance on a consistent monthly basis from July to December 2021, instead of waiting until tax filing season to receive all of their Child Tax Credit benefits.

In addition, the American Rescue Plan extended the full Child Tax Credit permanently to Puerto Rico and the U.S. Territories. For the first time, low-income families residing in Puerto Rico and the

U.S. territories will receive this vital financial assistance to better support their children's development and health and educational attainment.

Emergency Rental Assistance
The Emergency Rental Assistance program makes funding available to government entities to assist households that are unable to pay rent or utilities.

HOW FEDERAL RENTAL ASSISTANCE WORKS

Treasury provides emergency rental assistance funding to the Department of Hawaiian Home Lands, Tribally Designated Housing Entities, and state, local, territorial, and tribal governments to distribute assistance to qualifying landlords, utility providers, and renters, which helps struggling renters keep up with rent and other expenses related to housing. Many of these programs offer assistance to landlords, utility providers, and renters. Renters, utility providers, and landlords can find out what emergency rental assistance covers, how it works, and who is eligible on the interagency housing portal hosted by the Consumer Financial Protection Bureau (CFPB).

CIVIL RIGHTS COMPLAINTS

To file a program discrimination complaint about an Emergency Rental Assistance Program, send your complaint to:
   Director, Office of Civil Rights and
   Equal Employment Opportunity
   1500 Pennsylvania Ave., N.W.
   Washington, DC 20220

WHAT THE DEPARTMENT OF THE TREASURY WILL DO TO ENSURE NONDISCRIMINATION

The Department of the Treasury will conduct investigations of civil rights complaints filed against recipients of financial assistance under any of its programs. If discrimination is found, the Department of the Treasury can defer action on an application for federal financial assistance, issue a cautionary letter, or as an ultimate consequence deny funding. Independently of any possible actions to be taken by the Department of the Treasury, courts have interpreted that Title VI provides a private right of action.

REPORT FRAUD, WASTE, AND ABUSE
The Office of Inspector General offers the following guidance, which is also available at Report Fraud, Waste, and Abuse, Office of Inspector General (https://oig.treasury.gov/report-fraud-waste-and-abuse).

In addition to filing a complaint with ERA office, it is strongly recommended you also report Emergency Rental Assistance (ERA) fraud to the local agency responsible for disbursing Rental Assistance funds (the entity who accepts and processes ERA applications for rental assistance) or the District of Columbia, Tribe, Tribally Designated Housing Entity (TDHE), Department of Hawaiian Home Lands (DHHL), State, Local government, or Territorial Agency that oversees the program. That agency may be able to take immediate action regarding the issue or redirect funds appropriately.

Please be aware that local law enforcement is a valuable resource for many issues of the type you may also refer to this office. Local law enforcement may offer advantages such as the ability to interact quickly with the community, prosecute criminal offenses, and often has comprehensive victim, witness, and social services support programs, which may better offer real-time assistance. Your state, local, tribal, territorial, or DC law enforcement agency with primary law enforcement jurisdiction is usually the same agency that responds to 911 calls.

FUNDING TO STATES, LOCAL, TERRITORIAL, AND TRIBAL GOVERNMENTS
Even as the American economy continues its recovery from the devastating impact of the pandemic, millions of Americans face deep rental debt and fear evictions and the loss of basic housing security. COVID-19 has exacerbated an affordable housing crisis that predated the pandemic and that has deep disparities that

threaten the strength of an economic recovery that must work for everyone.

To meet this need, the Emergency Rental Assistance program makes funding available to government entities to assist households that are unable to pay rent or utilities.

ASSISTANCE FOR SMALL BUSINESSES

The COVID-19 public health crisis and resulting economic crisis have created a variety of challenges for small, micro, and solo businesses in communities across the country. The Department of Treasury is providing critical assistance to small businesses across the country, facilitating the urgent deployment of capital and support to help these organizations not just persevere, but recover on solid footing.

Small Business Tax Credit Programs

The American Rescue Plan extends a number of critical tax benefits, particularly the Employee Retention Credit and Paid Leave Credit, to small businesses.

EMPLOYEE RETENTION CREDIT

The American Rescue Plan extends the availability of the Employee Retention Credit for small businesses through December 2021 and allows businesses to offset their current payroll tax liabilities by up to $7,000 per employee per quarter. This credit of up to $28,000 per employee for 2021 is available to small businesses who have seen their revenues decline, or even been temporarily shuttered, due to COVID-19.

FOR FINANCIAL YEAR 2020

For 2020, the ERC is a tax credit against certain payroll taxes, including an employer's share of social security taxes for wages paid between March 12, 2020, and December 31, 2020. The tax credit is 50 percent of the wages paid up to $10,000 per employee, capped at $5,000 per employee. If the amount of the tax credit for an employer is more than the amount of the employer's share of social security tax owed, the excess is refunded—paid—directly to the employer.

If your business is eligible for the ERC for 2020 and you have not yet claimed the credit, you can file amended payroll tax forms to claim the credit and receive your tax refund.

Businesses that took out PPP loans in 2020 can still go back and claim the ERC, but they cannot use the same wages to apply for forgiveness of PPP loans and to count toward the ERC. If your business had payroll costs that were more than the amount covered by your PPP loan, you may be able to claim tax credits for those additional payroll costs.

FOR FINANCIAL YEAR 2021

The ERC is now available for all four quarters of 2021. The amount of the maximum tax credit has been increased to $7,000 per employee per quarter, and the level of qualifying business disruption has been reduced so that a 20 percent decline in gross receipts during a single quarter will make a business eligible, for a maximum benefit of $28,000 for the full year.

PAID LEAVE CREDIT

The American Rescue Plan extends through September 2021 the availability of Paid Leave Credits for small and midsize businesses that offer paid leave to employees who may take leave due to illness, quarantine, or caregiving. Businesses can take dollar-for-dollar tax credits equal to wages of up to $5,000 if they offer paid leave to employees who are sick or quarantining.

FOR FINANCIAL YEAR 2020

Beginning in early 2020 as part of the CARES Act, businesses with fewer than 500 employees were required to provide paid sick leave and paid family leave to employees who were dealing with certain consequences of the ongoing pandemic. Under the law, businesses are entitled to a tax credit equal to 100 percent of the paid sick leave and paid family leave provided to employees.

The 2020 sick leave rules required businesses to provide up to 80 hours of paid leave at either:
- the employee's regular wage, capped at $511/day up to a total of $5,110, if the employee was sick or quarantining
- two-thirds of the employee's regular wage, capped at $200/day up to a total of $2,000, if the employee was taking time to care for someone else who was quarantining or a child whose school or child care was closed due to COVID-19

The 2020 family leave rules required businesses to provide up to 10 additional weeks of leave for employees who are unable to work because they need to care for children whose school or normal child care is not available due to COVID-19. Those employees are entitled to two-thirds of their regular wages, capped at $200/day up to a total of $10,000.

Businesses that paid employees under these programs during the period from April 1, 2020, through December 31, 2020, can take the tax credit against their payroll taxes. If the amount of the credit exceeds a business's portion of its employment taxes, then the excess is refunded—paid—directly back to the business.

If your business provided paid leave to employees in 2020 and you have not yet claimed the credit, you can file amended payroll tax forms to claim the credit and receive your tax refund.

FOR FINANCIAL YEAR 2021

Although the law no longer requires businesses with 500 or fewer employees to offer paid leave as part of the continuing COVID-relief efforts, if a business does provide paid leave to its employees then it can claim these dollar-for-dollar tax credits for wages paid through September 30, 2021. These credits can be claimed against payroll taxes on a quarterly basis.

Emergency Capital Investment Program

The Emergency Capital Investment Programs support the efforts of low- and moderate-income community financial institutions.

COVID-19 Impact on the Global Economy

Established by the Consolidated Appropriations Act, 2021, the Emergency Capital Investment Program (ECIP) was created to encourage low- and moderate-income community financial institutions to augment their efforts to support small businesses and consumers in their communities.

Under the program, Treasury will provide up to $9 billion in capital directly to depository institutions that are certified Community Development Financial Institutions (CDFIs) or minority depository institutions (MDIs) to, among other things, provide loans, grants, and forbearance for small businesses, minority-owned businesses, and consumers, especially in low-income and underserved communities, that may be disproportionately impacted by the economic effects of the COVID-19 pandemic. Treasury will set aside $2 billion for CDFIs and MDIs with less than $500 million in assets and an additional $2 billion for CDFIs and MDIs with less than $2 billion in assets.

Paycheck Protection Program

The Paycheck Protection Program is providing small businesses with the resources they need to maintain their payroll, hire back employees who may have been laid off, and cover applicable overhead.

SMALL BUSINESS PAYCHECK PROTECTION PROGRAM

The Paycheck Protection Program established by the CARES Act is implemented by the Small Business Administration with support from the Department of the Treasury. This program provides small businesses with funds to pay up to eight weeks of payroll costs including benefits. Funds can also be used to pay interest on mortgages, rent, and utilities.

The Paycheck Protection Program prioritizes millions of Americans employed by small businesses by authorizing up to $659 billion toward job retention and certain other expenses.

Small businesses and eligible nonprofit organizations, veterans organizations, and tribal businesses described in the Small Business Act, as well as individuals who are self-employed or are independent contractors, are eligible if they also meet program size standards.

ASSISTANCE FOR STATE, LOCAL, AND TRIBAL GOVERNMENTS
Coronavirus State and Local Fiscal Recovery Funds

The American Rescue Plan provides $350 billion in emergency funding for eligible state, local, territorial, and tribal governments to respond to the COVID-19 emergency and bring back jobs.

The Coronavirus State and Local Fiscal Recovery Funds (SLFRF) program, a part of the American Rescue Plan, delivers $350 billion to state, local, and tribal governments across the country to support their response to and recovery from the COVID-19 public health emergency.

The SLFRF program provides governments across the country with the resources needed to:
- fight the pandemic and support families and businesses struggling with its public health and economic impacts
- maintain vital public services, even amid declines in revenue resulting from the crisis
- build a strong, resilient, and equitable recovery by making investments that support long-term growth and opportunity

Capital Projects Fund

The Coronavirus Capital Projects Fund (CCPF) takes critical steps to address many challenges laid bare by the pandemic, especially in rural America and low- and moderate-income communities, helping to ensure that all communities have access to the high-quality, modern infrastructure needed to thrive, including Internet access.

The Coronavirus Capital Projects Fund (Capital Projects Fund) will address many challenges laid bare by the pandemic, especially in rural America, tribal communities, and low- and moderate-income communities, helping to ensure that all communities have access to high-quality modern infrastructure, including broadband, needed to access critical services.

The American Rescue Plan provides $10 billion for payments to eligible governments to carry out critical capital projects that directly enable work, education, and health monitoring, including remote options, in response to the public health emergency.

Homeowner Assistance Fund

The American Rescue Plan provides nearly $10 billion for states, territories, and tribes to provide relief for the country's most vulnerable homeowners.

The purpose of the Homeowner Assistance Fund (HAF) is to prevent mortgage delinquencies and defaults, foreclosures, loss of utilities or home energy services, and displacement of homeowners experiencing financial hardship after January 21, 2020. Funds from the HAF may be used for assistance with mortgage payments, homeowner's insurance, utility payments, and other specified purposes. The law prioritizes funds for homeowners who have experienced the greatest hardships, leveraging local and national income indicators to maximize the impact.

The Homeowner Assistance Fund provides:
- a minimum of $50 million for each state, the District of Columbia, and Puerto Rico
- $498 million for Tribes or Tribally designated housing entities and the Department of Hawaiian Home Lands
- $30 million for the territories of Guam, American Samoa, the U.S. Virgin Islands, and the Commonwealth of the Northern Mariana Islands

Emergency Rental Assistance Program

The American Rescue Plan provides $21.6 billion for states, territories, and local governments to assist households that are unable to pay rent and utilities due to the COVID-19 crisis.

Even as the American economy continues its recovery from the devastating impact of the pandemic, millions of Americans face deep rental debt and fear evictions and the loss of basic housing security. COVID-19 has exacerbated an affordable housing crisis that predated the pandemic and that has deep disparities that threaten the strength of an economic recovery that must work for everyone.

To meet this need, the Emergency Rental Assistance program makes funding available to assist households that are unable to pay rent or utilities. Two separate programs have been established: ERA1 (https://home.treasury.gov/system/files/136/era-1-program-statute-section-501.pdf) provides up to $25 billion under the Consolidated Appropriations Act, 2021, which was enacted on December 27, 2020, and ERA2 (https://home.treasury.gov/system/files/136/era-2-program-statute-section-3201.pdf) provides up to $21.55 billion under the American Rescue Plan Act of 2021, which was enacted on March 11, 2021. The funds are provided directly to states, U.S. territories, local governments, and (in the case of ERA1) Indian tribes. Grantees use the funds to provide assistance to eligible households through existing or newly created rental assistance programs.

State Small Business Credit Initiative

The American Rescue Plan provides $10 billion to state and tribal governments to fund small business credit expansion initiatives.

On March 11, 2021, President Biden signed the American Rescue Plan Act, which provided $10 billion to fund the State Small Business Credit Initiative (SSBCI). The SSBCI will fund state, territory, and tribal government small business credit support and investment programs.

This program will build off the inaugural model developed in 2011 during the Obama–Biden Administration, in which nearly $1.5 billion in capital supported over $8 billion in new lending and investing activity across 142 different programs in its first five years. The new iteration will expand in scale and include:
- $500 million to support very small businesses with fewer than 10 employees
- $1.5 billion for states to support businesses owned by socially and economically disadvantaged people
- $1 billion for an incentive program to boost funding tranches for states that show robust support for

businesses owned by socially and economically disadvantaged individuals
- $500 million for technical assistance

Coronavirus Relief Fund

Through the Coronavirus Relief Fund, the CARES Act provides for payments to state, local, and tribal governments navigating the impact of the COVID-19 outbreak.

The CARES Act established the $150 billion Coronavirus Relief Fund.

Treasury has made payments from the fund to states and eligible units of local government, the District of Columbia and U.S. territories (the Commonwealth of Puerto Rico, the United States Virgin Islands, Guam, American Samoa, and the Commonwealth of the Northern Mariana Islands), and tribal governments (collectively "governments").

The CARES Act requires that the payments from the Coronavirus Relief Fund only be used to cover expenses that:
- are necessary expenditures incurred due to the public health emergency with respect to the COVID-19
- were not accounted for in the budget most recently approved as of March 27, 2020 (the date of enactment of the CARES Act), for the state or government
- were incurred during the period that begins on March 1, 2020, and ends on December 31, 2022

The Local Assistance and Tribal Consistency Fund

The Local Assistance and Tribal Consistency Fund is a general revenue enhancement program that provides additional assistance to eligible revenue-sharing counties and eligible tribal governments.

The American Rescue Plan appropriated $2 billion to Treasury across fiscal years 2022 and 2023 to provide payments to eligible revenue-sharing counties and eligible tribal governments for use on any governmental purpose except for a lobbying activity. Specifically, the American Rescue Plan reserves $250 million to allocate and pay to eligible tribal governments for each of fiscal years 2022 and 2023 and reserves $750 million to allocate and pay to eligible revenue-sharing counties for each of fiscal years 2022 and 2023. Under this program, recipients have broad discretion on uses of funds, similar to the ways in which they may use funds generated from their own revenue sources.

Treasury has launched the Local Assistance and Tribal Consistency Fund for all eligible recipients, including eligible tribal governments and eligible revenue-sharing counties.

ASSISTANCE FOR AMERICAN INDUSTRY

The COVID-19 public health crisis and resulting economic crisis have put many sectors of the American economy under unprecedented strain. The Department of Treasury is offering financial support to American industry, so they can better support American workers and play a pivotal part in driving the national recovery effort.

Airline and National Security Relief Programs

In response to industry-specific challenges created by the pandemic, the following programs were created for Treasury to provide assistance to passenger air carriers, cargo air carriers, aviation contractors, and national security businesses, under the CARES Act; the Consolidated Appropriations Act, 2021; and the American Rescue Plan Act of 2021.

The CARES Act included provisions for Treasury to provide payments to passenger air carriers, cargo air carriers, and certain contractors that must be exclusively used for the continuation of payment of employee wages, salaries, and benefits (PSP1). The Act authorized the Department of Treasury to provide such payroll support in such form, and on such terms and conditions, as determined appropriate.

The following amounts were allocated for payment:
- passenger air carriers: $25 billion
- cargo air carriers: $4 billion
- contractors: $3 billion

The Consolidated Appropriations Act, 2021, enacted on December 27, 2020, created the Payroll Support Program Extension (PSP2) for passenger air carriers and certain contractors.

The following amounts were allocated for payment:
- passenger air carriers: $15 billion
- contractors: $1 billion

The ARP was enacted on March 11, 2021, authorizing Treasury to provide additional assistance to passenger air carriers and contractors that received financial assistance under PSP2 (PSP3).

The following amounts were allocated for payment:
- passenger air carriers: $14 billion
- eligible contractors: $1 billion

Coronavirus Economic Relief for Transportation Services Program

The Coronavirus Economic Relief for Transportation Services (CERTS) Program is providing eligible transportation service companies with resources to help maintain payroll, hire back employees who may have been laid off, and cover applicable overhead and operational expenses.

The CERTS Program is now closed; the Covered Period has ended. All unexpended funds must be returned to Treasury. If a grantee has correctly completed its final reporting requirements in accordance with the terms and conditions of its grant agreement, no further action is needed, unless notified otherwise by Treasury.

Payroll Relief Programs

EMPLOYEE RETENTION CREDIT

Employers of all sizes that face closure orders or suffer economic hardship due to COVID-19 are incentivized to keep employees on the payroll through a 50 percent credit on up to $10,000 of wages paid or incurred from March 13, 2020, through December 31, 2020.

ADDITIONAL TAX CREDITS

The IRS is issuing tax credits in order to give small and mid-sized businesses the resources they need to cover the cost of providing paid sick and family leave wages.

PAYROLL TAX DEFERRAL

To enhance cash flow so that businesses can better maintain operations and payroll, employers and self-employed individuals can defer payment of the employer share of the Social Security tax they otherwise are responsible for paying to the federal government with respect to their employees. The deferred employment tax can be paid over the next two years—with half of the required amount to be paid by December 31, 2021, and the other half by December 31, 2022.[4]

A GUIDE TO COVID-19 ECONOMIC STIMULUS RELIEF*

*The following are the guidelines that were used for tax benefits during the pandemic in 2020.

Americans are increasingly feeling the impact of the coronavirus, both on their everyday lives and their financial well-being. As a result of the recently signed CARES Act, the majority of Americans started to see some financial relief starting in April through EIPs being issued by the Internal Revenue Service (IRS).

The IRS has worked to break down the most common questions about the EIPs, including how much you are eligible to receive and when you can expect to receive it.

When Can You Expect to Receive Your Payment?

The IRS began rolling out EIPs in April 2020. For most people, you would not have to do anything—the payment will be directly deposited into your bank account or sent to you by check or prepaid debit card. Be aware, however, that if it is sent by check, it might take a little longer.

Do You Qualify, and How Much Will You Receive?

If you receive certain social security, retirement, disability, survivors, railroad retirement, or veterans benefits, you may automatically qualify to receive a payment.

---

[4] "COVID-19 Economic Relief," U.S. Department of the Treasury, October 18, 2022. Available online. URL: https://home.treasury.gov/policy-issues/coronavirus. Accessed December 30, 2022.

COVID-19 Impact on the Global Economy

For most people, the IRS will use information from your 2019 or 2018 tax return or information that you provide to see if you qualify for an EIP.

To qualify for a payment, you must:
- be a U.S. citizen or U.S. resident alien
- not be claimed as a dependent on someone else's tax return
- have a valid Social Security Number (SSN). Or, if you or your spouse is a member of the military, only one of you needs a valid SSN
- have an adjusted gross income below a certain amount that is based on your filing status and the number of qualifying children under the age of 17 (If you are not required to file taxes because you have limited income, even if you have no income, you are still eligible for payment.)

You may be eligible based on the criteria below (refer to Table 42.1), even if you are not required to file taxes. If you qualify, your EIP amount will be based on your adjusted gross income, filing status, and the number of qualifying children under age of 17. You will receive either the full payment or a reduced amount at higher incomes.

Table 42.1. Eligibility Criteria for Tax Filing during COVID-19

Single or Married but Filing Separately	Head of a Household	Married Filing Jointly
You are eligible to receive the full payment if your adjusted gross income is below $75,000 and a reduced payment amount if it is more than $75,000. The adjusted gross income limit for a reduced payment is $99,000 if you do not have children and increases by $10,000 for each qualifying child under 17.	You are eligible to receive the full payment if your adjusted gross income is below $112,500 and a reduced payment amount if it is more than $112,500. The adjusted gross income limit for a reduced payment is $136,500 if you do not have children and increases by $10,000 for each qualifying child under 17.	You are eligible to receive the full payment if your adjusted gross income is below $150,00 and a reduced payment amount if it is above $150,000. The adjusted gross income limit for a reduced payment is $198,000 if you do not have children and increases by $10,000 for each qualifying child under 17.

Table 42.1. Continued

Single or Married but Filing Separately	Head of a Household	Married Filing Jointly
If your adjusted gross income is below $75,000, you will receive the full $1,200. You will also receive $500 for each child under the age of 17 you claim on your taxes.	If your adjusted gross income is below $112,500, you will receive the full $1,200. You will also receive $500 for each child under the age of 17 you claim on your taxes.	If your adjusted gross income is less than $150,000, you will receive the full $2,400. You will also receive $500 for each child under the age of 17 you claim on your taxes.
If your adjusted gross income is above $75,000, you will receive an amount that will be reduced by $5 for every $100 in adjusted gross income above $75,000.	If your adjusted gross income is above $112,500, you will receive an amount that will be reduced by $5 for every $100 in adjusted gross income above $112,500.	If your adjusted gross income is above $150,000, you will receive an amount that will be reduced $5 for every $100 in adjusted gross income above $150,000.
If your adjusted gross income is more than $99,000 and you do not claim any children under the age of 17, you would not receive an EIP. This limit will increase to $109,000 if you have one child, $119,00 if you have two children, and an additional $10,000 for each child after that.	If your adjusted gross income is more than $136,500 and you do not claim any children under the age of 17, you would not receive an EIP. This limit will increase to $146,500 if you have one child, $156,500 if you have two children, and an additional $10,000 for each child after that.	If your adjusted gross income is more than $198,000 and you do not claim any children under the age of 17, you would not receive an EIP. This limit will increase to $208,000 if you have one child, $218,000 if you have two children, and an additional $10,000 for each child after that.

You Receive Social Security Retirement, Disability, Survivors, Supplement Security Income, or Veterans Benefits. Do You Automatically Qualify for an Economic Impact Payment?

In some cases, if you receive certain benefits, you will automatically receive an EIP. Make sure you read further to know if this applies to you and to know if you need to send the IRS any additional information, and how you will be receiving your payment.

The IRS is working to make it easier for certain beneficiaries to receive the EIP by using information from benefit programs to automatically send payments.

You will qualify for this automatic payment only if:
- you were not required to file taxes in 2018 or 2019 because you had limited income
- you receive one of the following benefits:
  - Social Security retirement, survivors, and disability insurance (RSDI) from the Social Security Administration
  - Supplemental Security Income (SSI) from the Social Security Administration
  - Railroad Retirement and Survivors benefits from the U.S. Railroad Retirement Board
  - veterans disability compensation, pension, or survivor benefits from the Department of Veterans Affairs

If you qualify for an automatic payment, you will receive $1,200 ($2,400 if your spouse also receives the benefit). You will receive this automatically the same way you receive your benefits, either by direct deposit or by check. You will not need to take any further action to receive this.

If you qualified for automatic payment through a benefit program, but you also have dependent children under the age of 17, you may need to provide the IRS with information about your dependents to receive additional payment. You will receive an additional $500 per child under the age of 17. The IRS says you can claim the additional payment when you file your taxes next year.

If you receive one of these benefits but have either filed your taxes in 2018 or 2019, or plan to in 2019, because you receive additional income through a pension or another source, you will receive your EIP based on your 2019 tax return or your 2018 return if you have not filed for 2019.

No matter how you receive your payment, the IRS will send you a letter in the mail—to the most current address they have on file—about 15 days after they send your payment to let you know what to do if you have any issues and contact information for any questions.

What Steps Do You Need to Take to Receive an Economic Impact Payment?

If you receive certain social security, retirement, disability, survivors, railroad retirement, or veterans benefits, you may automatically qualify to receive a payment.

For most people, you will not need to take any action, and the IRS will automatically send you your payment. For some people who are eligible for a payment, the IRS will need more information from you first before they can send you money. You will do this using one of two different IRS portals. It is important that you provide this information using the right IRS portal so that the IRS can process your information quickly.

- If you already filed your 2018 or 2019 taxes, go to the IRS "Get My Payment" portal (www.irs.gov/coronavirus/get-my-payment) to check the status of your payment. This portal will let you know if your payment has been processed and let you know if the IRS needs more information before sending you your payment.
  - If your payment has already been processed, the IRS does not need any more information from you at this time.
  - If you paid additional taxes when you filed your tax return, it is possible that the IRS does not have your payment account information to direct deposit your payment. You can provide that directly in the portal so that they can process this information quickly and send you your payment. If the IRS does not have your direct deposit information and you do not provide it to them, your payment will be sent to you by check to the address they have on file.
- If you still need to file your 2018 or 2019 taxes but have not yet done so, you need to file your taxes before the IRS can send you your payment.
- If you do not typically file taxes because you have limited income which does not require you to file, you will need to submit information to the IRS first so that

they can send you your payment. You can do this by either:
- Going to the IRS nonfilers portal and submitting your personal information so that the IRS can send you your payment, or
- Filing a 2019 tax return. In most cases, you can do this for free.

How Will the IRS Send Your Payment?

If you receive certain social security, retirement, disability, survivors, railroad retirement, or veterans benefits, your payment will be distributed in the same method as your benefits.

EIPs will either be directly deposited into your bank account or a check or prepaid debit card will be mailed to you.

IF YOU RECEIVED A TAX REFUND

If you received a refund through direct deposit with your most recent taxes (2019 or 2018), the IRS has your bank account information on file, and they will send your EIP directly to that account.

IF YOU OWED TAXES

If you paid taxes with your most recent filing (2019 or 2018), you will receive a check or prepaid debit card to the address the IRS has on file.

IF YOU PROVIDED INFORMATION USING THE IRS NONFILERS PORTAL

If you provided your personal information to the IRS using the nonfilers portal (www.irs.gov/coronavirus/non-filers-enter-payment-info-here), your money will be direct deposited into the bank or credit union account or prepaid card that you provided when you submitted your information. If you did not provide payment account information, a check will be mailed to you to the address you provided.

No matter how you receive your payment, the IRS will send you a letter in the mail—to the most current address they have on file—about 15 days after they send your payment to let you know what to do if you have any issues, including if you have not received the payment.

Can You Provide the IRS with Your Account Information?

If you receive certain social security, retirement, disability, survivors, railroad retirement, or veterans benefits, your payment will be distributed in the same method as your benefits.

If you filed your taxes in 2018 or 2019 and owed taxes when you filed, you will receive a check or prepaid debit card in the mail. If you filed your taxes but received a refund that was directly deposited, you will receive the refund in the same account and will not be able to update this information at this time.

If you do not typically file taxes and you are providing your information to the IRS through their nonfilers portal, you can provide your account information directly in the portal for direct deposit.

If you are being asked to provide banking account information and would like to receive payment on your own prepaid card, enter your card's direct deposit routing and account number directly in the portal. Check your account online or call the card provider to find out if your prepaid account is eligible to receive direct deposit, which is the fastest way to receive the payment.

You Have Moved Since You Filed Your Taxes. How Can You Update Your Address?

If you received a refund through direct deposit with your latest tax return (either 2019 or 2018), the IRS will directly deposit your money into this account, and they would not need your updated address. If you have not filed your 2019 taxes yet, the IRS will receive your updated address through your tax return. The IRS is encouraging people to use these electronic methods for providing this information as they are unable to process other requests for an address change at this time due to the pandemic.

If You Still Need to File Your 2018 and 2019 Taxes, Can You Still Receive the Economic Impact Payment?

Yes. The IRS urges anyone with a tax filing obligation and who has not yet filed a tax return for 2018 or 2019, to file as soon as they can to receive an EIP. When you file your taxes, include your direct deposit information on the return so that the IRS can send you your payment quickly.

If you are required to file a tax return, there may be free or low-cost options for filing your return. If you need someone to help you to file, it is important to choose a reputable tax preparer that will file an accurate return. Mistakes could result in additional costs and complications in the future.

If your 2019 adjusted gross income was less than $69,000, you may be able to find one or more online tools to file your taxes for free. Review each company's offer to make sure you qualify for a free federal return. Some companies offer free state tax returns, but others may charge a fee.

Keep in mind that the IRS has extended the deadline for filing your 2019 taxes until July 15, 2020. If you are concerned about visiting a tax professional or local community organization in person to get help with your tax return, the IRS indicates the EIPs will be available throughout the rest of 2020.

You Are Not Typically Required to File Taxes. Can You Still Receive the Economic Impact Payment?

Yes, but you will need to visit IRS.gov and then go to www.irs.gov/coronavirus/non-filers-enter-payment-info-here. If you did not file a tax return in 2018 or 2019, this web portal allows you to submit basic personal information to the IRS so that you can receive payments. To receive your payment quickly, enter your account information so that your payment will be directly deposited in your bank or credit union account or prepaid card.

The tool will request the following basic information to check your eligibility, calculate, and send the EIPs:
- full names and Social Security numbers, including for spouse and dependents

- mailing address
- bank account type, account, and routing numbers

If you receive certain social security, retirement, disability, survivors, railroad retirement, or veterans benefits, you may automatically qualify to receive a payment.

You Do Not Have a Social Security Number. Can You Still Get an Economic Impact Payment?

In almost all cases, a person is only eligible to receive an EIP if they have a Social Security number (SSN).

One exception to this is if you are a member of the military and file a married filing jointly tax return. Your spouse is not required to have an SSN for you to get the EIP.

Another exception is you have dependent child under the age of 17 who is adopted and has an "Adoption Taxpayer Identification Number" (ATIN), you will receive the $500 child payment.

You Are a Representative Payee for a Social Security or Supplemental Social Security Income Beneficiary. What Do You Need to Know about the Economic Impact Payments?

The beneficiary's EIP will arrive in the same way they either receive their monthly benefits or their tax return for 2019 or 2018.

- If the beneficiary did not file a 2019 or 2018 tax return, they will receive their EIPs the same way they receive monthly Social Security or SSI payments. This may be through direct deposit to their banking account or Direct Express card or a mailed paper check.
- If the beneficiary did file a 2019 or 2018 tax return, the payment will be deposited to the same bank account or debit card as the most recent tax refund or mailed to the address on the beneficiary's last tax return.

DISCUSS THE ECONOMIC IMPACT OF PAYMENT WITH THE BENEFICIARY

A representative payee is only responsible for managing Social Security or SSI benefits. The EIP is not an SSA benefit and belongs to the beneficiary. Discuss the payment with the beneficiary, and if they request access to the funds, you are obligated to provide it.

THE ECONOMIC IMPACT PAYMENT DOES NOT AFFECT ELIGIBILITY FOR INCOME-TESTED BENEFITS

The EIP is a tax credit. That means it should not be counted as income and should not affect the beneficiary's eligibility for income-tested benefits. As long as the payment is spent within 12 months of the date it was received, it also would not count against resource limits for Medicaid, Medicare Savings Programs, SSI, SNAP, or Public Housing benefits.

NURSING HOMES AND ASSISTED-LIVING FACILITIES CANNOT TAKE THE ECONOMIC IMPACT PAYMENT FOR THE FIRST 12 MONTHS

Since the payment does not qualify as a resource for Medicaid purposes until 12 months after it was first received, nursing homes and assisted-living facilities should not require residents to sign over their payment until this period has passed. If you believe a nursing home or assisted living facility has improperly taken the payment from you or a loved one, file a complaint with your state's attorney general.

Can the Government Reduce or Garnish Your Economic Impact Payment?

Your EIP will not be subject to most types of federal offset or federal garnishment as a result of defaulted student loans or tax debt. However, the payments are still subject to garnishment if you are behind on child support.

The payments may also still be subject to state or local government garnishment and also to court-ordered garnishments.

You Received a Message from the IRS Asking for Your Personal Information. Is This a Scam?

Yes, this is a scam. With the rollout of EIPs there is an increased risk of scams. It is important to stay vigilant and aware of

unsolicited communications asking for your personal or private information—through mail, email, phone call, text, social media, or websites—that:
- ask you to verify your SSN, bank account, or credit card information
- suggest that you can get a faster payment if they fill out information on your behalf or if you sign over your check to them
- send you a bogus check, perhaps in an odd amount, and then ask you to call a number or verify information online in order to cash that check

Be aware that scammers are also able to replicate a government agency's name and phone number on caller ID. It is important to remember that the Internal Revenue Service will never ask you for your personal information or threaten your benefits by phone call, email, text, or social media.

If you receive an unsolicited email, text, or social media attempt that appears to be from the IRS or an organization associated with the IRS, such as the Department of the Treasury Electronic Federal Tax Payment System, notify the IRS at phishing@irs.gov.[5]

---

[5] "A Guide to COVID-19 Economic Stimulus Relief," Consumer Financial Protection Bureau (CFPB), July 7, 2020. Available online. URL: www.consumerfinance.gov/about-us/blog/guide-covid-19-economic-stimulus-checks. Accessed December 30, 2022.

Chapter 43 | COVID-19 Impact on Well-Being

Chapter Contents
Section 43.1—The Pandemic's Effects on Mental Health..........547
Section 43.2—Unintended Consequences Caused by the
            Pandemic..551
Section 43.3—Social Impact 556

Section 43.1 | The Pandemic's Effects on Mental Health

Both severe acute respiratory syndrome coronavirus 2 (SARS-CoV-2) and the COVID-19 pandemic have significantly affected the mental health of adults and children. In a 2021 study, nearly half of Americans surveyed reported recent symptoms of an anxiety or depressive disorder, and 10 percent of respondents felt their mental health needs were not being met. Rates of anxiety, depression, and substance use disorder have increased since the beginning of the pandemic. And people who have mental illnesses or disorders and then get COVID-19 are more likely to die than those who do not have mental illnesses or disorders.

Mental health is a focus of National Institutes of Health (NIH) research during the COVID-19 pandemic. Researchers at the NIH and supported by the NIH are creating and studying tools and strategies to understand, diagnose, and prevent mental illnesses or disorders and improve mental health care for those in need.

HOW COVID-19 CAN IMPACT MENTAL HEALTH

If you get COVID-19, you may experience a number of symptoms related to brain and mental health, including:
- cognitive and attention deficits (brain fog)
- anxiety and depression
- psychosis
- seizures
- suicidal behavior

Data suggest that people are likely to develop mental illnesses or disorders in the months following infection, including symptoms of posttraumatic stress disorder (PTSD). People with long COVID may experience many symptoms related to brain function and mental health.

HOW THE PANDEMIC AFFECTS DEVELOPING BRAINS

The impact of the COVID-19 pandemic on the mental health of children is not yet fully understood. NIH-supported research

is investigating factors that may influence the cognitive, social, and emotional development of children during the pandemic, including:
- changes to routine
- virtual schooling
- mask wearing
- caregiver absence or loss
- financial instability

NOT EVERYONE IS AFFECTED EQUALLY

While the COVID-19 pandemic can affect the mental health of anyone, some people are more likely to be affected than others. People who are likely to experience symptoms of mental illnesses or disorders during the COVID-19 pandemic include:
- people from racial and ethnic minority groups
- mothers and pregnant people
- people with financial or housing insecurity
- children
- people with disabilities
- people with preexisting mental illnesses or substance use problems
- health-care workers

People who belong to more than one of these groups may be at an even greater risk for mental illness.

TELEHEALTH'S POTENTIAL TO HELP

The pandemic has prevented many people from visiting health-care professionals in person, and as a result, telehealth has been more widely adopted during this time. Telehealth visits for mental health and substance use disorders increased significantly from 2020 to 2021 and now make up nearly half of all total visits for behavioral health.

Widespread adoption of telehealth services may help people who otherwise would not be able to access mental health support, such as people in rural areas or places with few providers.

YOU HAVE A PREEXISTING MENTAL ILLNESS. IS COVID-19 MORE DANGEROUS TO YOU?

COVID-19 can be worse for people with mental illnesses. Data suggest that people who reported symptoms of anxiety or depression had a greater chance of being hospitalized after a COVID-19 diagnosis than people without those symptoms.

The Centers for Disease Control and Prevention (CDC) reports that having mood disorders and schizophrenia spectrum disorders can increase a person's chances of having severe COVID-19. People with mental illnesses who belong to minority groups are also more likely to get COVID-19. And people with schizophrenia are significantly likely to get COVID-19 and die from it.

Despite these risks, effective treatments are available. If you have a preexisting mental illness and get COVID-19, talk to your health-care professional to determine the treatment plan that is appropriate for you.

WHAT SHOULD YOU DO IF YOU ARE EXPERIENCING SYMPTOMS OF A MENTAL ILLNESS OR DISORDER?

If you are experiencing symptoms of anxiety, depression, or any other mental illness or disorder, there are ways you can get help. For immediate help, do the following:

- Call 911.
- Call or text the 988 Suicide and Crisis Lifeline at 988.
- Call or text the Disaster Distress Helpline at 800-985-5990 (press 2 for Spanish).
- The Substance Abuse and Mental Health Services Administration can help you find mental health or substance use specialists.
- Talk to your health-care professional or mental health-care professional. Together, you can work on a plan to manage or reduce your symptoms.

THE NIH'S CURRENT RESEARCH ON THE MENTAL HEALTH IMPACTS OF COVID-19

The National Institute of Mental Health (NIMH) and other institutes of the NIH have created research initiatives to address mental health for people in general and for the most vulnerable people specifically. Examples of this research include the following:

- The NIMH launched a five-year research study called "RECOUP-NY" to promote the mental health of New Yorkers from communities hard-hit by COVID-19. The study will test the use of a new care model called "Problem Management Plus" (PM+) that can be used by nonspecialists.
- A study funded by the NIMH is examining the use of mobile apps to address mental health disparities.
- The Eunice Kennedy Shriver National Institute of Child Health and Human Development (NICHD) is funding research to understand the effects of mask usage for children, including any impacts on their emotional and brain development.
- The NIMH is funding research on the impacts of the pandemic on underserved and vulnerable populations and on the cognitive, social, and emotional development of children.
- The National Institute on Alcohol Abuse and Alcoholism (NIAAA) is funding research on how COVID-19 and SARS-CoV-2 affect the causes and consequences of alcohol misuse.
- A collaborative study supported by the NIMH and the National Center for Complementary and Integrative Health (NCCIH) enrolled more than 3,600 people from all 50 U.S. states to understand the stressors affecting people during the pandemic.[1]

---

[1] COVID-19, "Mental Health during the COVID-19 Pandemic," National Institutes of Health (NIH), August 24, 2022. Available online. URL: https://covid19.nih.gov/covid-19-topics/mental-health. Accessed January 2, 2023.

COVID-19 Impact on Well-Being

Section 43.2 | Unintended Consequences Caused by the Pandemic

The COVID-19 pandemic is a continuing global health crisis caused by the spread of the novel coronavirus, SARS-CoV-2, which first emerged in China in December 2019 and quickly spread to other countries. The pandemic remains a major public health concern, and its consequences have had significant implications for individuals and societies worldwide.

Efforts to address the pandemic's immediate health and economic impacts also led to a range of unintended consequences that have affected individuals and communities in various ways, such as disruptions to education, mental health, social interactions, access to health care, and other aspects of life.

One of the notable consequences of the COVID-19 pandemic is the disruption of regular treatment and care for those suffering from both chronic and acute illnesses. Unfortunately, during the pandemic, the health-care industry's focus was primarily on containing the spread of COVID-19. Recognizing the negative health consequences of pandemic lockdowns was not prioritized in the early months of the pandemic. Following are some unintended health consequences of the global pandemic response:

- **Delays in surgery**. During the pandemic, a significant number of surgeries were either delayed or postponed. According to an estimate by the U.K.'s COVIDSurg Collaborative, the overall surgery cancellation rate was more than three-fourths, resulting in only 30 percent of scheduled elective surgeries being performed in 2020. Thousands of people were forced to postpone surgery and live with untreated pain and/or disability.
- **Uninsured medical care**. Uninsured people were the most adversely affected in getting access to health care during the pandemic's peak in the United States. Uninsured workers such as drivers, cooks, and cashiers who cannot work remotely were at greater risk of exposure to the infection as they came into regular contact with the public. When uninsured workers are exposed to the virus, observing a quarantine period cut

them off from their income source, pushing them to financial difficulties. For those infected with COVID-19, the need to pay for treatment out of pocket further put them at a higher risk of accruing large medical bills.

- **Suicide rates and mental health crises.** Emotional stress peaked during the pandemic, with people forced to stay behind closed doors for months. Isolation from family, friends, and other social interactions proved overwhelming for many people already struggling with mental health issues. According to a Centers for Disease Control and Prevention (CDC) report, one in every four young adults aged 18–44 surveyed had suicidal thoughts during the pandemic, and more than 40 percent of respondents said the crisis had caused behavioral problems, leading to an increase in suicidality.

  The negative consequences of lockdowns and quarantines was demonstrated in China, where mental illness has emerged as a prominent crisis affecting millions of Chinese families. According to the World Health Organization (WHO), depression and anxiety disorders are China's two most common mental disorders, with 54 million and 41 million affected individuals, respectively. Recent studies have shown that the pandemic increased insomnia, depression, and anxiety among Chinese middle school students. Additionally, a survey conducted in 2020 found that nearly 35 percent of participants experienced psychological distress during the pandemic's peak that year.

  Additionally, public protests erupted across several Chinese cities, largely due to the government's "dynamic zero-COVID" policy, which resulted in ongoing lockdowns, extensive electronic surveillance of residents, mass testing, and border closings. As a result, citizens took to social media to express their discontent with the government and the resulting isolation and frustration of its efforts to contain COVID-19.

- **Substance abuse.** Social isolation contributed to substance abuse during the pandemic by many people, including former users who relapsed. According to estimates, for example, opioid overdose deaths in Maryland doubled during the pandemic in 2020 compared to previous years. According to the Overdose Detection Mapping Application Program (ODMAP), overdoses have increased by about 18 percent nationwide in the early months of the pandemic, resulting in thousands more overdose deaths.
- **Hunger due to the economic downturn and lockdowns.** The Chinese government's response to the COVID-19 outbreak in its initial stages was characterized by authoritarian measures and strict lockdowns. However, this response was not accompanied by adequate efforts to provide people with essential supplies such as food and other necessities. Officials prioritized virus control over their constituents' well-being, resulting in economic recession, chaos, and crisis. The government's pursuit of a zero-COVID policy with strict lockdowns contributed to suffering from hunger and other hardships.

  Americans faced hunger, too. According to the *Wall Street Journal*, nearly 20 percent of Americans with children at home could not afford to feed them adequately, and approximately 12.1 percent of adults had to live in households with insufficient food during the peak of the pandemic. Business closures exacerbated the economic consequences of the pandemic, causing widespread malnutrition and hunger.
- **Domestic violence.** Isolating people from the outside world and restraining them at home led to mental stress that contributed to an increase in domestic violence incidents. Pandemic confinement increased the likelihood of intimate partner violence too. According to the National Commission on COVID-19

and Criminal Justice, enforcing COVID-19 lockdown orders has resulted in an 8.1 percent increase in domestic violence cases in the United States. One factor in this increase was the inability of victims to avoid or escape their abusers due to lockdown restrictions.

Effective mitigation planning by governments or health authorities requires a complete understanding of the pandemic and the unintended consequences of attempts to contain it. When a policy decision results in negative effects, policymakers must reassess it, weigh its negative outcome against its benefits, and take remedial measures as appropriate. It is essential to acknowledge and address these unintended consequences to ensure that efforts to contain and recover from the pandemic do not harm the population as much or more than the disease itself.

References

Abramson, Ashley. "Substance Use during the Pandemic," Overdose Detection Mapping Application Program (ODMAP), March 1, 2021. Available online. URL: www.apa.org/monitor/2021/03/substance-use-pandemic. Accessed December 23, 2022.

"Ask the Expert: Protests in China over Lockdown Policies," Michigan State University, December 7, 2022. Available online. URL: https://msutoday.msu.edu/news/2022/Ask-the-expert-protests-in-China-over-lockdown-policies. Accessed December 23, 2022.

Baumbusch, Jennifer; Lloyd, Jennifer E. V.; Lamden-Bennett, Shawna R and Ou, Christine. "The Unintended Consequences of COVID-19 Public Health Measures on Health Care for Children with Medical Complexity," Wiley Online Library, January 18, 2022. Available online. URL: https://onlinelibrary.wiley.com/doi/10.1111/cch.12968. Accessed December 23, 2022.

"Care on Hold: COVID's Unintended Side Effects," Organisation for Economic Co-operation and Development (OECD), November 19, 2021. Available online. URL: www.oecd.org/coronavirus/en/data-insights/care-on-hold-covid-s-unintended-side-effects. Accessed December 23, 2022.

"Nearly 1 in 4 Young Adults in US Treated for MH during Pandemic, CDC Survey Finds," Wiley Online Library, September 12, 2022. Available online. URL: https://onlinelibrary.wiley.com/doi/full/10.1002/mhw.33365. Accessed December 23, 2022.

"New Analysis Shows 8% Increase in U.S. Domestic Violence Incidents Following Pandemic Stay-at-Home Orders," Council on Criminal Justice (CCJ), February 24, 2021. Available online. URL: https://counciloncj.org/new-analysis-shows-8-increase-in-u-s-domestic-violence-incidents-following-pandemic-stay-at-home-orders. Accessed December 22, 2022.

Nodell, Bobbi and Moran, Tony. "Study: Pandemic Halts, Delays 28 Million Elective Surgeries," University of Washington, May 19, 2020. Available online. URL: https://newsroom.uw.edu/postscript/study-pandemic-halts-delays-28-million-elective-surgeries. Accessed December 23, 2022.

"Prioritising COVID-19 over Everything: The Unintended Harm," The Lancet, July 1, 2022. Available online. URL: www.thelancet.com/journals/landia/article/PIIS2213-8587(21)00147-9/fulltext. Accessed December 23, 2022.

Yuan, Li. "The Army of Millions Who Enforce China's Zero-COVID Policy, at All Costs," The Economic Times, January 12, 2022. Available online. URL: https://economictimes.indiatimes.com/news/international/world-news/the-army-of-millions-who-enforce-chinas-zero-covid-policy-at-all-costs/articleshow/88862529.cms. Accessed December 23, 2023.

Section 43.3 | Social Impact

The COVID-19 pandemic upended many family dynamics, but one positive consequence of this upheaval is parents shared more dinners with and read to their children more often, according to the U.S. Census Bureau's 2020 Survey of Income and Program Participation (SIPP). Many families spent extra time together in the spring and summer of 2020 when lockdowns were in place in many parts of the United States.

Most interviews for the 2020 SIPP were conducted during March–June 2020. The data show that parental interactions with children changed from prior years: While parents shared more dinners and read to children more often in 2020, they also took them on fewer outings.

There were, however, big differences depending on parents' socioeconomic characteristics. Frequent outings with young children dropped for most parents but more so for parents with fewer economic resources. And parents who were married and more educated read more often to young children.

SURVEY OF INCOME AND PROGRAM PARTICIPATION AND PARENTAL INVOLVEMENT

The SIPP collects information on child well-being, including details on parental involvement with children. Specifically, it asks a reference parent (usually the mother) to identify the number of times in a typical week they had dinner with their children aged 0–17 and how many times another parent (usually the spouse or cohabiting partner of the reference parent) did.

The survey also asks how many outings the reference parent or other parent took their young children (aged 0–5) on and whether they or another family member read to them. All of these behaviors have been associated with improved child well-being and family dynamics. All estimates shown are at the reference-parent level at the time of the interview.

In recent decades, parents have been highly engaged with children. Since 1998, at least 80 percent of children often ate dinner with their parents (five or more times per week). Since 2014, about 80 percent of children were often taken on outings by their parents (two or more times per week) and at least 48 percent of young children were often read to by parents (five or more times per week).

IMPACT OF COVID-19 ON PARENTAL INVOLVEMENT

Most likely as a result of COVID-19 lockdowns in early 2020, the proportion of parents taking their young children on outings two or more times a week dropped from 87 percent in 2019 to 82 percent in 2020. The frequency of children's weekly outings with their other parent was not statistically different across those same years (about 67%).

In contrast, parents shared more weekly meals with children aged 0–17. There was only a one percentage point increase in shared dinners from 2018 (84%) to 2020 (85%). But the change was statistically significant and coupled with the dip in outings, resulted in shared meals becoming the most common type of parental involvement in 2020.

The proportion of shared meals between children and their other parent, as reported by the reference parent, also rose, from 56 percent in 2018 to 63 percent in 2020. Plus, parents or relatives read to children more often in 2020 than in prior years.

In 2020, 69 percent of parents reported reading to young children five or more times per week compared with 65 percent in 2018 and 64 percent in 2019.

PARENT–CHILD OUTINGS DROPPED IN ALMOST ALL SOCIO-ECONOMIC CATEGORIES

Across all but one (poverty) of the characteristics considered, the proportion of parents taking kids on frequent outings dropped four percentage points from 2019 to 2020. Frequent parent–child outings decreased in 2020 compared with 2019 for many reasons, including shutdowns and travel bans.

Many places that families typically visit such as restaurants and malls closed, and travel, both domestic and foreign, was discouraged or banned during the pandemic.

Families have struggled during COVID-19. Many have had to juggle work and childcare responsibilities while also facing food insufficiency and financial hardships such as job or wage loss. For example, unemployment, stimulus, and Child Tax Credit payments have been used to pay for the basics such as food, rent, and paying off debt, leaving little discretionary income for outings.

Solo parents—those with no spouse or cohabiting partner present—experienced an 11 percentage point drop in frequent outings with young children: 75 percent reported going on two or more outings a week in 2020 compared with 86 percent in 2019. Solo parents, by definition the sole parental figure living with young children, were especially hard-hit during the pandemic with limited time, financial resources, and support networks. Although younger solo parents are typically more involved than older solo parents with young children, young adults experienced some of the highest levels of job loss due to the COVID-19 downturn, which may have impacted their involvement with their children.

Even parents with more resources did not take their children on outings as frequently. That includes parents with more education and married parents who may alternate childcare responsibilities. Frequent outings among those socioeconomic groups dropped about four percentage points in 2020 compared with 2019.

Results for parents in poverty were not statistically different during the period examined (2019 and 2020), which may be due to no real changes or to nonresponse issues.

FREQUENT READING TO CHILDREN INCREASED AMONG ADVANTAGED PARENTS

The share of married parents who read to young children five or more times a week increased from 68 percent in 2019 to 73 percent in 2020.

Groups who read to their young children more frequently are as follows:
- native-born parents (66% in 2019 compared to 71% in 2020)
- parents who were above the poverty level (66% in 2019 compared to 70% in 2020)

COVID-19 Impact on Well-Being

- highly educated parents with a bachelor's degree or higher who read to their kids frequently at a higher rate than all parents in 2020: 81 percent compared to 69 percent

These characteristics are associated with certain advantages, such as higher income, residential and family stability, and white-collar jobs with flexible work schedules. That may have allowed these parents to leverage their resources to be more involved with children during the COVID-19 pandemic.

In 2020, parents who were solo (58%), foreign-born (62%), or poor (56%) or did not have a bachelor's degree (60%) read to young children less often than other parents (69%). Still, more than half of parents with fewer resources managed to read to young children five or more times a week in 2020.

PARENT CHARACTERISTICS IMPACTED BY NONRESPONSE BIAS

The 2020 SIPP had high nonresponse rates, meaning that many people who were asked to participate in the survey did not. Additionally, there was nonresponse bias, that is, the characteristics of those who responded were different from those who did not respond. Consequently, reference parents who reported on their involvement with children in the SIPP were likely to be older, foreign-born, married, more educated, and above the poverty level than in the two prior years. The proportions of parents who were foreign-born or married were not statistically different between 2019 and 2020, but the 2019 SIPP also experienced higher nonresponse rates due to the 2018–2019 lapse in federal funding that stopped operations and other factors.[2]

---

[2] "Pandemic Brought Parents and Children Closer: More Family Dinners, More Reading to Young Children," United States Census Bureau, April 12, 2022. Available online. URL: www.census.gov/library/stories/2022/01/parents-and-children-interacted-more-during-covid-19.html. Accessed January 2, 2023.

Chapter 44 | COVID-19 Impact on Education

Chapter Contents
Section 44.1—Education during the COVID-19
              Pandemic 563
Section 44.2—Distance Education during the
              COVID-19 Pandemic 570

Section 44.1 | Education during the COVID-19 Pandemic

COVID-19'S WIDESPREAD EFFECTS ON K-12 STUDENTS AND SCHOOLS
COVID-19's Costs in Instructional Time, Access, and Content

For the past year, many students have had to learn in front of screens at home and in other settings, affected by illness, loss, and economic hardship stemming from the global pandemic. Even with heroic efforts by teachers, staff, and school leaders—many of whom quickly developed online lessons, remote-teaching plans, and concrete strategies for meeting students' basic needs—challenges were profound.

Rural and high-poverty school districts faced especially stark challenges early in the pandemic maintaining one-on-one contact and regular check-ins between teachers and students in a virtual setting. More generally, learning time also dropped from prepandemic norms in many schools around the country. According to one nationally representative survey from May 2020, only 15 percent of districts expected their elementary students to be receiving instruction for more than four hours per day during remote learning, while 85 percent of districts expected instructional time to dip under four hours—more than an hour per day less than the prepandemic national average of five instructional hours per day. Even further, according to the same report, in nearly a fifth of districts surveyed (17%), the instruction students did receive in spring 2020 was designed not to teach new skills and understanding but to review what had already been taught—in a sort of pandemic holding pattern.

That picture improved, however, through the 2020–2021 school year. By January 2021, according to a nationally representative survey conducted by the National Center for Education Statistics (NCES), 31 percent of districts were reportedly offering more than five hours of live instruction for their fourth graders learning remotely, with 34 percent offering the same for eighth graders during remote learning. Those figures remained roughly constant through the spring of 2021. Meanwhile, the number of students receiving in-person instruction also rose steadily throughout the spring: from 38 percent of fourth graders and 28 percent of eighth graders learning in-person by January to 44 and 33 percent, respectively, by March. And, by the same time, 88 percent of schools nationwide were offering some form of in-person learning, whether full-time or in hybrid settings, with 54 percent of schools with fourth or eighth grades providing the option of learning in-person full-time to all students. Yet, despite the improving picture overall, Black, Latinx, and Asian students were all substantially less likely to be enrolled in full-time in-person instruction through the spring.

PARTICIPATION DISPARITIES IN FULL-TIME IN-PERSON INSTRUCTION

In-person instruction provides strong engagement between students and teachers, students and their peers, and direct access to the full range of academic and wraparound services that a school provides. However, students of color have been less likely to be enrolled in full-time in-person instruction during the pandemic. As recently as March 2021, 58 percent of White students attending schools that serve fourth graders—often but not always elementary schools—were enrolled in full-time in-person instruction, while only 36 percent of Black students, 35 percent of Latinx students, and 18 percent of Asian students in schools serving fourth graders were enrolled in full-time in-person instruction.

STRUGGLING TO LOG ON AND STAY CONNECTED DURING DISTANCE LEARNING

- **Technology barriers.** The pandemic's uneven effects on students began with the basics: logging into the virtual classroom. According to one survey, as of the summer of 2020, nearly a third of teachers in majority Black schools reported that their students lacked the technology necessary to take part in virtual instruction. Only one in five teachers said the same in schools where fewer than 10 percent of students were Black. Similar challenges have been reported for Latinx students. In an online survey of more than 60,000 secondary and 22,000 upper elementary students, 30 percent of Latinx respondents cited a lack of reliable Internet access as an obstacle to distance learning, compared to 23 percent of their surveyed classmates. That technology gap remained through the fall of 2020, though narrowing somewhat. By October 2020, almost one of every 10 Black and Latinx households still lacked consistent computer access, compared to only 6.7 percent of White households. And, while only 4.7 percent of White households reported inconsistent Internet access, more than twice as many Black households and one-and-a-half times that many Latinx households said the same. State and district efforts over the last year—boosted by Federal CARES Act funding—helped narrow these technology gaps, at least in the short term. By early 2021—prior to the passage of the American Rescue Plan—some gaps persisted, and they continued to be more common among lower-income families, again, disproportionately affecting Black and Latinx students.

- **Logging in to class**. Even when they had access, many students did not log into online portals for virtual classes, especially during the early weeks of the pandemic. And those participation rates—though not necessarily reflecting engagement—were disproportionately lower for many students of color. In Chicago, for example, Black students last spring registered among the lowest rates of virtual participation, with nearly 30 percent not logging in at all at one point during distance learning—compared to 14 percent of White students not logging in during the same period. And, in Seattle, Black boys in high school (grades 9–12) had among the lowest virtual participation rates for their grades, with nearly a quarter not logging in at all between March and June, compared to the 12 percent of all high schoolers who also did not log in.
- **Losing contact with school**. In addition, more families of color reportedly fell out of contact with their children's

schools during the pandemic, especially early on. In one nationally representative survey conducted in the spring of 2020, nearly 30 percent of principals from schools serving "large populations of students of color and students from lower-income households" said they had difficulty reaching some of their students and/or families—in contrast to the 14 percent of principals who said the same in wealthier, predominantly White schools. Throughout the 2020–2021 school year, similar concerns have been expressed in districts across the country about students that have gone "missing" from the classroom.

DISRUPTED LEARNING DURING THE PANDEMIC

The public health restrictions that shuttered schools last spring also seriously disrupted individualized services for many students with disabilities—a difficulty school districts and teachers have acknowledged. As the U.S. Government Accountability Office (GAO) detailed in the fall of 2020, the school districts they surveyed reported encountering a variety of logistical and instructional factors that made it more difficult to deliver special education services during distance learning. And, for students whose needs require hands-on, face-to-face interaction—such as occupational or physical therapy—COVID-19, in some cases, brought services to a standstill.

Parents and families of students with disabilities also reported disruptions in their children's services. In a survey widely cited by major media outlets, conducted in May 2020 with 1,594 parents contacted through Facebook by the advocacy group ParentsTogether, only 20 percent of respondents said their children were receiving the services called for by their individualized education programs (IEPs), and 39 percent reported receiving no services at all. As a nonrandom sample, this survey cannot support definitive general conclusions. With that caveat, it bears noting that parents of children with IEPs in the same survey were also more than twice as likely than parents of children without IEPs to say that their child was doing little to no remote learning (35–17%) and that distance learning was not going well (40–19%). By the summer of

2020, evidence emerged from not only this poll but also another larger-scale online survey of more than 80,000 secondary and upper elementary students that students with disabilities may have been facing more mental health challenges than their peers and more generally having less positive experiences with schoolwork than other students. Those disruptions and related challenges have reportedly persisted through the 2020–2021 school year.

There are also some early indications that the pandemic has exacerbated academic achievement disparities for students with disabilities. In the fall of 2020, for example, several school districts reported sharp spikes in the number of their students with disabilities failing their classes. Data from one Maryland district, for example, revealed that the number of sixth graders with disabilities earning failing marks in English had doubled from the previous year. Meanwhile, a Virginia district saw a 111 percent increase in the number of students with disabilities receiving Fs in two or more subjects in the first quarter of the 2020–2021 school year. And a California district similarly reported an across-the-board jump in the fall of 2020 in the number of Ds and Fs given to students with disabilities in its middle and high schools. More research will be needed to assess whether these reports are reflective of broader and enduring trends.

COVID-19'S DISPARATE IMPACTS ON STUDENTS IN HIGHER EDUCATION

Postsecondary students and the institutions they attend have faced unprecedented challenges to their academic and living conditions since March 2020. In short order, many colleges and universities pivoted to remote learning for spring and summer terms, with residential campuses sending most of their students home. The 2020–2021 academic year saw some students return to in-person instruction on campus; for others, instruction remained remote or hybrid.

But the images of closing residence halls and online commencements told only a part of the story. As discussed below, while you may not understand the full scope of the pandemic's effects for some time, early research shows that the disparities in student experience and by institutional sectors were stark. Undergraduate enrollment during the 13 months you looked at was down throughout the country, especially among community colleges that disproportionately serve the students with the fewest resources. Additionally, the number of students experiencing financial insecurity and mental health challenges increased significantly. At the start of the 2020–2021 academic year, many of America's students were leaving higher education (or not entering at all), losing jobs, taking fewer classes, juggling caregiving responsibilities, and being concerned about their financial well-being and work opportunities.

COVID-19 AND STUDENT ENROLLMENT: WIDESPREAD EFFECTS AND DISPARATE IMPACTS

Beginning in mid-March 2020, many—if not most—colleges and universities shifted quickly to an online learning environment. By fall 2020, out of nearly 3,000 colleges surveyed, 44 percent were fully or primarily online, while 27 percent were fully or primarily in-person. Plans for the spring 2021 term turned out to be similar: 43 percent of institutions indicated, as of January 31, 2021, that they planned to remain fully or primarily online, while only 18 percent planned to be fully or primarily in-person.

- **Abrupt changes in plans for 2020 high school graduates.** Changes took place occurred for graduating students with heightened drop-offs in college enrollment from high-poverty high schools. For students who graduated from high school in 2020, college enrollment was down in 2020. The National Student Clearinghouse reported a nearly seven percent drop in enrollment compared with 2019 graduates. Meanwhile, another national study of about 60,000 households conducted by the U.S. Bureau of Labor Statistics (BLS) found that by October 2020, 62.7 percent of 2020 high school graduates were enrolled in colleges or universities, down from 66.2 percent in 2019. Of those keeping with their college plans, over one-fifth changed their first-choice school, with most citing cost and location as the most

important factors for doing so. For 2020 graduates of high-poverty high schools, the turn away from college has been even greater: an 11.4 percent falloff in college enrollment compared to a 1.6 percent decline in 2019.
- **Steep drops in community college enrollment.** Community colleges were also hit hard, with enrollment among 2020 high school graduates down 13.2 percent in the fall of 2020. And, although overall enrollment in community colleges had been declining in recent years, the fall 2020 drop—by 10.1 percent—was almost 10 times steeper than the 1.4 percent decrease in overall enrollment reported in 2019. Spring 2021 enrollment continued the downward trend: Undergraduate enrollment slumped 5.9 percent from a year earlier, and community colleges remained the hardest hit, with enrollment off 11.3 percent from spring 2020. Enrollment by young college students (aged 18–20) who make up 40 percent of all undergraduates shrunk by 7.2 percent, the greatest of any age group, with the deepest declines occurring at community colleges, which were down 14.6 percent.
- **Reduced enrollment and retention for students who are caregivers.** The shift to online learning had a profound effect on students' lives, including their decisions to enroll or remain in school. That shift took a particularly heavy toll on students who had to juggle their own education while caring for children, elderly or sick parents, or others. A survey of more than 30,000 undergraduates conducted in the spring of 2020 found that student caregivers faced a range of heightened risks and demands, including greater-than-average financial hardship, food insecurity, and generalized anxiety. Those demands may also have created the potential for parents to sacrifice their own well-being to meet the caregiving needs of their children, especially among mothers who frequently assume the primary caregiving role. And there is already evidence that some students—both women and men—had to drop

out of classes, or not enroll at all, as they struggled to balance those responsibilities.[1]

Section 44.2 | Distance Education during the COVID-19 Pandemic

Nearly 93 percent of people in households with school-age children reported their children engaged in some form of "distance learning" from home, but lower-income households were less likely to rely on online resources.

The COVID-19 pandemic in the spring dramatically shifted the way children were being educated. Perhaps the most salient change was the closure of schools forcing students to continue their education from home. From May 28 to June 2, when many school districts across the country are normally in session, 80 percent of people living with children reported the children were using online resources. About 20 percent were using paper materials sent home by the school. (The categories overlap because respondents could select more than one category.)

The Household Pulse Survey (www.census.gov/data/experimental-data-products/household-pulse-survey.html) show that high-income households with children were using online resources at higher rates than those in lower-income households. For example, in households with income of $100,000 or more, 85.8 percent of people with children reported using online resources for distance learning.

By contrast, only 65.8 percent of people in households with income of less than $50,000 and 76.5 percent of households with income of $50,000–$99,999 reported that children were using online resources for distance learning.

Conversely, low-income households reported higher rates of using paper materials sent home from school than high-income

---

[1] "Education in a Pandemic: The Disparate Impacts of COVID-19 on America's Students," U.S. Department of Education (ED), August 15, 2021. Available online. URL: www2.ed.gov/about/offices/list/ocr/docs/20210608-impacts-of-covid19.pdf. Accessed December 16, 2022.

COVID-19 Impact on Education

households. Households with income less than $50,000 (21.1%) and households with income from $50,000 to $99,999 (19.1%) were significantly more likely to use paper materials sent home for distance learning than households with income of $100,000 or more (15.3%).

There were no significant percentage differences for the use of paper materials sent home from school in households with income less than $50,000 and $50,000–$99,999. People aged 18 and over in households with children in school who did not report their household income (4.9% of the total sample) are excluded.[2]

IMPLEMENT HIGH-QUALITY AND EFFECTIVE TUTORING

Tutoring can yield important results for students when done in effective ways. The best available evidence suggests that tutoring is most effective when districts and schools:

- **Use trained staff and educators as tutors.** Teachers, paraprofessionals, teaching candidates, and recently retired teachers are most likely to be effective, especially when given ongoing coaching and time to plan and collaborate with classroom teachers. However, others can be effective tutors when they receive preservice and ongoing training and professional development.
- **Regularly provide opportunities for tutoring.** Schedules that include frequent sessions—at least three times a week of at least 30–50 minutes—are most effective in accelerating learning.
- **Schedule tutoring sessions during the school day when possible.** Research shows that tutoring programs that occur during the school day have the largest effects. School leaders can ensure students still receive core instruction by creating space for tutoring by using double blocking or tutoring during study hall and flexible periods.

---

[2] "Schooling during the COVID-19 Pandemic," United States Census Bureau, December 21, 2021. Available online. URL: www.census.gov/library/stories/2020/08/schooling-during-the-covid-19-pandemic.html. Accessed February 23, 2022.

- **Align tutoring with an evidence-based curriculum.** Tutoring may be more effective when it is conducted alongside a high-quality curriculum and practices that support positive learning experiences during regular class time.

INTEGRATE AND PRIORITIZE THE SOCIAL, EMOTIONAL, AND ACADEMIC NEEDS OF ALL STUDENTS

Research shows that social, emotional, cognitive, and academic development are linked, and schools can promote student growth in each of these areas. For example, districts and schools can:
- implement evidence-based schoolwide programs and strategies to support social, emotional, and academic development, including tools such as Positive Behavioral Interventions and Supports (PBIS) and the CASEL School Guide
- design equitable learning environments for students by focusing on developing strong and trusting relationships, fostering belonging, creating rigorous and engaging and culturally responsive learning environments, and offering integrated support systems
- use evidence-based strategies to create school systems, structures, and practices that support all aspects of child development

PROVIDE STUDENTS WITH TAILORED LEARNING ACCELERATION OPPORTUNITIES

Learning acceleration is a strategy designed to get students on grade level by using evidence-based interventions to help close content and skill gaps as efficiently as possible. The goal of tailored acceleration is to ensure that all students attain college and career readiness regardless of where they may be starting. Research shows that learning acceleration is an important strategy for advancing equity and that students who experienced acceleration struggled less and learned more than students who started at the same point

but experienced remediation instead. To support learning acceleration, districts and schools can do the following:
- Provide teachers and staff with high-quality and ongoing professional development and coaching, including coaching on how to identify content and skills that need to be prioritized, design and select instructional strategies, and use data to inform instruction. Professional learning communities may provide such professional development and coaching. Professional learning communities are most effective when they use data to determine student and educator learning needs, identify shared goals for student and educator learning, support educators in their content instruction and classroom management strategies, select and implement appropriate evidence-based strategies to improve outcomes, and use evidence to monitor progress and improve when needed.
- Use school vacation time during the school year to support students with the greatest need. For example, Acceleration Academies are intensive, targeted, instructional programs conducted over vacation breaks to support student learning and help students address lost instructional time.
- Adopt and use high-quality instructional materials that appropriately challenge students, are culturally relevant, and are aligned with grade-level standards.

SUPPORT THE SUCCESSFUL TRANSITIONS OF STUDENTS FROM PRESCHOOL TO ELEMENTARY SCHOOL, ELEMENTARY SCHOOL TO MIDDLE SCHOOL, MIDDLE SCHOOL TO HIGH SCHOOL, AND HIGH SCHOOL TO POSTSECONDARY EDUCATION AND THE WORKFORCE

Students thrive when they have access to appropriately challenging programs and instructional materials that are aligned to rigorous standards and culturally and linguistically relevant. To better understand where students are and the support they need to succeed during key transitions in their education, schools can employ a data-driven decision-making process to identify and match students' needs to interventions and monitor their progress. To support these efforts, districts and schools can do the following:

- Establish an early warning indicator (EWI) and intervention system to promote targeted engagement strategies in response to data from EWIs. EWI systems can track attendance, assignment completion, discipline, and grades. When appropriately viewed at the school, grade, classroom, and student level to support student well-being, these data can strengthen a school's ability to provide specific and timely interventions. For example, schools can use on-track indicators to assess how well students are making the transition into middle and high school so that the schools can provide additional support as needed.
- Establish summer bridge programs that provide social, emotional, and academic support for students entering middle and high school to ensure that they are ready for middle and high school and set on a path toward success.
- States and districts can also leverage funding to improve access and success in college in high school programs. College in High School programs are an effective tool to increase access to college, improve persistence and completion in college, improve workforce readiness, and reduce the overall costs of college.

USE HIGH-QUALITY OUT-OF-SCHOOL TIME LEARNING EXPERIENCES TO SUPPORT STUDENTS' SOCIAL, EMOTIONAL, AND ACADEMIC NEEDS

Research has shown that learning can happen in many contexts. A wide range of programs can be delivered via Office of the Secretary (OST) programs, including work-based learning programs, youth development programs, and experiential or service-learning programs. High-quality evidence-based programs that are strongly rooted in the school context can also lead to positive social, emotional, and academic outcomes, greater self-confidence, increased civic engagement, better attendance, improved high school graduation, and decreased disciplinary actions. In designing and implementing high-quality OST programs, schools and districts can do the following:

- Align OST programs academically with the school curriculum so OST educators can build on skills and materials students are already learning.
- Create systems and processes to adapt instruction to individual and small group needs. OST groups of more than 20 students per staff member are shown to be less effective.
- Provide high-quality, engaging learning experiences to students with the goal of providing students with important opportunities for academic support and access to enrichment activities that develop social and emotional well-being and leadership skills.
- Ensure students with the most need for additional support have adequate opportunities to participate in OST programs.
- Regularly assess program performance using disaggregated results to improve or adjust the program as needed.
- Partner with community-based organizations and local intermediary organizations to increase access to high-quality OST opportunities. Partnerships may provide additional enrichment opportunities; expand the opportunity for students to interact with organization staff who may be more racially, culturally, and linguistically diverse; and create additional opportunities for community engagement.
- Support students with disabilities by providing Extended School Year (ESY) services under the Individuals with Disabilities Education Act (IDEA). These services can help accelerate learning for IDEA-eligible students with disabilities who, based on

their individual needs as determined by the student's individualized education program (IEP) team, need instruction beyond the regular school year in order to receive a free appropriate public education. American Rescue Plan (ARP) resources may be used to support the IDEA ESY authority or to provide summer learning and acceleration programs for students with disabilities who may not qualify for ESY.[3]

---

[3] "Supporting Learning Acceleration with American Rescue Plan Funds," U.S. Department of Education (ED), June 9, 2021. Available online. URL: www2.ed.gov/documents/coronavirus/learning-acceleration.pdf. Accessed December 16, 2022.

Chapter 45 | COVID-19 Impact on Health-Care Facilities

HEALTH CARE DELIVERY
Hospitals Reported Significant Challenges in Meeting the Needs of COVID-19 Patients and Uncertainty about Future COVID-19 Caseloads

Hospitals are at the forefront of health care delivery during the COVID-19 pandemic, and hospital administrators described the strain the pandemic has placed on patient care. In some cases, hospitals reported that underlying problems with health care delivery were exacerbated, such as challenges providing care for underserved patients and challenges for rural hospitals with limited resources.

THE VOLUME OF COVID-19 PATIENTS AND THE COMPLEXITY OF THEIR IMMEDIATE AND LONG-TERM NEEDS SIGNIFICANTLY STRAINED PATIENT CARE AND HOSPITAL OPERATIONS

Hospitals reported being overwhelmed by the volume of patients, especially during surges in COVID-19 infections. They explained that this put a severe strain on their bed capacity. Some hospitals reported that they operated at over 100-percent capacity during surges, and high occupancy continues for some hospitals. At the time of the survey, 40 responding hospitals had over 90-percent inpatient occupancy, and 56 had over 90 percent of their intensive care unit (ICU) beds occupied. One urban hospital, with a nearly full ICU the week before the survey, reported that it would do only urgent surgeries and discharged patients to their homes for recovery because of a shortage of recovery areas in the hospital.

Hospitals emphasized the great clinical challenges in treating COVID-19 patients, particularly those with severe illness and comorbidities. Hospital clinicians have had to keep up with emerging treatment protocols, often without sufficient specialty staff, such as infectious disease specialists, pulmonologists, respiratory therapists, and clinical nurses trained in treating COVID-19.

COVID-19 patients with longer-term effects will also need complex specialty care. Hospitals reported seeing patients with serious post-COVID conditions, such as pulmonary issues, pneumonia, heart problems, and blood clots. One hospital described "a tsunami of people going forward" who they predicted would experience long-term effects from COVID-19.

Administrators reported challenges in balancing the complex and resource-intensive care needed for COVID-19 patients with efforts to resume routine hospital care. Hospitals reported having difficulty integrating COVID-19 care into normal operations, chiefly because of concerns about infection control. As hospitals reopened more services for patients after the early months of the pandemic, such as resuming elective surgeries, they experienced increased challenges in keeping infected COVID-19 patients separated from noninfected patients. Complicating this further, hospitals explained that a new patient's COVID-19 positivity status may not be immediately known.

HOSPITALS REPORTED CHALLENGES IN DISCHARGING COVID-19 PATIENTS DURING THEIR RECOVERY, WHICH AFFECTED AVAILABLE BED SPACE THROUGHOUT THE HOSPITAL

Hospitals reported difficulty in discharging COVID-19 patients following the acute stage of their illness, resulting in longer hospital stays. Administrators reported challenges in transferring patients to postacute facilities such as nursing homes, rehabilitation hospitals, and hospice facilities. According to administrators, some postacute facilities were either unwilling or unable to accept patients because the facilities were concerned about potential COVID-19 infections. Others did not have bed capacity or staff to care for the patients.

Administrators reported that delays in discharge affected available bed space throughout the hospital and had other downstream effects. For example, hospitals reported that patient opportunities for specialized postacute care (e.g., rehabilitation) were delayed. Hospitals also reported that longer stays created bottlenecks throughout hospitals, including in ICUs and emergency departments. As an example, one hospital reported that 13 of its 17 emergency treatment rooms were occupied by COVID-19 patients waiting to be admitted to the hospital.

UNCERTAINTY ABOUT FUTURE COVID-19 CASELOADS AND THE IMPLICATIONS OF NEW VIRUS VARIANTS ADDS TO HOSPITALS' CHALLENGES

Administrators expressed concern about emerging issues such as new variants of the virus and vaccine efficacy. Hospitals worried that the new variants could bring additional challenges and changes to treatment needs, infection control, and best care practices. Administrators also had questions about the long-term efficacy of vaccines and worried about the possibility of future COVID-19 surges. One hospital administrator asked, "Are we out of the woods or will it come back again?" Another hospital expressed concern that COVID-19 may become a regular seasonal infection, such as influenza, which could present serious ongoing preparedness challenges given that COVID-19 is both more infectious and more deadly than the flu.

Hospitals reported that continuing fluctuations in the number of patients with COVID-19 made it difficult to plan for the future. Hospitals were cautious about taking steps toward resuming normal operations. For example, one hospital not treating any COVID-19 patients the week before the survey reported that it was hesitant to repurpose its antibody infusion room or to fill rooms designated for isolation because of the risk of another wave of COVID-19 cases despite other demands for this space.

Hospitals Reported That the Pandemic Led to Delayed Care and Feared That an Erosion of Trust in Hospital Safety Would Continue to Keep Patients from Seeking Needed Care

Administrators raised concerns about the public not receiving needed health care during the pandemic due to patients delaying and forgoing care, as well as to hospitals suspending elective care due to COVID-19. They reported that lack of care and reduced use of hospitals have had significant ramifications for patients and the hospitals that treat them.

HOSPITALS REPORTED THAT PATIENTS HAVE DELAYED OR FORGONE ROUTINE HEALTH CARE, WHICH HAS LED TO WORSENING OF PATIENT CONDITIONS

Many hospitals chose or were required, to suspend elective surgeries and other services at different points during the pandemic to preserve resources for emergencies and COVID-19 surges, but according to administrators, delayed care has persisted past these early suspensions. As causes of delaying and forgoing care, administrators cited patients' fear of contracting COVID-19 and practical concerns such as difficulty finding transportation during the pandemic. Hospitals described reduced patient volume across hospital departments and services, including emergency care, preventative care, chronic condition management, and surgeries. Delayed care included preventative and urgent care for serious conditions such as heart attacks or strokes. One administrator attributed some emergency room deaths at their hospital to patients not following up on their prior care needs.

Administrators predicted that such widespread delayed care would result in higher hospitalization rates and a need for more complex hospital care in the future. They explained that when patients miss routine exams and diagnostic tests, such as cancer screenings and cardiology tests, serious diagnoses may go unidentified. One administrator reported finding a sharp decline in cancer diagnoses during the pandemic and that patients were not presenting for examination at the onset of symptoms. Another administrator described seeing patients for diabetes and cardiac management who were sicker and required more care after postponing prior appointments. One administrator reported, "My only concern is how sick our patients are. There was a long period of time where patients were not receiving primary care. We see the impact here almost daily with the symptoms patients are presenting with."

HOSPITALS REPORTED THAT PUBLIC TRUST IN HOSPITAL SAFETY AND CREDIBILITY HAS ERODED DURING THE PANDEMIC

Hospital administrators perceived that some in their communities appeared to newly question whether hospitals are safe and can keep patients safe. Administrators reported that patients continue to be concerned about contracting COVID-19 in the hospital despite the protective procedures that hospitals have put in place to mitigate exposure. Some administrators speculated that this could be in part because of confusion over evolving public health guidelines during the pandemic.

Hospitals voiced concern that some patients were less likely to trust hospital care recommendations as credible, possibly because the patients received confusing and changing messages about COVID-19 during the pandemic. Administrators worried that lack of trust could contribute to patients further delaying and forgoing care. One administrator said, "Unless we can get everyone on the same page to get routine health care, we shudder at the burden of disease that may occur."

Hospitals Expressed Concern about Meeting the Increased Need for Mental and Behavioral Health Care That Has Emerged as an Outgrowth of the Pandemic

Administrators voiced concern that the pandemic has led to greater mental and behavioral health needs among patients. They explained that these added needs resulted from many factors, including lockdowns, social isolation, and burnout. Administrators anticipated that the needs for mental and behavioral health services at their hospitals would continue to grow. Administrators reported concern about meeting these needs and about how mental health challenges can exacerbate other health problems. One hospital reported concern for seniors in particular, observing that the elderly may be among the most vulnerable to depression associated with the pandemic.

Some hospitals believe that they may not have the capacity or resources to meet the increased needs for mental and behavioral health care. For example, one hospital closed a psychiatric unit that focused on elderly patients because it needed the unit's staff to help serve COVID-19 patients. In addition to inpatient care, hospitals often serve as a primary mental health provider in communities. Some administrators explained that their role includes conducting mental health screenings and treating mental and behavioral health issues as comorbidities to other medical conditions. Hospitals reported that there was a need for additional resources and specialists to provide this care before the pandemic and that the pandemic increased the need further. Additionally, administrators reported that it can be more difficult to treat COVID-19 patients who suffer from mental illness or behavioral challenges.

Rural Hospitals Reported That Long-Standing Operational Challenges Have Worsened during the Pandemic

Administrators reported that the COVID-19 pandemic has disproportionately hampered operations for rural hospitals. For example, they reported that the pandemic has worsened long-standing challenges in recruiting and retaining staff, limited bed capacity, lack of access to specialized services, and financial strain.

Some hospitals raised that strategies used by other hospitals to address resource challenges, such as sharing clinicians across systems, may not work for rural hospitals. One administrator reported that rural hospitals do not have access to back-up resources, observing, "As a rural community, we have a limited number of physicians. If one physician falls ill, we are done." A few rural hospitals reported attempts to provide more telehealth services to fill gaps in care, but their patients sometimes lacked access to the technology needed to use these services. They also reported that limited patient access to technology, such as broadband Internet access, affected other aspects of care, such as hampering outreach about vaccines.

Furthermore, administrators reported that a lack of available beds at many larger hospitals sometimes prevented them from transferring COVID-19 patients and other critically ill patients. Most rural hospitals are designed to provide urgent and routine care services for a wide geographic area and to transfer patients requiring specialty or intensive care to other hospitals. One rural hospital in Louisiana that does not have an ICU reported that it was contacting hospitals in neighboring states because they had the closest available ICU beds. Among your responding hospitals, 67 served rural communities, and 28 of these hospitals operated fewer than 15 inpatient beds.

Hospital Administrators Raised Concerns That the COVID-19 Pandemic Has Worsened Existing Disparities in Access to Care and Health Outcomes

Hospitals reported that the COVID-19 pandemic has exacerbated long-standing problems with access to care, particularly for rural communities and for low-income populations across geographic settings. Hospitals reported that many rural communities face health-care provider shortages, transportation challenges that make it difficult to access hospitals that may be hours away, and lack of Internet service to support using telehealth to reduce these barriers. Many low-income individuals face barriers to health care (even in nonrural settings), including lack of health insurance or transportation. Hospitals also reported that low-income individuals may be unable to afford Internet service or devices to support using telehealth to reduce these barriers.

In addition, hospitals raised concerns about disparities in health outcomes, including higher incidence rates and severity of COVID-19 infections in certain communities, concerns raised by others in the health-care community throughout the pandemic. According to the Centers for Disease Control and Prevention (CDC), communities that have high levels of poverty, crowded housing, and other attributes associated with higher social vulnerability have been likely to experience high rates of COVID-19. Among responding hospitals, 41 were located in counties where 20 percent or more of the population had household incomes below the federal poverty level, and 113 hospitals serve communities with higher social vulnerability than the national average according to the CDC's Social Vulnerability Index.

Administrators from hospitals in communities with higher social vulnerability reported deep concern about worse outcomes for many of their patients. Hospitals also reported clinical challenges in treating patients with certain comorbidities that disproportionately affect people of color, such as heart and lung ailments and chronic illnesses such as diabetes, and that patients with these comorbidities are at higher risk of severe illness from COVID-19. These patients may enter hospitals at a more severe stage of illness and require a higher level of care. In some cases, hospitals explained that they lack this advanced care capacity or may lack the resources to treat a large number of vulnerable patients. Hospitals reported that patients who have low incomes are also less likely to have access to primary care that could prevent disease worsening.

Hospitals Reported the Adoption and Use of Telehealth Was Beneficial and a Change They Want to Retain despite Some Challenges

Administrators reported that telehealth has become an important care delivery modality for their hospitals during the COVID-19 pandemic, increasing patient access to care while reducing risk and workload for hospital staff. Hospitals described a wide range of situations for which they implemented or expanded telehealth services, including connecting remote specialists to help severely ill patients in ICUs, conducting follow-up visits for patients recovering from COVID-19, conducting mental health services, and providing education for at-home care.

Although administrators were overwhelmingly positive about the benefits of telehealth, they reported three key challenges in delivering care with this method. First, telehealth cannot cover all aspects of health care delivery and by its very nature lacks the in-person interaction valued by some providers and patients. Second, technology created challenges for telehealth care delivery.

Hospitals reported that some patients do not have the devices or Internet access to conduct telehealth visits, particularly in underserved communities. One administrator worried that telehealth visits do not work equally well for all communities. Although some patients are able to conduct video calls, others must rely on audio-only telephone calls, particularly the elderly and those in underserved communities. Third, some hospitals reported that they received lower payments for some services provided through telehealth than they would have received for in-person services, and they did not believe the payments reflected the value of those telehealth services.

STAFFING
Hospitals Reported That Increased Workloads and the Stress of Treating Seriously Ill and Dying COVID-19 Patients Have Led to Staff Burnout and, in Some Cases, Trauma

Hospitals reported that increased hours and responsibilities and other stressors caused by the COVID-19 pandemic resulted in staff being exhausted, mentally fatigued, and sometimes experiencing possible posttraumatic stress disorder (PTSD). Hospitals reported that for the past year, staff have worked longer hours, extra shifts, and mandatory overtime. In addition, some reported that caring for higher level and critically ill patients who might have been transferred to other facilities prior to the pandemic caused additional stress on staff who felt ill-equipped to handle such care on a continuing basis. Furthermore, hospitals reported that staff were "wearing many hats"—balancing multiple clinical and administrative responsibilities to cover the staffing gaps. Other staff were pulled away from their normal duties to complete new COVID-19-related tasks. For example, hospitals reported dedicating staff to meet COVID-19 data entry and reporting requirements, with one administrator describing it as "very labor intensive." Another hospital reported pulling staff from their regular duties to manage the thousands of incoming telephone calls when the community learned that the hospital had received vaccine doses.

Several hospitals reported that the COVID-19-related deaths that staff witnessed especially weighed on their mental health. One administrator observed that with family unable to be present at patient bedsides, it has been heartbreaking for nurses to be the last person a dying patient sees. Furthermore, administrators reported that hospital staff experienced COVID-19 deaths among their coworkers, which took a toll on those remaining and continuing the work. One representative from a hospital network described a monthly gathering for staff to mourn colleagues who passed away from COVID-19. Adding to this emotional distress, hospitals explained that some staff have had to separate from their families for extended periods to protect their family members from infection.

Administrators at one major teaching hospital (where, the week before the survey, nearly 50 percent of ICU patients had COVID-19) reported that treating COVID-19 formerly involved everyone on staff but now involves only certain staff while others get to go back to "normal." The administrators explained that staff still treating COVID-19 patients experienced more fatigue attributable to loss of the teamwork that existed in earlier months of the pandemic and a strong desire to return to normalcy like some of their colleagues.

Hospitals Reported That High Turnover and Competition for Medical Staff Have Created Staffing Shortages That in Some Cases Affect Patient Care

Hospitals reported that they were experiencing higher than normal turnover among medical staff, resulting in concerning staffing shortages. Among your responding hospitals, 38 reported to the U.S. Department of Health and Human Services (HHS) Protect that they faced a critical staffing shortage during the week before the pulse survey. Turnover was particularly high among nurses, according to the hospitals. One hospital in a high-poverty and socially vulnerable community in Texas (which was operating at 100-percent ICU occupancy the week before the survey) reported that its annual average for nurse turnover increased from two percent prior to the pandemic to 20 percent in 2020. Hospitals also reported losing other types of staff in the past year, including respiratory therapists, certified nursing assistants, phlebotomists, laboratory technicians, and other support staff vital to hospital operations.

Many hospitals attributed the increased turnover of staff to stress and burnout caused by COVID-19, leading some staff to retire early or seek jobs outside of health care. Hospitals also cited competition for health-care workers and the opportunity to earn more money by leaving a hospital to join a staffing agency.

SOME HOSPITALS REPORTED STRUGGLING WITH THE UNEXPECTED INCREASE IN COMPETITION FOR MEDICAL STAFF

Administrators reported an increase in competition for medical staff, particularly nurses, among hospitals and staffing agencies. Many hospitals reported that they were unable to compete with staffing agency salaries, with one administrator describing the competition over health-care workers as a "wage war." Hospitals that lost nurses reported that they often experienced increased staffing costs from the higher hourly rates charged by staffing agencies.

Smaller hospitals and rural hospitals reported that it was particularly hard for them to compete for staff with large urban hospitals and that the inability to compete led to further shortages. An administrator from a critical access hospital stated that they always had a few nursing vacancies that they could not fill, even with offering bonuses. As another administrator explained, recruiting providers in a rural community is always difficult but had gotten harder during the pandemic.

HOSPITALS REPORTED THAT STAFFING SHORTAGES POSED CHALLENGES IN MAINTAINING PATIENT SAFETY AND QUALITY OF CARE

Hospitals raised concerns that the quality of care has suffered as a result of losing nursing staff. Several administrators reported that staffing shortages have forced them to assign substantially more patients per staff, such as one administrator who reported that their hospital had to cut its staff-to-patient ratio in half for some periods during the pandemic, to 1-to-12 from 1-to-6. Reduced staff-to-patient ratios can lead to mistakes when less attention is given to each patient. Hospitals also reported that staffing shortages have resulted in staff having to work longer hours, extra shifts, and mandatory overtime for the past year. Representatives from one hospital network reported that it had seen an increase in central line infections, which can be life-threatening. They attributed the increase in these infections to not having sufficient staff and reported that staff's fatigue led to process failures. Another hospital reported that feedback scores from patients on communication and quality had decreased and attributed that to tired and frustrated staff.

Some hospital administrators reported quality of care concerns even when they bolstered staffing levels with traveling nurses, reporting that these nurses are not as familiar with the hospital's particular processes as nurses with longer tenures. For example, one hospital attributed a rise in its hospital-acquired infections to the hiring of agency staff not trained in that hospital's infection control processes.

HOSPITALS EXPRESSED CONCERNS THAT A SHRINKING RECRUITMENT POOL FOR NURSES COULD CONTINUE TO WORSEN STAFFING SHORTAGES

Hospitals raised concerns that nationwide shortages of nurses and other health-care workers, already a concern before the COVID-19 pandemic, had worsened as a result of the pandemic. Administrators from several hospitals believed that the pandemic has deterred people from entering the medical profession, with fewer students seeking degrees in medical disciplines. As one hospital administrator said, "We cannot overstate the staffing gap that exists now that's likely to get worse over the next few years." An administrator from one teaching hospital reported that the hospital would typically recruit nurses who have completed training at the hospital, but this year only 100 nurses were expected to graduate and the hospital had 200 open nursing positions.

Furthermore, several hospitals expressed concern that because of the pandemic, newly graduated nurses may not have gained sufficient clinical experience with other ailments and that hospitals lacked resources to adequately train new nurses. One administrator explained that some nursing students have been unable to graduate because they could not complete their clinical training.

VACCINATIONS
Hospitals Reported That Vaccination Efforts Were Positive Steps toward Pandemic Recovery but Exacerbated Challenges with Clinical Staff Shortages and Hospital Finances

Hospital staff were among the earliest to get vaccinations, which helped to reduce risk of infection to front-line health-care workers and to limit the spread of COVID-19 within the hospital. Hospitals reported that they have set up the infrastructure necessary to administer COVID-19 vaccines to their communities. These efforts include creating mass vaccination sites and reallocating clinical staff to administer vaccines.

Many hospitals reported that they were ready to vaccinate on a large scale as soon as vaccine supply became more available. As one administrator explained, hospitals are well-positioned to administer vaccines, given that they have the needed space, exam rooms, clinical expertise, and workflow processes. Hospitals viewed their vaccination efforts as a positive step toward pandemic recovery. For example, one hospital noted that providing vaccinations was important to economic recovery.

Some hospitals reported that vaccination efforts sometimes exacerbated existing challenges with clinical staff shortages and hospital finances. Some hospitals reported needing to divert clinical staff away from patient care to administer vaccines, which has "strained an already stressed system" as one administrator explained. Hospitals reported shifting nurses from other departments, including ICUs, operating rooms, emergency departments, and obstetrics, to administer vaccines and sometimes at remote locations.

Hospitals reported that it takes a considerable amount of staff time to operate vaccination clinics. One administrator explained that it took 25 staff members working an eight-hour shift to distribute 600 vaccines. Hospitals also reported frustration with inefficiencies in required data reporting. For example, one hospital reported that to meet federal, state, and local reporting requirements, it had to enter vaccine data into three separate systems. It characterized such data entry as "cumbersome" and "redundant," noting that "none of the three systems are talking to each other, [despite the fact that] they are inputting the exact same data into each system."

Hospitals also reported that costs associated with vaccine administration have strained hospital financial resources. Beyond staffing, hospitals explained that costs include equipment for storing vaccines (e.g., freezers) and supplies to administer vaccines. Although a few hospitals reported using the Coronavirus Aid, Relief, and Economic Security (CARES) Act funding to offset the expense of vaccinating the community, others reported that this support did not cover all of the hospital expenses for operating vaccination sites. (Note that after the pulse survey, the Centers for Medicare & Medicaid Services (CMS) increased the Medicare payment amount for administering the COVID-19 vaccine to offset costs associated with establishing or operating vaccination sites and hiring additional staff.)

Differences in Government Guidelines regarding Vaccine Eligibility and Prioritization Created Challenges for Hospitals

Hospitals reported receiving varying information from different levels of government about who is eligible to receive the COVID-19 vaccine and when they are eligible. Federal, state, and local governments have prioritized different population groups to receive vaccines. The CDC's Advisory Committee on Immunization Practices made recommendations that prioritized health-care workers and long-term care facility residents, but states have discretion to adjust the guidelines based on their populations, vaccine supply, and capacity to vaccinate.

Hospitals reported that differences in vaccination priorities across jurisdictions have made it more complicated to determine who is eligible, which can be time-consuming and resource-intensive for hospitals. For example, hospitals serving communities at state borders must vary their vaccination approach based on each state's priorities. One hospital explained, "We are near Indiana and Michigan, and depending on what side of [the] street you are on, it affects what rules apply." A further complication is that within states, counties and cities may determine their own priority populations that can vary across each jurisdiction. For example, one hospital network noted that "vaccine 1b eligibility criteria and allocation varies to a great extent across Illinois, Wisconsin, Cook County, and City of Chicago."

Hospitals Reported That Some Hospital Staff and Members of the Community Were Hesitant to Get Vaccinated

Hospitals noted that they were struggling to convince some staff of the importance and safety of the vaccine. Administrators from several hospitals reported more than a third of their staff had declined to be vaccinated as of the date of the survey. Administrators attributed this lack of willingness to take the COVID-19 vaccine to multiple causes. For example, they explained that some staff distrusted the rapid vaccine development and approval process and others had concerns that the vaccines may not be effective.

Hospitals also raised concerns about hesitancy among members of their communities and reported working to combat misinformation about the vaccine. Hospitals worried that fewer vaccinations would allow the virus to continue circulating longer than necessary. Some administrators reported that the public lacked complete information about vaccines, which appeared to increase hesitancy to be vaccinated. For example, one administrator reported hearing a variety of concerns, from questions about the long-term side effects of the vaccines to false assertions that vaccines carry microchips.

Hospitals Reported Challenges in Ensuring Access to Vaccinations for Rural, Senior, and Low-Income Populations

Administrators reported that vaccinating rural communities presented unique challenges in ensuring access. Hospitals in rural areas, including critical access hospitals, reported that rural areas often have few vaccination sites and lengthy travel between sites. For example, in some rural communities, the hospital may be the nearest vaccination site for patients who live hours away. Hospitals noted that this distance can make it difficult to vaccinate residents who do not have reliable transportation. Officials from one critical access hospital noted that many rural areas have a higher proportion of low-income residents, who may not have reliable transportation for long travel. Additionally, hospitals explained that those without a car have difficulty traveling to mass vaccination sites.

Hospitals reported taking extra steps to ensure that senior and low-income populations could access vaccinations. Vaccination appointments have been commonly scheduled online, and hospitals reported that this creates barriers for individuals who lack internet service, devices, or capabilities needed to access and navigate online scheduling. For these patients, hospitals reported needing to use different scheduling options, such as calling elderly patients directly to schedule vaccination appointments. Some hospitals also reported going into the community to vaccinate, such as by setting up vaccine clinics in parking lots in certain neighborhoods.

Hospitals Reported Frustration with the Unpredictable and Insufficient Supply of Vaccines

Hospitals reported that the supply of vaccines they receive has been unpredictable, and they often get little advance notice about changes to shipment quantities. Administrators explained that quantities of vaccine shipped to hospitals varied from week to week and did not always match the amount they expected. Hospitals reported that this inconsistency led to inefficient use of resources and caused hospitals to cancel patient appointments at the last minute.

Several administrators expressed frustration about building infrastructure and planning for mass vaccinations only to have that capacity be underutilized due to inconsistent supply. For example, one hospital reported that it has capacity to vaccinate 5,000 people a week but received only 2,000 doses a week. Another hospital reported creating three vaccine locations within its system and allocated staff to provide 6,000–8,000 vaccines a week but had no vaccines at the time of their survey on February 21, 2021. (Note: Since the time of the pulse survey conducted the week of February 22–26, 2021, the Food and Drug Administration (FDA) issued an emergency use authorization for a third vaccine for the prevention of COVID-19, helping to lead to an increase in daily vaccinations.)

SUPPLIES
Hospitals Reported Difficulty Maintaining a Steady Supply of Affordable, High-Quality PPE

Hospitals reported that they were no longer experiencing the extreme shortages of PPE that occurred at the beginning of the COVID-19 pandemic, but some still lacked dependable supply chains for PPE. Hospitals noted that supplies of surgical gloves and N95 masks were particularly unpredictable. One problem reported with gloves was that only large sizes could be purchased, often the wrong size for many hospital staff. During the week before the pulse survey, 19 of your responding hospitals reported to HHS Protect that they could not order and obtain N95 masks. Furthermore, some hospitals reported sanitizing and reusing PPE to preserve supplies.

Many hospitals reported difficulty in identifying reputable vendors to provide a consistent supply of PPE. As one administrator described, "We are routinely changing vendors because we cannot get [PPE] from our normal manufacturers and vendors." Some administrators expressed that it was inefficient for individual hospitals to be searching for vendors and that there should be more centralized supply chain management.

When hospitals must switch to N95 masks produced by different manufacturers, staff often must repeat mask fit-testing, which one administrator reported occurred for their hospital four or five times. Even when hospitals found PPE vendors, administrators reported inconsistent delivery, including orders that were canceled, delayed, or incorrect. One hospital noted that it was difficult to anticipate when their orders would be backordered or canceled. This made it challenging to build up supplies, and hospitals reported concerns about having enough PPE supplies for surges or waves of COVID-19 infections in the future.

Some hospitals reported receiving poor-quality PPE, and others reported inflated prices. For example, one hospital reported that when they purchased PPE made outside the United States, many of the supplies did not meet U.S. standards. A few hospitals described the PPE that they received as "counterfeit" or discovered the PPE was inadequate for use after testing it. Some hospitals also indicated that they experienced substantial price increases for PPE. One administrator said, "We used to pay about $1 per [N95] mask. Now it is $8 to $9 per mask."

FINANCES
Hospitals Reported That Their Operational Costs Have Risen Dramatically While Their Revenues Have Declined, Threatening Their Financial Stability

Many hospitals identified financial stability as a concern resulting from the COVID-19 pandemic. Administrators pointed to a variety of increased costs that their hospitals encountered during the pandemic, including higher costs associated with staffing and PPE, as well as COVID-19 patient care, testing, and vaccinations. Some hospitals also reported increased administrative costs associated with new data reporting requirements for COVID-19 cases, testing, and vaccinations. Some hospitals expressed that the combination of their higher costs coupled with declining revenues raised concerns about whether they would be able to remain in operation.

Hospitals that serve disproportionately underinsured and uninsured populations and rural communities reported being particularly concerned about financial instability. These hospitals also tend to serve more patients enrolled in Medicaid, which often reimburses at lower rates than private insurance. Several hospitals noted that they faced financial challenges prior to the pandemic and worried that it would be hard to recover financial stability after the pandemic ends. As an administrator of a hospital serving a community with high poverty rates described, "We were one of the [hospitals in] danger of disappearing... now we have to restart in a different world, and I do not know if we can get it back."

Hospitals reported a significant decline in revenue resulting from suspending elective procedures. In March 2020, the CMS recommended the suspension of elective surgeries and other procedures to help conserve PPE and other supplies needed to respond to the pandemic. The next month, in April 2020, the CMS issued additional recommendations to guide practices as state, tribal, and local health-care entities considered safely resuming elective surgeries and other procedures. However, hospitals reported that non-COVID-19-related services have remained low, with fewer patient visits for both routine and emergency care and fewer elective procedures (compared to before the pandemic). As a result of fewer patient visits, one administrator said their hospital was operating at a 25-percent reduction in revenue. As discussed earlier in the report, hospitals surmised that fear of contracting COVID-19 was the main cause of patients avoiding coming to the hospital, even for medically necessary treatment.

Some administrators expressed that based on their experience, Medicare fee-for-service reimbursement did not always cover their costs associated with some COVID-19 patients. For example, one hospital estimated that it was potentially losing $3,000 per COVID-19 patient. Medicare reimburses hospitals a predetermined amount

COVID-19 Impact on Health-Care Facilities

based on the COVID-19 diagnosis and any other diagnoses for the patient and provides additional payment increases to hospitals as part of the CARES Act. However, administrators believed that these reimbursement amounts often did not cover their added staff and equipment costs associated with COVID-19 patients who have prolonged ICU hospital stays.

Medicare alternative payment models that base payment on value, risk, and outcomes presented a different set of financial challenges, according to hospital administrators. Although one administrator expressed satisfaction with payments under such models, other hospitals noted concerns that they could be penalized under alternative payment models, specifically in calculations of future incentive payments. For example, one hospital worried that caring for COVID-19 patients, who often have lengthy hospital stays and increased risk of hospital-acquired infections, could negatively affect their quality metrics, potentially costing "hundreds of thousands of dollars" in missed incentive payments.

Hospitals Expressed Uncertainty about Rules on Repayment of Prior Federal Loans

Several administrators expressed concern about whether they would have to repay the federal financial assistance that they had already received. Hospitals noted that loans from the Medicare Accelerated and Advance Payment Programs were essential in facing cash flow disruptions during the early days of the pandemic. However, they anticipated problems repaying the loans when the first payments become due starting late March 2021. Some hospitals also said that guidance on CARES Act funds, such as Paycheck Protection Program (PPP) loans, seemed to have changed over time, leaving them uncertain about the current rules for repayment.[1]

---

[1] Office of Inspector General, "Hospitals Reported That the COVID-19 Pandemic Has Significantly Strained Health Care Delivery," U.S. Department of Health and Human Services (HHS), March 1, 2021. Available online. URL: https://oig.hhs.gov/oei/reports/OEI-09-21-00140.pdf. Accessed January 3, 2023.

Chapter 46 | Impact of COVID-19 on Travel and Tourism

Early outbreaks of COVID-19 affected large populations in New York and New Jersey in the spring of 2020, leading the Centers for Disease Control and Prevention (CDC) to issue a domestic travel advisory for those states. In the rest of the country, the economy was already beginning to feel the economic impacts of the pandemic, especially on tourism and related industries that rely on people traveling.

Not surprisingly, regions with the most severe COVID-19 outbreaks and the largest share of tourism jobs were disproportionately affected at the start of the pandemic, and the Census Bureau's Quarterly Workforce Indicators (QWI) show the extent of the employment and earnings impacts from state to state.

Travel, tourism, and outdoor recreation jobs make up approximately 4–5 percent of total private employment in most states. However, Hawaii and Nevada are outliers with much larger shares of 14.4 and 21.0 percent in the second quarter of 2019, respectively. In addition to Nevada and Hawaii, Wyoming (7.3%), Montana (7.2%), and Florida (7.1%) make up the five states with the largest employment share in travel, tourism, and outdoor recreation.

DROP IN TOURISM AT ONSET OF PANDEMIC

Quarterly Workforce Indicators data can be used to show year-over-year changes in travel, tourism, and outdoor recreation employment. Note that you calculate year-over-year changes rather than quarterly changes due to the seasonality of these industries.

The states with the greatest declines in travel, tourism, and outdoor recreation employment were Rhode Island (decline of 37.9%), Vermont (37.4%), Connecticut (36.4%), Massachusetts (32.1%), New York (31.5%), and Washington (24.9%). These states reflect the locations of initial outbreaks at the start of the pandemic and the disproportionate impact it had on travel and tourism in these areas.

EARNINGS LOSSES IN TOURISM JOBS

Workers employed in travel, tourism, and outdoor recreation at the beginning of the second quarter of 2020 also experienced significant earnings losses during the quarter (up to 40%) compared to those employed at the start of the second quarter of 2019. These earnings losses reflect lost hours or weeks of work during the quarter as well as any layoffs later in the quarter. Again, the impact on earnings varied widely across states.

States that saw the largest earnings decreases among these workers were Nevada (decline of 42.9%), Hawaii (41.9%), West Virginia (37.5%), the District of Columbia (34.3%), and Missouri (30.3%). States with the largest employment losses, however, were not always the same states that saw the largest percentage of earnings declines during this time period.

FEMALE WORKERS

Women were likely to lose either employment or earnings in the second quarter of 2020 relative to other workers in the industry. Nationally, the share of female employment in travel, tourism, and outdoor recreation was just over 50 percent, with some variation across states. However, women experienced larger employment and earnings declines than men. Notably, the decline in average earnings for women was considerably more pronounced than the decline in employment at the beginning of the quarter. Women accounted for well over 50 percent of travel, tourism, and outdoor recreation job losses in most states and for more than 60 percent of employment losses in several states.

Impact of COVID-19 on Travel and Tourism

MORE JOBS/EARNINGS LOSSES FOR YOUNG WORKERS

Young workers were more likely to lose either employment or earnings in the second quarter of 2020 relative to other workers in the industry. The largest declines in both employment and earnings in these industries were among workers younger than 25 years old. These young workers accounted for just under 20 percent of national employment in travel, tourism, and outdoor recreation with some variation across states. Yet they typically accounted for a larger fraction of employment declines in some states. In Florida, Pennsylvania, Texas, and Virginia, for example, young workers accounted for up to 35 percent of the total decline in travel, tourism, and outdoor recreation employment. But they made up a smaller share of employment losses in Western states.[1]

---

[1] "Tourism and Related Industries Declined Sharply in Northeastern States in Spring 2020, Women and Young Workers More Affected Nationwide," United States Census Bureau, June 23, 2021. Available online. URL: www.census.gov/library/stories/2021/06/initial-impact-of-covid-19-on-travel-tourism-outdoor-recreation-varied-widely-across-states.html. Accessed December 15, 2022.

Chapter 47 | Impact of the Pandemic on Population Estimates of Major Cities

While the COVID-19 pandemic has not officially ended, the U.S. Census Bureau's first release of population estimates for cities and towns in this decade reveals how population growth trends shifted during the first year of the pandemic. Some of the fastest-growing cities before the pandemic grew at a much slower rate after it started, changing the rankings among the top 15 gainers. While many rankings of cities and towns remained roughly the same, there were notable differences in the magnitudes of change.

The new estimates show that some fast-growing cities in 2019 grew at a slower rate in 2021. At the same time, others grew at a faster pace during the pandemic. Overall, growth slowed in the nation's biggest cities, and some states experienced an uptick in population due to migration to the South and West in the first year after the pandemic hit.

HOW CITY GROWTH RATES CHANGED

As of July 1, 2021, six of the top 15 fastest-growing cities (or towns) with populations of 50,000 or more were also among the top fastest-growing in the prepandemic July 1, 2019, estimates. While the list was mostly similar, growth slowed for some.

Leander, Texas, top-ranked in 2019 with a 12.0 percent increase from 2018, slipped to second place with a 10.1 percent growth from 2020 to 2021. In Idaho, Meridian's growth fell from 7.2 percent in 2019 to 5.2 percent in 2021, slipping from 6th to 13th in the rankings.

DIFFERENT CITIES EXPERIENCING DECLINE

San Francisco was not among the 15 fastest-declining cities in 2019 but topped the list in 2021 with a 6.3 percent drop in population from the previous year. Six of the cities on the declining list in 2021 were in California. And major cities, including Boston and Washington, DC, also made the list. Even though only one city—Cupertino, California—was one of the 15 fastest-declining in both 2019 and 2021, the magnitude of the drop (in its population growth rate) nearly tripled. Overall, the prepandemic population losses from 2018 to 2019 were much lower than after the pandemic hit.

For instance, Petaluma, California, had the largest percentage population decline from July 1, 2018, to July 1, 2019, a drop of 2.1 percent. But that drop would not even have ranked among the top 15 in 2020–2021, after the start of the pandemic. These rates of population decline of five percent or more in a single year were nearly unprecedented. Population decline can result from a variety of causes, including natural disasters such as hurricanes and wildfires. For example, Hurricane Laura, a destructive Category 4 hurricane in August 2020, may have contributed to the population losses of Lake Charles, Louisiana, the second-fastest declining city with a decrease of 5.0 percent from 2020 to 2021.

POPULATION GAINS

One year into the pandemic, Phoenix, Arizona—the city with the largest numeric increase from 2018 to 2019—moved into second place, switching places with San Antonio. Its population gain of 13,626 was roughly half what it had added in 2019.

In addition, San Antonio and Fort Worth, Texas, and Meridian, Idaho, while still among the 15 cities with the largest numeric increases, all showed notably smaller increases. Collectively, the total population increase for the nation's 15 largest-gaining cities was a little over 187,100 people before the pandemic hit, compared to about 129,000 a year into it.

Impact of the Pandemic on Population Estimates of Major Cities

POPULATION LOSSES

While New York City remained the city with the largest numeric decrease, its population decline in 2021 (305,465) was nearly six times its numeric decrease in 2019 (53,624). Chicago, Illinois, had a similar experience. Still ranked third with a numeric decrease of 45,175 in 2021, its population dropped by only 7,447 (six times less) in 2019. All told, the cities with the largest numeric drop in population had a combined loss of nearly 609,800 a year into the pandemic, compared to about 102,700 between 2018 and 2019.

SMALL TOWN POPULATION TRENDS

The 2021 population estimates also provide a regional perspective on growth in cities and towns of all sizes.

On average, small towns with populations of less than 5,000 experienced uneven growth across U.S. regions:
- In the Northeast, the populations of small towns decreased on average by 0.2 percent.
- In the Midwest, small towns experienced no change on average.
- In the South, small towns grew on average by 0.4 percent.
- In the West, small towns saw the largest growth, with an average increase of 1.1 percent.

HOW THE U.S. CENSUS BUREAU CALCULATES ESTIMATES

Unlike the decennial census, which aims to count every person living in the United States, the annual population and housing unit estimates for states, counties, cities, and towns are developed using various administrative data sources, such as birth and death certificates and tax return statistics on people who changed residences. The decennial census serves as a starting point for each decade of subcounty population estimates.

Cities and towns are more likely than larger geographies to annex land or disincorporate. The U.S. Census Bureau applies these types of legal boundary changes to the decennial census to create an updated base for population and housing units. Such geographic updates are made annually so that each new time series of estimates the U.S. Census Bureau produces begins from a newly updated geographic base. This "estimates base" created from the census is essential to accurately distributing the population.[1]

---

[1] "New Data Reveal Most Populous Cities Experienced Some of the Largest Decreases," United States Census Bureau, May 26, 2022. Available online. URL: www.census.gov/library/stories/2022/05/population-shifts-in-cities-and-towns-one-year-into-pandemic.html. Accessed December 27, 2022.

Chapter 48 | The COVID-19 Pandemic and Employment

HOW DOES THE PANDEMIC AFFECT THE MAJOR LABOR MARKET MEASURES?

The most obvious impact of the pandemic is visible in the estimates of employment and unemployment that are highlighted in the Employment Situation news release each month.

Among the unemployed, the number of people on temporary layoff spiked at the onset of the pandemic and remains above the level before the pandemic. However, some workers who were not at work during the entire reference week were not classified as unemployed on temporary layoff, especially in the initial months of the pandemic. Rather, they were classified as employed but absent from work. U.S. Bureau of Labor Statistics (BLS) and United States Census Bureau analyses of the underlying data suggest that this group included some workers affected by the pandemic who should have been classified as unemployed on temporary layoff. The degree of misclassification was highest in the early months of the pandemic and has been considerably lower in recent months.

In addition to the employment and unemployment measures, there are other ways the household survey estimates show the impacts of the pandemic on the labor market. For example, there are estimates of the number of people who were absent from work, either for the entire survey reference week or, for certain workers, for part of the week.

The pandemic may have affected the number of hours some people worked during the survey reference week. Some people may have worked during the reference week, but not as many hours as they usually work. Some people may have worked more hours than usual. For example, the number of people working part time for economic reasons rose at the onset of the pandemic, clearly reflecting slack work or business conditions due to the pandemic. Other effects can be seen in the number of people at work part time for noneconomic reasons.

The number of people not in the labor force who currently want a job has been elevated during the pandemic as the impact of the pandemic likely kept many individuals from engaging in labor market activity. Beginning in May 2020, the household survey has information on people who did not look for work because of the pandemic.

Other new questions were added to the household survey in May 2020 to measure the effects of the pandemic on the labor market. These questions ask whether people were unable to work because their employers closed or lost business, whether they were paid for that missed work, and whether people teleworked or worked from home because of the pandemic.

WHAT IS THE DIFFERENCE BETWEEN A FURLOUGH AND A LAYOFF?

Some people use the terms furlough and layoff interchangeably, and others find them to be distinct. The household survey does not have a formal measure or definition of furlough.

The survey identifies different reasons people are unemployed, including being on temporary layoff. This measure includes people who were "furloughed" although that is not a term used in the survey questionnaire. (The manual provided to survey interviewers discusses how to code responses from people who report that they are furloughed. This guidance was prepared several years ago and was tailored to the use of "furlough" as a term describing budget-related layoffs, typically among government organizations.)

The COVID-19 Pandemic and Employment

Unemployed people on temporary layoff are those who:
- said they were laid off or were not at work during the survey reference week because of layoff (temporary or indefinite) or slack work/business conditions
- who have been given a date to return (or expect to be recalled within the next six months)
- who could have returned to work if they had been recalled (except for their own temporary illness)

Unlike other unemployed people, those on temporary layoff do not need to look for work to be classified as unemployed. Pay status is not a criterion to be unemployed on temporary layoff. People absent from work due to temporary layoff can be classified as unemployed on temporary layoff, whether or not they are paid for the time they are off work.

The monthly household survey does not include any information on whether people on temporary layoff return to their employers. The monthly survey provides a snapshot of the labor market and is not designed to track people's work experience over time.

HOW ARE PEOPLE WHO WERE ABSENT FROM THEIR JOBS COUNTED IN THE HOUSEHOLD SURVEY?

The monthly household survey has two measures that show the number of people who missed work during the survey reference week. One addresses people who did not work at all in the reference week, and the other addresses people who usually work full-time but were at work part-time (1–34 hours) during the reference week.

It is important to note that these household survey data do not reflect all cases of people who missed work during the month. The two measures refer to work missed only during the survey reference week. The data on people who miss part of the week are restricted to instances where people who usually work full time (35 hours or more per week) worked 1–34 hours. Thus, a person who usually works 50 hours per week but missed eight hours would not be included in this measure since they still worked more than

35 hours. Also, this measure does not reflect work missed by people who usually work part time.

HOW MANY PEOPLE WERE NOT AT WORK DURING THE REFERENCE WEEK?

People who say they have a job but were not at work during the survey reference week may be classified as employed or unemployed depending on the reason they missed work. For example, people who missed work due to vacation or illness are classified as employed. People who were temporarily laid off and expecting recall (and available to return to their job if recalled) are classified among the unemployed on temporary layoff. Under the guidance provided to the household survey interviewers, most workers who indicate that they were not working during the entire reference week due to pandemic-related business closures or cutbacks should be classified as unemployed on temporary layoff.

There are many reasons why employed people may not work for the entire survey reference week. BLS tabulates data on employed people not at work whose main reason for being absent was vacation, own illness, childcare problems, other family or personal obligations, labor dispute, bad weather, maternity or paternity leave, school or training, civic or military duty, and other reasons. Vacation and a person's own illness are typically the most common reasons people are not at work. People who were not at work to care for a sick family member should be counted in the other family or personal obligations category.

Since March 2020, the number of employed people included in the "not at work for other reasons" category has been higher than usual. BLS and U.S. Census Bureau analyses of the underlying data suggest that this group includes some workers affected by the pandemic who should have been classified as unemployed on temporary layoff. However, the degree of misclassification was highest in the early months of the pandemic.

WHAT IS THE MISCLASSIFICATION ISSUE?

Other than those who were themselves ill, under quarantine, or self-isolating due to health concerns, most people who did not

The COVID-19 Pandemic and Employment

work during the survey reference week due to the coronavirus pandemic should have been, and were, classified as unemployed on temporary layoff. However, since March 2020, some people who were not at work during the entire reference week for reasons related to the coronavirus pandemic were not included in this category but were instead misclassified as employed but not at work for other reasons.

Such a misclassification is an example of nonsampling error and can occur when respondents misunderstand questions or interviewers record answers incorrectly. (A similar misclassification occurred with federal workers in both the 2013 and 2019 partial federal government shutdowns.)

The misclassification hinges on a question about the main reason people were absent from their jobs. If people who were absent due to temporary, pandemic-related business closures or cutbacks were recorded as absent due to "other reasons," they could have been misclassified. According to special guidance provided to interviewers, most people absent due to temporary, pandemic-related business closures or cutbacks should be recorded in the "on layoff (temporary or indefinite)" category. (This response option is generally not available for people identified as business owners.)

Recording these answers as "on layoff (temporary or indefinite)" ensures that people are asked the follow-up questions needed to classify them as unemployed although it does not necessarily mean they are classified as unemployed on temporary layoff. People unemployed on temporary layoff must have been given a date to return to work (or expect to be recalled within the next six months) and also be available to return if recalled (except for their own temporary illness).

The degree of misclassification was highest in the early months of the pandemic and has been considerably lower in recent months. Census Bureau training on this question improved interviewers' understanding of the special instructions. When interviewers record a response of "other reason," they also add a few words describing that other reason. The BLS and U.S. Census Bureau staff extensively reviewed these brief descriptions and found that the share of responses that may have been misclassified was much smaller after the initial months of the pandemic.

According to usual practice, the data from the household survey are accepted as recorded. To maintain data integrity, no ad hoc actions are taken to reassign survey responses to the labor force questions.

WHAT WOULD THE UNEMPLOYMENT RATE BE IF THE MISCLASSIFIED WORKERS WERE INCLUDED AMONG THE UNEMPLOYED?

If the misclassified workers who were recorded as employed but not at work for the entire survey reference week had been classified as unemployed on temporary layoff, the overall unemployment rate would have been higher than reported. Each month since March 2020, the BLS has presented a calculation that includes the upper bound of the estimate of potentially misclassified workers among the unemployed in the monthly impact summary that accompanies the Employment Situation news release. This kind of exercise requires some assumptions. For example, first one needs to determine how many workers might be misclassified.

Because the exact extent of the misclassification is unknown, you had to make assumptions to construct these estimates. Specifically, you assumed that all of the increase in the number of employed people who were not at work for other reasons compared with the average for the same month in recent years was due solely to misclassification. You also assumed that all of these people expected to be recalled and were available to return to work.

Following this approach, for example, there were 1.4 million workers with a job but not at work who were included in the "other reasons" category in September 2020, about 773,000 higher than the prepandemic average for September 2016–2019. If you assume that this 773,000 increase was entirely due to misclassification and that all of these misclassified workers expected to be recalled and were available for work, the number of unemployed people in September (on a not seasonally adjusted basis) would increase from 12.3 million to 13.1 million. The number of people in the labor force would remain at 160.1 million in September (not seasonally adjusted) as people move from employed to unemployed but stay in the labor force. The resulting unemployment rate for September would be 8.2 percent (not seasonally adjusted), compared with the official estimate of 7.7 percent (not seasonally adjusted). Estimates of people with a job but not at work are not available on a seasonally adjusted basis, so seasonally adjusted data, such as the unemployment rate mentioned in the Employment Situation news release, are not used in this exercise. (Repeating this exercise, but combining the not seasonally adjusted data on additional people with a job but "not at work in the other reasons" category with the seasonally adjusted estimates for unemployed people and the labor force for September yields 8.3 percent, compared with the official seasonally adjusted rate of 7.8 percent.) See the calculations in the monthly impact summaries (www.bls.gov/covid19/effects-of-covid-19-pandemic-and-response-on-the-employment-situation-news-release.htm#summaries) for other months.

These broad assumptions represent the upper bound of your estimate of misclassification—the largest estimate of unemployment and correspondingly the highest unemployment rate. However, these assumptions probably overstate the size of the misclassification error. It is unlikely that everyone who was misclassified expected to be recalled and was available to return to work. It is also unlikely that all of the increase in the number of employed people not at work for "other reasons" was due to misclassification. Some people may be correctly classified in the "other reasons" category. For example, someone who owns a business (and does not have another job) is classified as employed in the household survey.

Regardless of the assumptions made as to the degree of misclassification, the trend in the unemployment rate is the same—for example, the rate increased in March and April and eased in later months.

WHY PEOPLE WERE WORKING PART-TIME

The number of people working part time for economic reasons rose at the onset of the pandemic, clearly reflecting slack work or business conditions due to the pandemic. These individuals, who would have preferred full-time employment, were working part time because their hours had been reduced or they were unable to find full-time jobs. (This group includes people who usually work full-time and people who usually work part-time.) This measure is highlighted in the Employment Situation news release each month.

Employed people who usually work full-time (35 hours or more per week) but indicated that they had worked fewer than 35 hours in the survey reference week are asked why they worked part-time that week. Depending on the reason provided, these workers are then grouped into those at work part-time for economic or noneconomic reasons. Economic reasons include working reduced hours due to slack work or business conditions, seasonal work, or starting or ending a job during the week. Noneconomic reasons include illness, vacation, holidays, schooling, childcare problems, labor dispute, bad weather, and other reasons.

HOW MANY PEOPLE WERE UNABLE TO WORK BECAUSE THEIR EMPLOYER CLOSED OR LOST BUSINESS DUE TO THE PANDEMIC?

New questions were added to the household survey in May 2020 to measure the effects of the pandemic on the labor market, including whether people were unable to work because their employers closed or lost business and whether they were paid for that missed work. This question was asked each month from May 2020 to September 2022.

All people were asked if, at any time in the last four weeks, they were unable to work because their employer closed or lost business due to the coronavirus pandemic. This question was designed to include both those who did not work at all and those who worked fewer hours. People who reported that they were unable to work were asked if they received any pay from their employer for the hours they did not work in the last four weeks.

These data do not include all people who were unable to work because of the pandemic. The fact that someone is employed at the time of the survey does not necessarily mean they are working for the same employer that closed or lost business. Also, no information was collected about how much pay people received, such as whether they were paid for all of the time not worked.

Beginning with the report for August 2020 and continuing through September 2022, key indicators from these data were highlighted in the Employment Situation news release.

HOW MANY PEOPLE WERE NOT LOOKING FOR WORK BECAUSE OF THE PANDEMIC?

The unemployed are people who are actively looking for work or those on temporary layoff expecting to be recalled to work. Because of the importance of job search in the definition of unemployment, the BLS added a supplemental question to the monthly household labor force survey to identify people who did not look for work because of the pandemic.

Beginning in May 2020, people not in the labor force were asked "Did the coronavirus pandemic prevent you from looking for work in the past four weeks?" This question was asked each month from May 2020 to September 2022. The number of people not in the labor force who did not look for work because of the pandemic was highlighted in the Employment Situation news release.

HOW MANY PEOPLE TELEWORKED BECAUSE OF THE PANDEMIC?

The household survey does not routinely ask about teleworking. However, a supplemental question on whether people teleworked or worked from home because of the pandemic was added to the household survey in May 2020. This question was asked each month from May 2020 to September 2022.

These data refer to employed people who teleworked or worked at home for pay at some point in the last four weeks specifically because of the coronavirus pandemic. People did not have to telework for the entire time that they worked to be counted among those who telework. By design, people whose telework was unrelated to the pandemic, such as employed people who worked entirely from home before the pandemic, should not be included in this measure. The number of people who teleworked because of the pandemic was highlighted in the Employment Situation news release.

HOW ARE THESE DATA DIFFERENT FROM THE UNEMPLOYMENT INSURANCE CLAIMS DATA?

Every week, the Employment and Training Administration (ETA) of the U.S. Department of Labor (DOJ) reports the number of people filing initial and continued claims for Unemployment Insurance

(UI) benefits. Individuals file initial claims to request a determination of basic eligibility for the UI program. A continued claim is filed after an initial claim to receive benefits for a particular week of unemployment. Because the UI claims data are weekly series, they can capture the impact of economic shocks more quickly than the BLS monthly household and establishment surveys, particularly when these shocks hit between survey reference periods.

Data users must be cautious about trying to compare or reconcile the UI claims data with the official unemployment figures derived from the household survey. The unemployment data gathered through the household survey in no way depend upon the eligibility for or receipt of UI benefits. There are conceptual, coverage, and scope differences between the two data sources.

In many cases, UI claims data exclude people who would be identified as unemployed in the household survey. For example, the UI claims data generally exclude:
- unemployed people who exhausted their benefits without finding work
- unemployed people who have not yet earned benefit rights because they have not met their state's work and wage requirements, such as new entrants and reentrants to the labor force
- unemployed people who voluntarily quit their previous jobs
- unemployed people who were fired for cause from their previous jobs
- otherwise eligible unemployed people who either delay filing for benefits or choose not to file for benefits

In other cases, the UI claims data include people who would not meet the household survey definition of unemployed. Some regular state UI programs allow individuals to collect partial benefits when their work hours have been reduced. These working people would be classified as employed in the household survey, and many might be included among those working part-time for economic reasons, a category of workers that grew considerably at the onset of the pandemic.

The COVID-19 Pandemic and Employment

In addition, the Families First Coronavirus Response Act (FFCRA), specifically the Division D-Emergency Unemployment Insurance Stabilization and Access Act of 2020 (EUISAA), signed into law on March 18, 2020, allowed state UI programs to temporarily modify or suspend the "actively seeking work" requirement in response to the pandemic. With the exception of those unemployed on temporary layoff, people without a job who are not actively seeking work are not classified as unemployed in the household survey. Rather, they are classified as not in the labor force.

Thus, the number of claimants in the regular state UI programs includes both people who would be considered employed and people who would be considered not in the labor force in the household survey. ETA's weekly claims report does not include information on whether claimants are collecting partial benefits or actively seeking work.

With respect to geographic scope, the U.S. totals published by ETA include claims reported by Puerto Rico and the U.S. Virgin Islands, both of which maintain regular state UI programs. The household survey covers the 50 states and the District of Columbia and does not include Puerto Rico or the Virgin Islands.

Furthermore, the Coronavirus Aid, Relief, and Economic Security (CARES) Act, signed into law on March 27, 2020, created two new programs for unemployment compensation in response to the coronavirus pandemic. These programs are Pandemic Unemployment Assistance (PUA) and Pandemic Emergency Unemployment Compensation (PEUC). The PUA program provides up to 39 weeks of benefits to individuals who are self-employed, seeking part-time employment, or otherwise would not qualify for or have exhausted all rights to regular unemployment compensation, extended benefits, or PEUC. The PEUC program provides up to 13 weeks of benefits to individuals who have exhausted or have no rights to regular benefits and who are able, available, and actively seeking work. Additionally, states must offer flexibility in meeting the "actively seeking work" requirement if individuals are unable to search for work because of illness, quarantine, or movement restriction.

COVID-19 and the Coronavirus Sourcebook, First Edition

The number of people claiming benefits under these new programs are listed in ETA's UI weekly claims report separately from the number of people claiming benefits under the regular state UI programs, with a one-week lag. As with the regular state UI programs, claimants under these new programs would cut across the household survey classifications of employed, unemployed, and not in the labor force.[1]

---

[1] U.S. Bureau of Labor Statistics (BLS), "Effects of COVID-19 Pandemic on the Employment Situation News Release and Data," U.S. Department of Labor (DOL), September 1, 2022. Available online. URL: www.bls.gov/covid19/effects-of-covid-19-pandemic-and-response-on-the-employment-situation-news-release.htm. Accessed December 27, 2022.

Chapter 49 | How to Approach a Possible Outbreak in the Future

PANDEMIC PREPAREDNESS: PLANNING AND RESOURCES
For the first time in the history, you have the opportunity—due to advances in science and technology—not just to refill your stockpiles but also to transform your capabilities. However, you need to start preparing now.

The United States must fundamentally transform its ability to prevent, detect, and rapidly respond to pandemics and high-consequence biological threats. This would include investments in critical scientific goal areas—vaccines, therapeutics, diagnostics, and early warning—as well as associated investments in strengthening disease surveillance, health systems, surge capacity, personal protective equipment (PPE) innovation, biosafety and biosecurity, regulatory capacity, and global pandemic preparedness.

Pandemic Preparedness Goals
- transforming your medical defenses, including dramatically improving vaccines, therapeutics, and diagnostics
- ensuring situational awareness about infectious disease threats, for both early warning and real-time monitoring
- strengthening public health systems, both in the United States and internationally to be able to respond to emergencies, with a particular focus on protecting the most vulnerable communities

- building core capabilities, including personal protective equipment, stockpiles and supply chains, biosafety and biosecurity, and regulatory improvement
- managing the mission, with the seriousness of purpose, commitment, and accountability of the Apollo Program (program on biodefense)

All of these efforts must, from the outset, include a strong emphasis on reducing inequities and increasing access by all Americans to the resulting advances. Importantly, the COVID-19 pandemic has exposed fundamental issues with the nation's public health that go far beyond pandemic preparedness. These issues include the need to increase overall public health funding, strengthen the public health workforce, eliminate barriers to access, improve data systems, address disparities, improve communication, and improve coordination across federal, state, local, and tribal authorities.

PANDEMIC PREPAREDNESS: MANAGING THE MISSION

The mission of transforming U.S. pandemic preparedness and biodefense capabilities should be managed with the seriousness of purpose, commitment, and accountability of an Apollo Program. There should be a centralized "Mission Control," acting as a single, unified program management unit, that draws on expertise from multiple U.S. Department of Health and Human Services (HHS) agencies, including the National Institutes of Health (NIH), Centers for Disease Control and Prevention (CDC), Biomedical Advanced Research and Development Authority (BARDA), U.S. Food and Drug Administration (FDA), and Centers for Medicare & Medicaid Services (CMS), as well as other departments such as U.S. Department of Defense (DoD), U.S. Department of Energy (DoE), and U.S. Department of Veterans Affairs (VA; e.g., the Countermeasures Acceleration Group (formerly, "Operation Warp Speed") is led by a single joint program management unit).

Mission Control should have the responsibility and authority to:
- develop and update plans with objective and transparent milestones

How to Approach a Possible Outbreak in the Future

- regularly assess and publicly report on mission progress
- shift funding to ensure that goals are achieved
- coordinate linkages across performers in government, academia, philanthropy, and industry
- conduct periodic exercises to evaluate national pandemic preparedness by deploying national capabilities, including rapid product development

Mission Control should seek the input of outside experts on critical issues and consider establishing working groups that focus on scientific and technical assessments, improving public health, and ensuring that the capabilities serve all communities, especially the most vulnerable.

PANDEMIC PREPAREDNESS: COST AND ECONOMIC CASE

An effective program to ensure that the United States is prepared for future pandemics and other major biological threats will require significant annual investment over a sustained period.

However, the required investment is modest relative to other efforts to create the capabilities needed to protect the nation against important threats: The annualized cost would be much smaller than what the United States spends on missile defense ($20 billion/year) and on preventing terrorism ($170 billion/year). In addition to protecting American lives, the annual investment is strongly justified from an economic standpoint: If major pandemics similar to COVID-19, costing the United States roughly $16 trillion, occur at a frequency of every 20 years, the annualized economic impact on the United States would be $800 billion per year. Even for somewhat milder pandemics, the annualized cost would likely exceed $500 billion.

Investing a modest amount annually to avert or mitigate the huge toll of future pandemics and other biological threats is an economic and moral imperative. It is hard to imagine a higher economic—or human—return on national investment. In any realistic accounting of costs and benefits, modest investments in pandemic preparedness should not be viewed as a cost but instead as providing a large return on investment.

PANDEMIC PREPAREDNESS: TRANSFORMING YOUR CAPABILITIES
Transform Your Medical Defenses
- **Vaccines**. Rapidly make effective vaccines against any human virus family.
  - Design, test, and review by 100 days after the pandemic threat appears (for COVID-19 = May 2020).
  - Produce enough vaccine for the United States by 130 days and the entire world by 200 days.
  - Simplify vaccine distribution (e.g., eliminate the need for cold storage).
  - Simplify vaccine administration (e.g., replace sterile injection, with skin patches and nasal sprays).
- **Therapeutics**. Develop life-saving medicines suitable for any virus family.
  - Develop medicines to block key virus functions (as done for HIV).
  - Enable rapid production of neutralizing antibodies (currently too slow).
  - Develop medicines to prevent severe immune overreactions (useful in public health).
- **Diagnostics**. Develop simple, inexpensive, accurate tests for any virus available within weeks.
  - Develop technologies to meet sustained demand, including daily home testing for all, if required.
  - Use new diagnostics in routine care, to serve public health, drive down costs, and expand capacity.

Ensure Situational Awareness
- **Early-warning systems**. Rapidly detect new viral outbreaks with pandemic potential.
  - Detect new threats by genome sequencing of patients with unexplained fevers in the United States and abroad.
  - Detect new viral threats by wastewater sampling.
  - Create early-warning networks to aggregate and analyze global data.

How to Approach a Possible Outbreak in the Future

- **Real-time monitoring**. Follow existing viral outbreaks for spread and evolution.
  - Improve tracking by combining diagnostic, epidemiological, sequencing, and environmental data.
  - Improve analysis and forecasting.

Strengthen Public Health Systems
- **U.S. public health**. Modernize infrastructure to prevent and contain biological threats.
  - Strengthen the public health workforce.
  - Invest in public health laboratories and public health digital infrastructure.
  - Prioritize vulnerable communities.
- **Global health**. Establish international infrastructure and financing for pandemic preparedness.
  - Create local capacity and international systems.
  - Catalyze sustainable international financing.

Build Core Capabilities
- **PPE**. Increase effectiveness, comfort, affordability, and manufacturability.
- **Stockpiles and supply chains**. Ensure the United States' ability to produce vital supplies.
- **Preventing catastrophic biological events**. Accelerate biosafety, biosecurity, and deterrence.
- **Regulatory improvement**. Ensure regulatory capacity for vaccines, therapeutics, and diagnostics.

Manage the Mission
- **Mission control**. Manage this national responsibility with the seriousness of purpose, commitment, and accountability of an Apollo Program and coordinate work with the international scientific community.[1]

---

[1] "American Pandemic Preparedness: Transforming Our Capabilities," Whitehouse.gov, September 1, 2021. Available online. URL: www.whitehouse.gov/wp-content/uploads/2021/09/American-Pandemic-Preparedness-Transforming-Our-Capabilities-Final-For-Web.pdf?page=29. Accessed January 4, 2023.

Chapter 50 | COVID-19: Moving from Pandemic to Endemic

Generally, a pandemic is a disease that has spread throughout many regions or around the whole world, affecting vast populations. In contrast, an endemic disease is always present but limited to a specific region with a predictable spread rate and periodic outbreaks. This can also include diseases present globally that are controlled or follow predictable patterns, such as the flu.

It is estimated that COVID-19 will transition from a pandemic to an endemic disease at different times in different parts of the world, with occasional outbreaks.

From the data published by the Centers for Disease Control and Prevention (CDC), in the United States, on June 23, 2021, the total cases per week were 82,186, with the total case rate per 100,000 being 10,243, which peaked on January 19, 2022, with weekly cases going up to 5,630,736 and total case rate per 100,000 to 20,982. On March 30, 2022, just in 10 weeks, the total cases per week dropped drastically to 193,733, with the total case rate per 100,000 to 24,452, essentially because of the implementation of restrictive measures such as vaccination programs, quarantine policies, and changes in people's behavior, which included increased handwashing, wearing masks, and social distancing.

Other reasons for the decline might include a portion of the population becoming immune to the disease following exposure to the virus (herd immunity) and the virus itself undergoing genetic changes, or mutations, that make it less virulent, leading to lower rates of disease spread and progression.

THE PATH FROM PANDEMIC TO ENDEMIC

The transition from a pandemic to an endemic state depends on various factors. The four essential aspects of the transition include the following:

- **Vaccines**. Initial vaccine programs addressed the first strain of the virus. Continuing to fight the disease this way requires efforts to develop new vaccines that cover a broader range of emerging COVID variants, availability of the vaccines, and effective administration of vaccine shots, especially boosters given at prescribed intervals. Consideration should also be given to broad-spectrum coverage ranging from young children to older adults with vaccine efforts prioritizing high-risk populations.
- **Treatments**. Current treatment modalities have proven effective as doctors better understand COVID-19 and how to treat it. Many attempted treatments, such as the antimalarial drug, hydroxychloroquine, are still considered ineffective although some clinical trials are investigating its usefulness. Improving the treatment methodology should remain a top priority for the transition into endemicity.
- **Health-care systems**. Health-care systems must prepare for future outbreaks. Pandemics, when cases rise rapidly, can overburden health-care facilities, such as hospitals and urgent care centers, but proper preparation can ease this strain. Management strategies to ensure continuity of care unrelated to the pandemic, such as regular medical checkups and elective surgeries, are required so that non-COVID-19 patients are not neglected during an outbreak or the endemic state.
- **At-risk populations**. Those living in densely populated areas, the economically disadvantaged, and those

with limited access to health care as well as those with high-risk comorbidities, such as diabetes, respiratory disease, or weakened immune systems, must be given special consideration in health-care response plans. Authorities should inform them about proper precautions to lower their risk.

PRACTICAL IMPLICATIONS OF ENDEMIC COVID

Although the endemic stage may eventually occur naturally in the United States and other countries, local governments have critical roles to play in determining its course over time. Individuals may transmit COVID-19 virus anywhere people congregate, so governments and public facilities should implement reasonable safety practices and policies, such as handwashing, mask wearing, and social distancing, as needed to effectively reduce the risk of transmission.

Part of the endemic stage will include people accepting that COVID-19 infection and the vaccinations and safety practices that reduce its risks have become a normal part of life.

ROLE OF OMICRON IN THE TRANSITION OF PANDEMIC TO ENDEMIC

The Omicron variant, which spread faster than earlier COVID variants, may seem to have delayed the transition to the endemic stage of COVID-19 infection. In reality, the Omicron surge induced natural immunity among people, also called "herd immunity." Furthermore, evidence suggests that antibodies produced by Omicron infection provide enhanced protection against other new emerging variants. Thus, the Omicron variant has been a positive catalyst in the overall transition from pandemic to endemic status.

COVID-19 cannot be eradicated. It will remain a part of life for years to come. The transition to endemicity will happen, depending on decreasing transmission rates among individuals, vaccination and booster efforts, and adoption of safe practices set by local authorities.

References

Charumilind, Sarun; Craven, Matt; Lamb, Jessica; Singhal, Shubham and Wilson, Matt. "Pandemic to Endemic: How the World Can Learn to Live with COVID-19," McKinsey & Company, October 28, 2021. Available online. URL: www.mckinsey.com/industries/healthcare-systems-and-services/our-insights/pandemic-to-endemic-how-the-world-can-learn-to-live-with-covid-19. Accessed January 4, 2023.

Cook, Gina; Gentzler, Doreen and Fantis, Patricia. "From Pandemic to Endemic: What to Expect from the Next COVID Phase," NBCUniversal Media, LLC, December 10, 2021. Available online. URL: www.nbcwashington.com/news/local/from-pandemic-to-endemic-what-to-expect-from-the-next-covid-phase/2905344. Accessed January 4, 2023.

"COVID Will Likely Shift from Pandemic to Endemic–but What Does That Mean?" The Conversation, September 20, 2021. Available online. URL: https://theconversation.com/covid-will-likely-shift-from-pandemic-to-endemic-but-what-does-that-mean-167782. Accessed January 4, 2023.

Kumar, Pooja; Parthasarathy, Ramya, and Yau, Bill. "Pandemic to Endemic: Where Do US Public-Health Systems Go from Here?" McKinsey & Company, June 30, 2022. Available online. URL: www.mckinsey.com/industries/public-and-social-sector/our-insights/pandemic-to-endemic-where-do-us-public-health-systems-go-from-here. Accessed January 4, 2023.

McNamara, Damian, MA. "Could Omicron Hasten the Transition from Pandemic to Endemic?" WebMD, LLC, January 6, 2022. Available online. URL: www.webmd.com/covid/news/20220106/omicron-pandemic-endemic. Accessed January 4, 2023.

Miller, Korin. "COVID-19 Will Likely Become an Endemic Disease–but When Will That Happen?" Health.com October 27, 2021. Available online. URL: www.health.

com/condition/infectious-diseases/coronavirus/endemic-covid. Accessed January 4, 2023.

Mozes, Alan. "Pandemic to Endemic: Is a New Normal Near?" U.S. News & World Report L.P., January 25, 2022. Available online. URL: www.usnews.com/news/health-news/articles/2022-01-25/pandemic-to-endemic-is-a-new-normal-near. Accessed January 4, 2023.

"Trends in Number of COVID-19 Cases and Deaths in the US Reported to CDC, by State/Territory," Centers for Disease Control and Prevention (CDC), March 10, 2022. Available online. URL: https://covid.cdc.gov/covid-data-tracker/#trends_weeklycases_totalcasesper100k_00. Accessed December 22, 2022.

Part 7 | Additional Help and Information

Chapter 51 | Glossary of Terms Related to COVID-19 and Other Communicable Diseases

antibody: A protein produced by the immune system that recognizes and binds to a specific antigen.

antigen: A substance that triggers the immune system to produce antibodies.

antigen test: A test that detects specific proteins on the surface of the virus.

asymptomatic: Describing someone who is infected with a virus but is not showing any symptoms.

community spread: The transmission of a virus within a community without a clear link to a specific source of infection.

comorbidities: The presence of one or more additional health conditions in a person with a primary disease.

contact tracing: The process of identifying, assessing, and managing people who have been in close contact with an infected person.

containment: The use of measures such as isolation and quarantine to prevent the spread of a virus.

coronavirus: A large family of viruses that can cause illness in animals and humans (e.g., SARS-COV-2 is one type of coronavirus that causes COVID-19).

This glossary contains terms excerpted from documents produced by several sources deemed reliable.

COVID-19: An infectious disease caused by the severe acute respiratory syndrome coronavirus 2 (SARS-COV-2), which was first identified in Wuhan, China, in 2019 and has since spread globally, causing a pandemic.

epidemic: An outbreak of a disease that occurs over a wide geographic area and affects an exceptionally high proportion of the population.

epidemiology: The branch of medicine concerned with the incidence, distribution, and control of diseases in a population.

false negative: A test result that incorrectly indicates that a person does not have a disease when they actually do.

herd immunity: The resistance to the spread of a disease within a population when a high proportion of individuals are immune to the disease.

immune system: The body's natural defense against infection and disease.

immunity: The ability of the body to resist infection or disease through the presence of antibodies or memory cells.

incubation period: The time between exposure to a virus and the onset of symptoms (e.g., the incubation period for COVID-19 is typically 2–14 days).

infection: The invasion of the body by harmful microorganisms, such as bacteria, viruses, or parasites.

intensive care unit (ICU): A specialized hospital unit that provides advanced medical and nursing care for critically ill patients.

isolation: Separating people who have a contagious disease from those who are healthy.

long COVID: A term used to describe a range of symptoms that persist for weeks or months after the acute phase of the illness.

MERS-CoV: A strain of the coronavirus that causes Middle East respiratory syndrome.

Middle East respiratory syndrome (MERS): It is a viral respiratory illness caused by the Middle East respiratory syndrome coronavirus (MERS-CoV).

mortality rate: The number of deaths in a specific population over a given period of time.

mutation: A change in the genetic material of a virus that can lead to changes in its characteristics or behavior.

N95 mask: A type of respirator that is designed to protect the wearer from airborne particles.

Glossary of Terms Related to COVID-19 and Other Communicable Diseases

outbreak: A sudden increase in cases of a disease above what is normally expected in a specific area or among a specific group of people.

pandemic: An outbreak of a disease that occurs over a wide geographic area and affects an exceptionally high proportion of the population.

pathogen: An organism or substance that causes disease.

personal protective equipment (PPE): Equipment worn to reduce exposure to a variety of risks including but not limited to infectious materials, respiratory hazards, toxic chemicals, and flying objects.

pneumonia: An infection of the lungs that can be caused by a variety of microorganisms, including SARS-COV-2.

polymerase chain reaction (PCR) test: A laboratory test that can detect the genetic material of the virus in a sample of respiratory secretions.

presymptomatic: Describing someone who is infected with a virus and will develop symptoms but currently has no symptoms.

prognosis: The likely outcome or course of a disease.

quarantine: A period of isolation for people who have been exposed to a contagious disease but have not yet developed symptoms.

reinfection: The occurrence of a new infection with a virus after a person has already recovered from a previous infection.

remdesivir: An antiviral drug that has been authorized for emergency use to treat COVID-19.

respiratory: Relating to the lungs and breathing.

risk factors: People with underlying medical conditions, such as diabetes, chronic lung disease, and weakened immune systems, are at a higher risk of severe illness from COVID-19.

SARS-COV-2: The virus that causes COVID-19, which is a type of coronavirus.

SARS-COV-2 spike protein: A protein on the surface of the virus that binds to the ACE2 receptor on human cells and allows the virus to enter and infect the cells.

self-isolation: Separating oneself from others to prevent the spread of a virus, typically after being exposed to a confirmed or suspected case of the virus.

social distancing: Measures taken to reduce close contact between people in order to slow the spread of a virus.

symptomatic: Describing someone who is showing symptoms of a disease.

symptoms: The physical and/or emotional characteristics of a medical condition.

t-cell: A type of white blood cell that plays an important role in the immune response to viral infections.

transmission: The spread of a virus from one person to another. Transmission of SARS-COV-2 primarily occurs through respiratory droplets when an infected person talks, coughs, or sneezes.

vaccination: The administration of a vaccine to help the immune system develop protection from disease.

vaccine: A biological product that provides active acquired immunity to a particular disease.

ventilator: A machine that helps a person breathe by delivering air into the lungs through a tube inserted into the windpipe.

viral loads: The amount of viral genetic material present in a person's blood or other bodily fluids.

virus: A tiny infectious agent that can only replicate inside the living cells of an organism.

zoonotic: A disease that can be transmitted from animals to humans.

Chapter 52 | Directory of Organizations That Provide Information about COVID-19 and Other Communicable Diseases

GOVERNMENT ORGANIZATIONS

Centers for Disease Control and Prevention (CDC)
1600 Clifton Rd.
Atlanta, GA 30329-4027
Toll-Free: 800-232-4636
(800-CDC-INFO)
TTY: 888-232-6348
Website: www.cdc.gov

Centers for Medicare & Medicaid Services (CMS)
7500 Security Blvd.
Baltimore, MD 21244
Toll-Free: 877-267-2323
Phone: 410-786-3000
Toll-Free TTY: 866-226-1819
TTY: 410-786-0727
Website: www.cms.gov

About This Chapter: Resources in this chapter were compiled from several sources deemed reliable; all contact information was verified and updated in March 2023.

Consumer Financial Protection Bureau (CFPB)
1700 G St., N.W.
Washington, DC 20552
Toll-Free: 855-411-2372
TTY/TDD: 855-729-2372
Website: www.consumerfinance.gov

MedlinePlus
8600 Rockville Pike
Bethesda, MD 20894
Website: www.medlineplus.gov

National Center for Complementary and Integrative Health (NCCIH)
9000 Rockville Pike
Bethesda, MD 20892
Toll-Free: 888-644-6226
Website: www.nccih.nih.gov
Email: info@nccih.nih.gov

National Institute of Allergy and Infectious Diseases (NIAID)
5601 Fishers Ln., MSC 9806
Bethesda, MD 20892-9806
Toll-Free: 866-284-4107
Phone: 301-496-5717
TDD: 800-877-8339
Fax: 301-402-3573
Website: www.niaid.nih.gov
Email: ocpostoffice@niaid.nih.gov

National Institute of Neurological Disorders and Stroke (NINDS)
31 Center Dr.
Rm. 8A07, MSC 2540
Bethesda, MD 20892-2540
Toll-Free: 800-352-9424
Phone: 301-496-5751
Fax: 301-402-2186
Website: www.ninds.nih.gov
Email: braininfo@ninds.nih.gov

National Institutes of Health (NIH)
9000 Rockville Pike
Bethesda, MD 20892
Phone: 301-496-4000
TTY: 301-402-9612
Website: www.nih.gov

Occupational Safety & Health Administration (OSHA)
200 Constitution Ave., N.W.
Rm. N3626
Washington, DC 20210
Toll-Free: 800-321-6742 (OSHA)
Website: www.osha.gov

Office of Disease Prevention and Health Promotion (ODPHP)
1101 Wootton Pkwy., Ste. 420
Rockville, MD 20852
Website: www.health.gov

Office of Inspector General (OIG)
330 Independence Ave., S.W.
Washington, DC 20201
Website: www.oig.hhs.gov
Email: Public.Affairs@oig.hhs.gov

Directory of Organizations

U.S. Bureau of Labor Statistics (BLS)
2 Massachusetts Ave., N.E.
Postal Square Bldg.
Washington, DC 20212-0001
Phone: 202-691-5200
Website: www.bls.gov

U.S. Department of Education (ED)
400 Maryland Ave., S.W.
Washington, DC 20202
Toll-Free: 800-872-5327
(800-USA-LEARN)
Phone: 202-401-2000
Website: www2.ed.gov

U.S. Department of Health and Human Services (HHS)
200 Independence Ave., S.W.
Hubert H. Humphrey Bldg.
Washington, DC 20201
Toll-Free: 877-696-6775
Website: www.hhs.gov

U.S. Department of Homeland Security (DHS)
2707 Martin Luther King Jr. Ave., S.E.
Washington, DC 20528-0525
Phone: 202-282-8000
Website: www.dhs.gov

U.S. Department of the Treasury (USDT)
1500 Pennsylvania Ave., N.W.
Washington, DC 20220
Phone: 202-622-2000
Fax: 202-622-6415
Website: www.treasury.gov
Email: inquiries@usmint.treas.gov

U.S. Food and Drug Administration (FDA)
10903 New Hampshire Ave.
Silver Spring, MD 20993-0002
Toll-Free: 888-463-6332
(888-INFO-FDA)
Website: www.fda.gov

U.S. Government Accountability Office (GAO)
441 G St., N.W.
Washington, DC 20548
Phone: 202-512-3000
Website: www.gao.gov
Email: contact@gao.gov

U.S. Senate Committee on Health, Education, Labor, and Pensions
428 Senate Dirksen Office Bldg.
Washington, DC 20510
Phone: 202-224-5375
Website: www.help.senate.gov

United States Census Bureau
4600 Silver Hill Rd.
Washington, DC 20233
Toll-Free: 800-923-8282
Phone: 301-763-4636 (INFO)
TTY: 800-877-8339
Website: www.census.gov

PRIVATE ORGANIZATIONS

American Academy of Family Physicians (AAFP)
11400 Tomahawk Creek Pkwy.
Leawood, KS 66211
Toll-Free: 800-274-2237
Website: www.aafp.org
Email: aafp@aafp.org

American Academy of Pediatrics (AAP)
345 Park Blvd.
Itasca, IL 60143
Toll-Free: 800-433-9016
Fax: 847-434-8000
Website: www.aap.org

American Association for the Advancement of Science (AAAS)
1200 New York Ave., N.W.
Washington, DC 20005
Phone: 202-326-6400
Website: www.aaas.org

American College of Obstetricians and Gynecologists (ACOG)
409 12th St., S.W.
P.O. Box 96920
Washington, DC 20024
Toll-Free: 800-673-8444
Phone: 202-638-5577
Website: www.acog.org
Email: communications@acog.org

American Lung Association
55 W. Wacker Dr., Ste. 1150
Chicago, IL 60601
Toll-Free: 800-586-4872
(800-LUNGUSA)
Website: www.lung.org
Email: info@lung.org

American Society for Microbiology (ASM)
1752 N St., N.W.
Washington, DC 20036
Phone: 202-737-3600
Website: www.asm.org
Email: service@asmusa.org

Breast Cancer Research Foundation (BCRF)
28 W. 44th St., Ste. 609
New York, NY 10036
Toll-Free: 866-346-3228
Fax: 646-497-0890
Website: www.bcrf.org
Email: bcrf@bcrf.org

Cleveland Clinic
9500 Euclid Ave.
Cleveland, OH 44195
Toll-Free: 800-223-2273
Phone: 216-444-2200
Website: my.clevelandclinic.org

Directory of Organizations

Health Affairs
1220 19th St., N.W., Ste. 800
Washington, DC 20036
Phone: 202-408-6801
Fax: 301-654-2845
Website: www.healthaffairs.org
Email: info@healthaffairs.org

Immunize.org
2136 Ford Pkwy., Ste. 5011
Saint Paul, MN 55116
Phone: 651-647-9009
Fax: 651-647-9131
Website: www.immunize.org
Email: admin@immunize.org

Infectious Diseases Society of America (IDSA)
4040 Wilson Blvd., Ste. 300
Arlington, VA 22203
Phone: 703-299-0200
Website: www.idsociety.org

International Monetary Fund (IMF)
700 19th St., N.W.
Washington, DC 20431
Phone: 202-623-7000
Fax: 202-623-4661
Website: www.imf.org
Email: publicaffairs@imf.org

Mayo Clinic
13400 E. Shea Blvd.
Scottsdale, AZ 85259
Toll-Free: 800-446-2279
Phone: 480-301-8000
Website: www.mayoclinic.org

National Bureau of Economic Research (NBER)
1050 Massachusetts Ave.
Cambridge, MA 02138
Phone: 617-868-3900
Website: www.nber.org
Email: info@nber.org

National Comprehensive Cancer Network (NCCN)
3025 Chemical Rd., Ste. 100
Plymouth Meeting, PA 19462
Phone: 215-690-0300
Fax: 215-690-0280
Website: www.nccn.org
Email: perri@nccn.org

National Conference of State Legislatures (NCSL)
444 N. Capitol St., N.W., Ste. 515
Washington, DC 20001
Phone: 202-624-5400
Website: www.ncsl.org

Northeast Document Conservation Center (NEDCC)
100 Brickstone Sq.
4th Fl.
Andover, MA 01810-1494
Phone: 978-470-1010
Fax: 978-475-6021
Website: www.nedcc.org
Email: info@nedcc.org

Pan American Health Organization (PAHO)
525 23rd St., N.W.
Washington, DC 20037
Phone: 202-974-3000
Fax: 202-974-3663
Website: www.paho.org

Regulatory Affairs Professionals Society (RAPS)
5635 Fishers Ln., Ste. 400
Rockville, MD 20852
Phone: 301-770-2920
Fax: 301-841-7956
Website: www.raps.org
Email: raps@raps.org

INDEX

INDEX

INDEX

Page numbers followed by "n" refer to citation information and by "t" indicate tables

A

acute disseminating encephalomyelitis (ADEM), nervous system 89
acute illnesses, COVID-19 pandemic 551
acute kidney injury (AKI), critical care management of COVID-19 267
acute necrotizing leukoencephalopathy, nervous system 80
acute respiratory distress syndrome (ARDS)
  COVID-19 and flu 54
  managing COVID-19 263
  nervous system 82
ADA *see* Americans with Disabilities Act
ADEM *see* acute disseminating encephalomyelitis
Adoption Taxpayer Identification Number (ATIN), COVID-19 economic stimulus relief 542
AKI *see* acute kidney injury
allergic reactions, COVID-19 vaccine 358, 391
American Academy of Family Physicians (AAFP), contact information 638
American Academy of Pediatrics (AAP), contact information 638
American Association for the Advancement of Science (AAAS), contact information 638
American College of Obstetricians and Gynecologists (ACOG), contact information 638
American Lung Association, contact information 638
American Society for Microbiology (ASM), contact information 638
Americans with Disabilities Act (ADA)
  COVID-19 safety considerations 198
  long COVID 447
  prevention and control at workplace 216
aneurysm, critical care management of COVID-19 265
anosmia
  coronavirus and nervous system 84
  post-COVID conditions 420
antibodies
  COVID-19 tests 62
  COVID-19 vaccine 371, 406
  Omicron variant 36
  overview 75–78
  pandemic preparedness 620
  treatment for COVID-19 259
  2009 H1N1 Pandemic 474

antibody test
    COVID-19 antibodies 76
    COVID-19 vaccine 408
    herd immunity 413
    multisystem inflammatory syndrome (MIS) 264
antigen tests
    COVID-19 59
    COVID-19 treatment in hospital 266
    post-COVID conditions 424
    SARS-CoV-2 239
antiretroviral therapy (ART), human immunodeficiency virus (HIV) 114
anxiety
    coronavirus and nervous system 86
    disparities in COVID-19 130
    impact on the education 569
    long COVID 46
    pandemic and mental health 547
    post-COVID health condition 419
    SARS-CoV-2 251
    see also depression
ARDS *see* acute respiratory distress syndrome
ART *see* antiretroviral therapy
arthralgia, post-COVID health condition 420
artificial ventilation, coronavirus and nervous system 81
asthma
    children and teens with disabilities 368
    chronic lung diseases 104
    overview 121–123
    SARS-CoV-2 240
    spiritual and psychosocial support 320
asymptomatic infections, COVID-19 vaccine benefits 381
ATIN *see* Adoption Taxpayer Identification Number
autism, children and teens with disabilities 369
autoimmunity, post-COVID conditions 421
autonomic nerves, coronavirus and nervous system 83
avian flu virus, 1957–1958 pandemic 469

B

bivalent boosters, COVID-19 vaccine benefits 385
blood clots
    coronavirus infection symptoms 55
    COVID-19 and health-care facilities 578
    COVID-19 vaccines safety 358
blood stem cell, preexisting medical conditions 108
bone marrow transplants, preexisting medical conditions 108
brain
    cerebrovascular disease 108
    coronavirus and nervous system 79
    neurological symptoms 45
    pandemic and mental health 547
    post-COVID health condition 419
brain development, pandemic and mental health 550
brain fog
    employees support 440
    neurological symptoms 45
    pandemic and mental health 547
    post-COVID health condition 419
breakthrough infection
    antibodies and COVID-19 76
    COVID-19 vaccine benefits 382
    Delta variant 33
    SARS-CoV-2 246
Breast Cancer Research Foundation (BCRF), contact information 638

Index

breast milk
    caring newborns 183
    pregnancy 102
    safety COVID-19 vaccination 373
breastfeeding
    overview 182–184
    pregnancy 102
    safety COVID-19 vaccination 377

C

C-reactive protein (CRP)
    multisystem inflammatory syndrome (MIS) 264
    SARS-CoV-2 240
cancer
    COVID-19 infection spread 13
    COVID-19 vaccines 369
    deaths due to COVID-19 147
    immunocompromised people 116
    impact on health-care facilities 580
    Middle East respiratory syndrome (MERS) 20
    people with preexisting medical conditions 104
    SARS-CoV-2 240
candidate vaccine virus, 1957–1958 pandemic (H2N2) virus 472
Centers for Disease Control and Prevention (CDC)
    contact information 635
    publications
        antibodies and COVID-19 78n
        breastfeeding and caring for newborns with COVID-19 184n
        caring for people with post-COVID conditions 438n
        caring for someone 182n
        cleaning and disinfecting at home 172n
        coronavirus and health coverage 327n
        coronavirus risk factors 92n, 95n
        COVID-19 after vaccination 384n
        COVID-19 case investigation and contact tracing 282n
        COVID-19 community mitigation measures 301n
        COVID-19 epidemiology 16n
        COVID-19 statistics 137n
        COVID-19 surveillance and data analytics 285n
        COVID-19 symptoms 44n
        COVID-19 test results 62n, 73n
        COVID-19 treatment in outpatients 255n
        COVID-19 vaccination 359n, 386n, 393n, 394n
        COVID-19 vaccine monitoring systems for pregnant people 401n
        COVID-19 vaccine myths and facts 408n
        COVID-19 vaccine safety in children and teens 402n
        COVID-19 vaccines for specific groups of people 379n
        COVID-19 vaccines work 382n
        earlier outbreaks caused by the coronavirus 18n
        effectiveness and benefits of getting a COVID-19 vaccine 382n
        endemics, epidemics, and pandemics 460n
        excess deaths associated with COVID-19 149n
        finding a COVID-19 vaccine or booster 350n
        global response to COVID-19 (2020–2023) 311n

Centers for Disease Control and Prevention (CDC) publications, *continued*
  guidance for COVID-19 prevention and control in schools 192n
  HIV and COVID-19 115n
  immunocompromised people 120n
  long COVID or post-COVID conditions 50n, 417n
  Middle East respiratory syndrome (MERS) 21n
  monitoring COVID-19 vaccine effectiveness 383n
  pandemics in history 482n
  people with moderate to severe asthma 123n
  people with preexisting medical conditions 110n
  personal protective equipment (PPE) 291n
  post-COVID conditions 276n, 428n
  post-COVID conditions and health-care provider appointments 434n
  pregnant and recently pregnant people 102n
  preventing COVID-19 transmission in schools 196n
  quarantine and isolation 181n
  self-testing at home or anywhere 65n
  side effects after getting a COVID-19 vaccine 392n
  similarities and differences between flu and COVID-19 56n
  spiritual and psychosocial support to people with COVID-19 at home 322n
  spread of COVID-19 infection 15n
  stay up-to-date with COVID-19 vaccines including boosters 368n
  staying away from people when you have COVID-19 168n
  telehealth and telemedicine during COVID-19 343n
  vaccine adverse event reporting system (VAERS) 398n
  variants of the coronavirus 32n
Centers for Medicare & Medicaid Services (CMS), contact information 635
central nervous system (CNS), neurological complications of COVID-19 82
cerebral palsy (CP), disparities in COVID-19 130
cerebrovascular disease, neurological complications of COVID-19 88
CF *see* cystic fibrosis
CFS *see* chronic fatigue syndrome
chemoprophylaxis, 2009 H1N1 pandemic 478
chest pain
  COVID-19 in pregnant people 102
  long COVID conditions 45
  neurological complications of COVID-19 84
  post-COVID conditions 419
  SARS-CoV-2 243
  spiritual and psychological support 320
chronic bronchitis, COVID-19 in people with preexisting medical conditions 105
chronic COVID, post-COVID conditions 417
chronic disorder, neurological complications of COVID-19 79

Index

chronic fatigue syndrome (CFS)
  long COVID condition 46
  neurological complications of COVID-19 86
  post-COVID condition 419
  post-COVID condition symptom 273
chronic kidney disease (CKD)
  COVID-19 in people with preexisting medical conditions 104
  Middle East respiratory syndrome (MERS) 20
  SARS-CoV-2 240
  SARS-CoV-2 in workers 216
  workplace COVID-19 prevention and control 204
CKD *see* chronic kidney disease
Cleveland Clinic, contact information 638
close contact
  breastfeeding and new mothers 183
  case investigation and contact tracing 279
  cloth face coverings 164
  coronavirus 5
  coronavirus outbreaks 17
  COVID-19 and flu 53
  COVID-19 home tests 64
  COVID-19 prevention and control in schools 194
  COVID-19 test result 73
  COVID-19 vaccines 361
  immunocompromised people 118
  infection in pets and animals 124
  personal protective equipment (PPE) 288t
  prevention and control at workplace 204
  public events and gatherings 223
  spiritual and psychological support 321
cloth face coverings
  overview 161–168
  prevention and control at workplace 204
CMV *see* cytomegalovirus
CNS *see* central nervous system
cognitive impairment
  acute COVID-19 250
  multisystem inflammatory syndrome in adults (MIS-A) 265
  neurological complications of COVID-19 84
  post-COVID conditions 419
  supporting employees with long COVID 439
common-source outbreak, epidemics 458
community transmission
  community mitigation for lower-resource countries 291
  COVID-19 safety in schools 197
  COVID-19 vaccines 364
  prevention and control at workplace 211
computed tomography (CT)
  assessment and testing tools for post-COVID conditions 428
  SARS-CoV-2 240
congenital heart disease, people with preexisting medical conditions 108
Consumer Financial Protection Bureau (CFPB)
  contact information 636
  publication
    COVID-19 economic stimulus relief 544n
contact tracing
  community mitigation 294t
  control measures 228
  overview 279–282

contact tracing, *continued*
  prevention and control at
    workplace 208
  prevention and control in
    schools 191
  prevention strategy 307
  telemedicine 339
contact/wet time, disinfect safely 171
convalescent plasma
  COVID-19 in
    immunocompromised
    people 119
  Delta variant 34
  outpatient treatments for
    COVID-19 255
cough
  acute COVID-19 249
  coronavirus 5
  COVID-19 symptoms 43, 176
  COVID-19 test result 72
  COVID-19 transmission 14
  masks and face coverings 164
  neurological complications 82
  1918 pandemic (H1N1 virus) 465
  1957–1958 pandemic (H2N2)
    virus 473
  personal protective equipment
    (PPE) 289t
  post-COVID conditions 419
  pregnant people 101
  prevention and control at
    workplace 204
  prevention and control in
    schools 187
  SARS-CoV-2 239
  spiritual and psychological
    support 321
COVID-19
  publications
    breathing and COVID-19 334n
    chronic viral infection and long
      COVID 332n

    mental health during
      COVID-19 550n
COVID-19 testing
  community-based COVID-19
    testing sites 71
  overview 59–62
COVID-19 treatment guidelines
  publications
    critical care management of
      adults with COVID-19 270n
    SARS-CoV-2 infection 252n
CP *see* cerebral palsy
creatine phosphokinase, laboratory
  testing for post-COVID
  conditions 425
CRP *see* C-reactive protein
CT *see* computed tomography
cystic fibrosis (CF), people with
  preexisting medical conditions 105
cytokines, COVID-19 critical care
  management 264
cytomegalovirus (CMV), chronic viral
  infection 331

D

decision support system (DSS),
  telemedicine 338
delirium
  nervous system 80
  COVID-19 treatment 267
Delta variant, overview 32–35
dementia
  COVID-19 excess deaths 139
  neurological disorders 88
  preexisting medical
    conditions 105
depression
  neuropsychiatric impairment 251
  pandemic and mental health 547
  post-COVID conditions 46, 426t
  pregnancy 101

Index

developmental disabilities
    children and teens 369
    preexisting medical conditions 106
diabetes
    children and teens with
        disabilities 368
    COVID-19 control and
        prevention 205
    epidemics 458
    health-care facilities 584
    neurological disorder 88
    pandemic to endemic 625
    preexisting medical
        conditions 105
    SARS-CoV-2 infection 240
disinfect
    asthma 121
    hand hygiene and respiratory
        etiquette 189
    Middle East respiratory syndrome
        (MERS) 19
    overview 171–173
disposable face masks, social
    distancing 161
distance education, pandemic 570
distance learning *see* distance
    education
dizziness
    neurological symptoms 46
    post-COVID conditions 424
    pregnancy 102
domestic violence, pandemic 553
Down syndrome
    disparities in COVID-19 130
    preexisting medical
        conditions 106
DSS *see* decision support system
dysautonomia
    neurological disorders 88
    post-COVID conditions 273, 426t
dysgeusia, post-COVID
    conditions 420

dyspnea
    post-COVID conditions 426t
    SARS-CoV-2 239
    telemedicine 343

E

EAP *see* employee assistance program
early care and education (ECE)
    programs, COVID-19 prevention
        and control 185
EBV *see* Epstein-Barr virus
ECE *see* early care and education
    programs
ECG *see* electrocardiogram
echocardiogram, post-COVID
    conditions evaluation 427
ECMO *see* extracorporeal membrane
    oxygenation
Economic Impact Payments (EIP),
    COVID-19 economic stimulus
    relief 519
ED *see* erectile dysfunction
EHR *see* electronic health record
EIP *see* Economic Impact Payments
electrocardiogram (ECG), post-
    COVID conditions
    evaluation 427
electronic health record (EHR)
    Clinical Immunization Safety
        Assessment (CISA)
        project 393
    surveillance resources 285
emergency plan, pandemic
    preparation 461
Emergency Rental Assistance (ERA),
    COVID-19 economic
    relief 522
Emergency Unemployment Insurance
    Stabilization and Access Act
    (EUISAA), pandemic and
    employment 615

Emergency Use Authorization (EUA)
    alternative therapies 255
    antibodies 77
    COVID-19 home tests 67
    Novavax COVID-19 vaccine 356t
emotional development, effects of pandemic 548
emphysema, people with preexisting medical conditions 105
employee assistance program (EAP), supporting employees with long COVID 442
employee resource group (ERG), supporting employees with long COVID 442
encephalopathy
    multisystem inflammatory syndrome in adults (MIS-A) 265
    neurological disorders 89
endemics, pandemics in history 457
epicenter, basics of COVID-19 24
epidemic
    described 457
    H1N1 pandemic 474
    zoonotic origin 10
epidemic curve, pandemics in history 459
epidemiologic investigation, endemics 457
Epstein-Barr virus (EBV), chronic viral infection 331
ERA *see* Emergency Rental Assistance
erectile dysfunction (ED), post-COVID conditions 420
ERG *see* employee resource group
EUA *see* Emergency Use Authorization
EUISAA *see* Emergency Unemployment Insurance Stabilization and Access Act
EWI *see* early warning indicator

excess deaths
    H3N2 virus 473
    overview 138–149
    pandemic impact 486
extracorporeal membrane oxygenation (ECMO), acute infection in brain 81

F

face masks
    contact tracing strategies 196
    coronavirus 5
    personal protective equipment (PPE) 289t
    protect yourself from COVID-19 infection 161
    SARS-CoV-2 213
    see also N95
face shield, SARS-CoV-2 212
facial nerve palsies, COVID-19 and neurological disorders 89
Families First Coronavirus Response Act (FFCRA)
    pandemic and employment 615
    screening workers 207
fatigue
    conditions after acute COVID-19 249
    coronavirus 6
    COVID-19 symptoms 43
    health-care facilities 585
    long COVID 439
    long-term neurological complications 82
    palliative care 323
    post-COVID health condition 419
    side effects of COVID vaccine 390
FDA *see* U.S. Food and Drug Administration
fertility, COVID-19 vaccine 370, 407

Index

fever
  coronavirus 6
  COVID-19 exposure 176
  COVID-19 symptoms 43
  COVID-19 test result 72
  COVID-19 vaccine 358, 407
  SARS-CoV-2 infection 239
  screening workers 207
  situational awareness 620
  staying healthy 102
  symptomatic management 255
  vaccine side effects 378
FFCRA *see* Families First Coronavirus Response Act
FFRs *see* filtering facepiece respirators
fibrinogen, coagulation disorders 425
fibromyalgia, post-COVID conditions 273
filtering facepiece respirators (FFRs)
  Occupational Safety and Health Administration (OSHA) 164
  personal protective equipment (PPE) 212
flu
  coronavirus and nervous system 89
  COVID-19 vaccine 377, 406
  1918 pandemic 462
  2009 H1N1 pandemic 474
  versus COVID-19 50

G

GAD-7 *see* Generalized Anxiety Disorder-7
GBS *see* Guillain-Barré syndrome
GDP *see* gross domestic product
Generalized Anxiety Disorder-7 (GAD-7), post-COVID conditions 426t
gloves
  cleaning and disinfecting 122
  contact tracing strategies 196
  disinfect safely 171
  health-care facilities 592
  natural zoonotic spillover 10
  psychosocial support 321
glycoprotein, vaccine formula 353t
gross domestic product (GDP), global economy 493
Guillain-Barré syndrome (GBS)
  coronavirus and nervous system 80
  multisystem inflammatory syndrome (MIS) 265

H

H1N1 *see* hemagglutinin type 1 and neuraminidase type 1
hand sanitizers
  breastfeeding 182
  cleaning and disinfecting home 173
  immunocompromised people 117
  infection in pets and animals 125
  Middle East respiratory syndrome (MERS) 21
  spiritual and psychosocial Support 320
HCP *see* health-care personnel
headache
  chronic clinical presentation 7
  COVID-19 symptoms 43
  COVID-19 vaccines 358
  Delta variant 35
  flu symptoms 51
  neurological symptoms 45
  neuropsychiatric impairment 250
  post-COVID conditions 273, 419
  pregnancy 102
  SARS-CoV-2 infection 240
  severe acute respiratory syndrome (SARS) 17
  side effects after COVID-19 vaccine 389
  spread of COVID-19 72

Health Affairs, contact
  information 639
health insurance policies,
  pandemics 461
health-care personnel (HCP)
  face masks 165
  personal protective equipment
    (PPE) 286
  pharmacies 70
health-care provider
  community mitigation 291
  community-based testing site 70
  COVID-19 exposure 175
  COVID-19 vaccination 368
  face masks 164
  fraudulent coronavirus test 315
  long COVID condition 44
  medical management 259
  post-COVID conditions 273, 429
  preexisting medical conditions 106
  side effects of COVID-19
    vaccine 391
  spread of COVID-19 infection 14
  telehealth 334
  vaccine safety and
    monitoring 368, 393
heart failure
  cardiopulmonary injury 250
  coronavirus and nervous
    system 81
  excess deaths 147
  preexisting medical conditions 106
heart palpitations, long COVID 439
heart rate
  neurological complications 82
  post-COVID conditions 423
heating, ventilation, and air
  conditioning (HVAC) settings,
  COVID-19 prevention and control
  in schools 188
hemagglutinin type 1 and
  neuraminidase type 1 (H1N1) virus

pandemics 461
  SARS-CoV-2 10
HEPA *see* high-efficiency particulate
  air filters
hepatitis A, epidemics 459
hepatitis B
  epidemic patterns 459
  epidemiology 15
  SARS-CoV-2 infection 245
herd immunity
  COVID-19 cases and deaths 153
  overview 409–413
  pandemic to endemic 623
high blood pressure
  preexisting medical conditions 105
  neurological disorder 88
high-efficiency particulate air (HEPA)
  filters, prevention and control in
  schools 189
HIV *see* human immunodeficiency
  virus
hospitalization
  acute clinical presentation 6
  antibodies and COVID-19 76
  COVID-19 cases and deaths 153
  COVID-19 vaccines 357, 375, 383
  Delta variant 34
  disparities in COVID-19 129
  epidemiology 16
  flu illness 54
  health coverage 325
  H1N1 pandemic 475
  neurological complications 86
  post-COVID condition 419
  pregnancy 100
  SARS-COV-2 reinfection 247
  surveillance and data analytics 284
human immunodeficiency virus (HIV)
  long COVID 331
  overview 111–115
  people with disabilities 130
  preexisting medical conditions 106

Index

human-to-human transmission, zoonotic spillovers 9
HVAC *see* heating, ventilation, and air conditioning settings
hygiene
    control and prevention strategy 307
    control measures 221
    filtering facepiece respirators (FFRs) 213
    Occupational Safety and Health Administration (OSHA) 163
    pandemics 462
    prevent illness 172
    quarantine and isolation 182
    SARS-CoV-2 209
    spread of COVID-19 infection 14
hypoxemia, SARS-CoV-2 infection 241
hypoxia, coronavirus and nervous system 81

I

IAQ *see* indoor air quality
ICU *see* intensive care unit
IFSP *see* individualized family service plan
immune system
    chronic viral infection 331
    COVID-19 and disability 449
    COVID-19 infections 13
    COVID-19 pandemic 625
    COVID-19 vaccines 381
    described 75
    herd immunity 410
    human immunodeficiency virus (HIV) 112
    neurological problems 89
    protein subunit vaccines 354
Immunize.org, contact information 639
immunocompromised
    coronavirus self-test kits 64t

COVID-19 risk factors 93
COVID-19 vaccinations 117
COVID-19 vaccine and booster 360
in vitro fertilization, COVID-19 vaccine and pregnancy 371
individualized family service plan (IFSP), COVID-19 in schools 190
indoor air quality (IAQ), COVID-19 prevention and control in schools 188
Infectious Diseases Society of America (IDSA), contact information 639
inflammation
    blood clots 80
    COVID-19 in adults 264
    COVID-19 vaccination 402
    flu and COVID-19 54
    physical or mental impairment 448
inflammatory markers
    post-COVID conditions 425
    SARS-CoV-2 240
influenza *see* flu
influenza A (H1N1) Pandemic Disease Mexico 2009 (pdm09) virus, pandemics in history 473
influenza A virus
    lung alveolus chip 333
    1918 influenza pandemic 461
    1968 pandemic (H3N2) virus 473
influenza B virus, 1957–1958 pandemic (H2N2) virus 466
influenza pandemic, H1N1pdm09 virus 475
influenza vaccine, H1N1pdm09 virus 467
Insomnia Severity Index (ISI), post-COVID conditions 426t
intensive care unit (ICU)
    blood clots 81
    breastfeeding 373

COVID-19 and the Coronavirus Sourcebook, First Edition

intensive care unit (ICU), *continued*
    critical care management of COVID-19 263
    telemedicine during COVID-19 339
International Monetary Fund (IMF), contact information 639
intimate partner violence (IPV), unintended consequences 553
IPV *see* intimate partner violence
ISI *see* Insomnia Severity Index
isolation
    at-home COVID-19 test 65
    breastfeeding 183
    children and teens with disabilities 369
    contact tracing strategies 194
    COVID-19 and pregnancy 100
    COVID-19 caseloads 579
    1918 flu pandemic 462
    personal protective equipment (PPE) 289t
    public events and gatherings 223
    telemedicine 336
    unintended consequences 552

J

J&J/Janssen *see* Johnson & Johnson's Janssen
Johnson & Johnson's Janssen (J&J/Janssen), COVID-19 vaccine 350

L

layoff
    COVID-19 and employment 605
    travel and tourism 598
    unemployment insurance claims 615
leukemia, epidemic patterns 458

lockdowns
    COVID-19 control measures 219
    social impact 557
    spread of COVID-19 25
    unintended consequences 551
long COVID
    chronic viral infection 331
    coronavirus and nervous system 82
    described 44
    mental health 547
    physical or mental impairment 448
    post-acute COVID-19 248
    supporting employees 439
long-haul COVID, post-COVID health condition 417

M

magnetic resonance imaging (MRI), post-COVID conditions 428
mask
    breakthrough infection 384
    Delta variant 33
    health-care provider 326
    influenza virus 464
    mental health 548
    overview 161–166
    pandemic to endemic 625
    personal protective equipment (PPE) 288t, 592
    post-COVID conditions 418
    prevention in schools 193
    SARS-CoV-2 5
    transmission risk 91
mast cell activation syndrome (MCAS), post-COVID conditions 273, 418
Mayo Clinic, contact information 639
MCAS *see* mast cell activation syndrome
MD *see* muscular dystrophy

Index

ME/CFS *see* myalgic encephalomyelitis/chronic fatigue syndrome
MedlinePlus
   contact information 636
   publication
      palliative care 324n
menstruation
   COVID-19 vaccination 371
   post-COVID conditions 273
mental illnesses, pandemic effects 547
mental stress, pandemic consequences 553
MERS *see* Middle East respiratory syndrome
MERV-13 *see* minimum efficiency reporting values 13 air filters
methicillin-resistant *Staphylococcus aureus* (MRSA), epidemiology 14
Middle East respiratory syndrome (MERS)
   coronavirus family 5
   defined 18
   post-COVID conditions 419
minimum efficiency reporting values 13 (MERV-13) air filters, COVID-19 prevention and control in schools 188
MIS *see* multisystem inflammatory syndrome
MIS-C *see* multisystem inflammatory syndrome in children
monitoring
   antibodies 62
   asymptomatic infection 243
   COVID-19 economic relief 529
   COVID-19 vaccine safety 392
   human immunodeficiency virus (HIV) 112
   pandemic preparedness 621
   telehealth 335
   transmission scenarios 299
   variants 31
   worker screening 207
mood disorders, mental health 107, 549
morbidity rates, herd immunity 410
mortality
   economic impact 487
   herd immunity 410
   influenza pandemic 462
   SARS-CoV-2 242
   see also excess deaths
motor nerves, defined 83
MRI *see* magnetic resonance imaging
MRSA *see* methicillin-resistant staphylococcus aureus
multisystem inflammatory syndrome (MIS)
   autoimmune conditions 421
   post-COVID conditions 47, 383
multisystem inflammatory syndrome in children (MIS-C)
   COVID-19 complications 55
   SARS-CoV-2 241
muscular dystrophy (MD), COVID-19 vaccines 368
muscular weakness, SARS-CoV-2 88
myalgic encephalomyelitis/chronic fatigue syndrome (ME/CFS)
   post-COVID conditions 46, 273, 419
   SARS-CoV-2 86
myocarditis
   autoimmune conditions 421
   COVID-19 vaccine risks 358
   heart attack 81
   multisystem inflammatory syndrome (MIS) 265

N

N95
   contingency 288t
   control and prevention 212
   coronavirus risk factors 91

N95, *continued*
   COVID-19 exposure 176
   COVID-19 self-test kits 64
   health-care facilities 592
   social distancing 164
   see also personal protective equipment (PPE)
NAAT *see* nucleic acid amplification test
National Bureau of Economic Research (NBER), contact information 639
National Center for Complementary and Integrative Health (NCCIH)
   contact information 636
   publication
      alternative treatments for COVID-19 318n
National Comprehensive Cancer Network (NCCN), contact information 639
National Conference of State Legislatures (NCSL), contact information 639
National Institute of Allergy and Infectious Diseases (NIAID), contact information 636
National Institute of Neurological Disorders and Stroke (NINDS)
   contact information 636
   publication
National Institutes of Health (NIH), contact information 636
natural immunity
   COVID-19 vaccines 404
   Omicron 625
   see also herd immunity
nausea
   clinical spectrum 239
   COVID-19 test result 72
   disability 450
   pregnant people 102
   severe acute respiratory syndrome (SARS) 19
   side effects of COVID-19 vaccine 390
   COVID-19 symptoms 43
nerve fibers, coronavirus and nervous system 89
nerve injury, SARS-CoV-2 virus 80
nervous system
   critical illness 263
   disabled children and teens 369
   flu and COVID-19 54
   overview 79–90
1918 influenza pandemic, H1N1 virus 461
noninfected patients, health-care facilities 578
Northeast Document Conservation Center (NEDCC), contact information 639
nucleic acid amplification test (NAAT)
   clinical spectrum 239
   SARS-CoV-2 59

O

obesity
   children and teens with disabilities 369
   epidemics 458
   neurological disorders 88
   SARS-CoV-2 infection 240
   2009 H1N1 pandemic 479
   workplace preventions 205
Occupational Safety and Health Administration (OSHA)
   contact information 636
   publications
      COVID-19 control and prevention at workplaces 217n
      COVID-19 guidance on social distancing at work 167n
      face masks and social distancing 166n

Index

Office of Disease Prevention and
    Health Promotion (ODPHP),
    contact information 636
Office of Inspector General (OIG)
    contact information 636
    publication
        COVID-19 impact on health-
            care facilities 595n
older adults
    COVID-19 and severe illness 53
    COVID-19 risk factors 92
    COVID-19 test result 72
    COVID-19 vaccines 381
    pandemic and endemic COVID-19
        624
    preexisting medical
        conditions 103
Omicron
    COVID-19 boosters 357
    COVID-19 cases and deaths 151
    educating school staff 193
    incubation period 6
    pandemic and endemic COVID-19
        625
    SARS-CoV-2 infection 36, 247
    weakened immune system 93
OTC *see* over-the-counter
over-the-counter (OTC)
    COVID-19 testing 60
    COVID-19 vaccine side
        effects 372, 391
    emergency medical attention 181
    negative test results 177
    pulse oximetry 243
overweight, preexisting medical
    conditions 107

P

palliative care
    overview 323–324
    post-intensive care syndrome
        (PICS) 270

palpitations
    employees with long COVID 439
    long COVID condition 45
    post-COVID health condition 420
    SARS-CoV-2 infection 249
Pan American Health Organization
    (PAHO), contact information 640
pancreas, cystic fibrosis (CF) 105
pandemic
    COVID-19 9, 624
    COVID-19 control measures 219
    COVID-19 excess deaths 138
    COVID-19 testing 71
    economy 490
    education 563
    employment 605
    epicenter 24
    face masks and social
        distancing 161
    herd immunity 409
    overview 455–482
    SARS-CoV-2 206
    spiritual and psychosocial
        support 319
    telehealth and telemedicine 334
    see also endemics; epidemic
Pandemic Unemployment Assistance
    (PUA), pandemic
    preparedness 617
paralyze, SARS-CoV-2 virus 81
paresthesia, post-COVID
    conditions 420
Parkinson disease (PD), neurological
    disorders 89
pathogens
    epidemiology 15
    face masks and social
        distancing 165
    global response to COVID-19 305
    personal protective equipment
        (PPE) 213
pathophysiologic processes, post-
    COVID conditions 421

Patient Protection and Affordable Care Act, long COVID as a disability 447
Paxlovid, interim COVID-19 treatment 253
PCR *see* polymerase chain reaction
PD *see* Parkinson disease
PEG *see* polyethylene glycol
PEM *see* post-exertional malaise
people with disabilities
    disparities in COVID-19 130
    long COVID 48
    mental health 548
    post-COVID conditions 275
    preexisting medical conditions 103
    public events and gatherings 223
pericarditis
    COVID-19 vaccines safety 358, 402
    multisystem inflammatory syndrome (MIS) 265
    post-COVID conditions 423
personal protective equipment (PPE)
    cleaning and disinfecting home 171
    overview 286–291
    prevention and control at workplace 203
    telehealth and telemedicine 334
PFTs *see* pulmonary function tests
physical activity
    overweight and obesity 107
    stringency index 221
physical distancing
    community mitigation 296
    coronavirus self-test kits 63
    COVID-19 safety in schools 198
    face masks and social distancing 163
    prevention and control at workplace 209
    telehealth and telemedicine 337
physical impairment, long-term COVID disability 448

physical therapy
    education in a pandemic 566
    telehealth and telemedicine 336
PICS *see* post-intensive care syndrome
plague, endemics 457
pneumonia
    asymptomatic or presymptomatic infection 243
    central nervous system (CNS) 85
    COVID-19 deaths 146
    health care delivery 578
    human immunodeficiency virus (HIV) 114
    influenza 468
    multisystem inflammatory syndrome (MIS) 54
    renal and hepatic dysfunction 267
    severe acute respiratory syndrome (SARS) 17
pointsource outbreak, epidemic patterns 458
polio
    COVID-19 herd immunity 411
    endemics 457
polyethylene glycol (PEG), vaccine formulation for children 352t
polymerase chain reaction (PCR)
    coronavirus 7
    COVID-19 medical management 262
    COVID-19 testing 59
    Omicron variant 36
    pandemics in history 472
post-acute COVID syndrome, post-COVID conditions 417
post-acute COVID-19 *see* post-acute COVID syndrome
post-COVID conditions
    coronavirus risk factors 94
    COVID-19 impact on health-care facilities 578
    COVID-19 vaccine effectiveness 33

Index

post-COVID conditions, *continued*
  overview 44–50
  post-COVID conditions 271
  post-COVID health condition 417
  SARS-CoV-2 248, 429
post-exertional malaise (PEM)
  long COVID condition 45
  testing for post-COVID conditions 426
post-intensive care syndrome (PICS)
  long COVID condition 47
  COVID-19 illness or hospitalization 422
posttraumatic stress disorder (PTSD)
  COVID-19's impact on mental health 547
  hospital staffing 585
  post-intensive care syndrome (PICS) 269
postsecondary students, COVID-19's impact on higher education 567
posttreatment Lyme disease syndrome, post-COVID conditions 273
postural orthostatic tachycardia syndrome (POTS)
  neurological complications of COVID-19 83
  post-COVID conditions 419
POTS *see* postural orthostatic tachycardia syndrome
PPE *see* personal protective equipment
practical nurse, 1918 pandemic 466
pre-exposure prophylaxis (PrEP), human immunodeficiency virus (HIV) 111
pregnancy
  COVID-19 risk factors 99
  COVID-19 vaccines 370
  SARS-CoV-2 infection 240
  vaccine safety monitoring systems 393

pregnancy registry, vaccine safety and monitoring 393
PrEP *see* pre-exposure prophylaxis
PrEP *see* preexposure prophylaxis
propagated outbreak, epidemics 459
psychological consequences, post-COVID conditions 417
psychologist, medications and preventive care 110
PTSD *see* posttraumatic stress disorder
PUA *see* Pandemic Unemployment Assistance
public health crisis
  assistance for American industry 519
  1918 pandemic 462
pulmonary fibrosis
  preexisting medical conditions 105
  post-COVID conditions 421
pulmonary function tests (PFTs), testing for post-COVID conditions 427
pulse oximetry
  SARS-CoV-2 infection 239
  telemedicine practice 342
pulse survey
  distance education 570
  hospital staffing 586
  post-COVID conditions 420
  telehealth and telemedicine 334

Q

QOL *see* quality of life
quality of life (QOL)
  long COVID 48
  palliative care 323
  post-COVID conditions 271, 417
  vital signs 426t
quarantine
  community mitigation 291
  contact tracing 279

quarantine, *continued*
   early care and education (ECE) 194
   economic relief 525
   global pandemic 490
   global response to COVID-19 305
   health coverage 325
   overview 181–182
   pandemics of the past 462
   stringency index 219
   telehealth and telemedicine 336
   unintended consequences 551
Quarterly Workforce Indicators (QWI), travel and tourism 597
QWI *see* Quarterly Workforce Indicators

R

rabies, endemics 457
Ready.gov
   publication
      pandemics in history 461n
Regulatory Affairs Professionals Society (RAPS), contact information 640
Rehabilitation Act
   athletics programs in schools 198
   long COVID 447, 452
   SARS-CoV-2 infection 216
remdesivir
   interim COVID-19 treatment 253
   medical management of COVID-19 260
renal failure
   causes of death 147
   post-COVID conditions 423
renal replacement therapy (RRT), multisystem inflammatory syndrome (MIS) 265
respirators
   COVID-19 vaccines 117
   face masks and social distancing 161

personal protective equipment (PPE) 212, 289
reaction
rural hospitals, COVID-19 and healthcare facilities 577

S

sanitize, cleaning and disinfecting home 169
SARS *see* severe acute respiratory syndrome
SARS-CoV-2 *see* severe acute respiratory syndrome coronavirus 2
SARS-CoV-2 infection
   clinical trials 239
   control and prevention strategy 308
   laboratory testing 424
   multisystem inflammatory syndrome (MIS) 264
   workplace 209
SARS-CoV-2 reinfection
   post-COVID health 421
   viral infections 246
SCD *see* sickle cell disease
schizophrenia, mental illnesses 549
school nurses, post-COVID 435
screening
   assessment tools 426t
   COVID-19 safety considerations 199
   COVID-19 testing 59
   diagnosis of COVID-19 7
   hospitalization 582
   telemedicine 338
   testing sites for COVID-19 71
   workplace 207
Section 1557, long COVID 447
Section 504
   long COVID 447
   students with disabilities 190

Index

seizures
  mental health 547
  multisystem inflammatory syndrome (MIS) 265
  nervous system 80
  respiratory disease 85
  U.S. Food and Drug Administration (FDA) 314
  vaccination 402
self-test *see* home test
self-test kits, COVID-19 testing 60
sensory nerves, long-term neurological complications 83
serial testing, SARS-CoV-2 60
serological tests
  contact tracing 228
  control and prevention strategy 306
severe acute respiratory syndrome (SARS)
  earlier outbreaks 17
  see also Middle East respiratory syndrome (MERS)
severe acute respiratory syndrome coronavirus 2 (SARS-CoV-2), contact tracing 279
severe illness
  breastfeeding 183
  community mitigation 291
  COVID-19 infection 16
  COVID-19 vaccines 369
  Delta variant 32
  human immunodeficiency virus (HIV) 111
  immune system 76
  long COVID 47
  pregnancy 99
  SARS-CoV-2 infection 244
  worldwide COVID-19 154
shortness of breath
  clinical spectrum 239
  COVID-19 test 72
  long COVID syndrome 439
  long-term neurological complications 84
  Middle East respiratory syndrome (MERS) 18
  persistent symptoms 249
  symptoms of COVID-19 43
sickle cell disease (SCD), preexisting medical conditions 107
skin pigmentation, clinical spectrum 241
sleep
  coronavirus and nervous system 86
  long COVID 46
  persistent symptoms 250
  post-COVID 273
  support employees with long COVID 439
  vaccine 407
SLRF *see* State and Local Fiscal Recovery Funds
smell
  COVID-19 symptoms 7
  COVID-19 test 72
  Delta variant 35
  long COVID 46
  neurological complications 84
  persistent symptoms 250
  transmission scenarios 297
social distancing
  Omicron variant 37
  pandemic 623
  protecting the health 167
  see also quarantine
social impact, overview 556–559
social isolation
  control measures 223
  COVID-19 vaccines 369
  pandemic 553
Social Security Number (SSN), Economic Impact Payments (EIP) 535

source investigation, contact tracing 195, 280
spike protein
  COVID-19 vaccine 354
  Delta variant 33
SSBCI *see* State Small Business Credit Initiative
SSN *see* Social Security Number
State and Local Fiscal Recovery Funds (SLFRF), economic relief 528
State Small Business Credit Initiative (SSBCI), economic relief 530
statistics
  control and prevention 283
  education in pandemic 563
  H2N2 virus 468
  outbreak 23
  U.S. Census Bureau 603
stress
  asthma 123
  cardiac injury 266
  COVID-19 impact 585
  H1N1PDM09 virus 480
  neurological complications 86
  people with preexisting medical conditions 110
  post-COVID 273
  quarantine restrictions 226
  supporting people with post-COVID conditions 436
  telemedicine 341
  unintended consequences 552
stroke
  coronavirus and nervous system 81
  COVID-19 impact 580
  critical care 267
  post-COVID conditions 423
  preexisting medical conditions 108
substance abuse, unintended consequences 553
substance use disorder (SUD)
  mental health 547
  post-COVID conditions 275
  preexisting medical conditions 108
swine flu, influenza pandemic 469
swollen lymph nodes, COVID-19 vaccine 389
syphilis, epidemic patterns 459

T

taste
  community mitigation strategies 297
  contagious respiratory illnesses 51
  COVID-19 symptoms 43
  Delta variant 35
  peripheral neuropathy 83
  SARS-CoV-2 infection 239, 243
  spread of COVID-19 72
TB *see* tuberculosis
technology barriers, distance learning 564
telehealth
  described 335
  health coverage 325
  immunosuppressive medications 118
  long-standing problems 583
  medical management of COVID-19 259
  mental health 548
  post-COVID conditions 275
  prevention strategy 309
telemedicine
  described 337
  pandemic effect on the global economy 509
  pandemics 461
  personal protective equipment (PPE) 288t
  post-COVID conditions 431
  pregnancy 101
  SARS-CoV-2 infection 244
  technology during pandemic 335

Index

telework
  long COVID 441
  pandemic and employment 606
  pandemics protection 460
  screening workers for COVID-19 209
thalassemia, preexisting medical condition 107
thrombosis with thrombocytopenia syndrome (TTS), COVID-19 vaccines 358
Trades Union Congress (TUC), long COVID condition 440
transverse myelitis, coronavirus and nervous system 88
troponin, post-COVID conditions 425
TTS *see* thrombosis with thrombocytopenia syndrome
tuberculosis (TB)
  epidemiology 15
  immunocompromising conditions 245
TUC *see* Trades Union Congress
type 1 diabetes, preexisting medical condition 105
type 2 diabetes, preexisting medical condition 105

U

U.S. Bureau of Labor Statistics (BLS)
  contact information 637
  publication
    COVID-19 and employment 616n
U.S. Department of Education (ED)
  contact information 637
  publications
    COVID-19 safety considerations 201n
    distance education during COVID-19 570n
U.S. Department of Health and Human Services (HHS)
  contact information 637
  publications
    community-based testing sites for COVID-19 71n
    COVID-19 treatments and therapeutics 255n, 260n
    disparities in COVID-19 131n
    interim COVID-19 treatment in outpatients 255n
    long COVID as a disability 452n
U.S. Department of Homeland Security (DHS)
  contact information 637
  publications
    COVID-19 8n
    variants of the coronavirus 35n, 39n
U.S. Department of the Treasury
  publication
    COVID-19 economic relief 534n
U.S. Food and Drug Administration (FDA)
  contact information 637
  COVID-19 in animals 126
  emergency use authorizations (EUAs) 313
  influenza antiviral drugs 55
  influenza historical timeline 468
  mission management 618
  negative test results 177
  neurological disorders 89
  Pfizer-BioNTech vaccine 351
  publications
    cleaning and disinfecting at home 173n
    coronavirus self-test kits 70n

U.S. Food and Drug Administration (FDA), *continued*
    COVID-19 infections in pets and animals 127n
    face masks and social distancing 163n
    fraudulent coronavirus tests, vaccines, and treatments 316n
    medical management of COVID-19 263n
    pulse oximetry 241
    vaccine adverse event reporting system (VAERS) 392
U.S. Government Accountability Office (GAO)
    contact information 637
    publication
        COVID-19 herd immunity 413n
U.S. Senate Committee on Health, Education, Labor, and Pensions
    contact information 637
    publication
        origins of the COVID-19 pandemic 12n
UI *see* unemployment insurance
unemployment insurance (UI)
    COVID-19 economic relief 520
    COVID-19 pandemic 485
unintended consequences, global health crisis 551
United States Census Bureau
    contact information 637
    publications
        COVID-19 economic impact 518n
        COVID-19 impact on mortality and economy 490n
        impact of COVID-19 on travel and tourism 599n
        impact of the pandemic on population estimates of major cities 604n
        schooling during COVID-19 571n
        social impact of COVID-19 559n
unpaid leave, supporting employees with long COVID 442

V

vaccination
    COVID-19 pandemic 24
    COVID-19 self-tests 63
    COVID-19 vaccine safety 401
    early care and education (ECE) 186
    finding a COVID-19 vaccine or booster 350
    gross domestic product (GDP) 494
    infection risk 590
    influenza historic timeline 469
    medical management 261
    neurological problems 90
vaccine adverse event reporting system (VAERS), COVID-19 vaccination 391
vaccine safety
    COVID-19 vaccination 374
    human immunodeficiency virus (HIV) 111
    neurological problems 89
    overview 392–394
vaccine technologies, COVID-19 vaccine effectiveness 383
VAERS *see* vaccine adverse event reporting system
varicella zoster virus (VZV), latent infections 245
vectorborne disease, epidemic patterns 459

Index

ventilation
  COVID-19 and flu 53
  COVID-19 prevention 108
  COVID-19 prevention and control in schools 188
  hypoxia 81
  intensive care unit (ICU) 267
  Occupational Safety and Health Administration (OSHA) 163
  personal protective measures 297
  preventive actions 321
ventilators
  COVID-19 infection spread 13
  influenza historic timeline 467
viral infection
  COVID-19 symptoms 79
  health coverage 325
  SARS-CoV-2 reinfection 246
viral test
  antigen test 424
  COVID-19 antibodies 77
  COVID-19 testing 59
  COVID-19 vaccine 408
vital organs, coronavirus and nervous system 81
vitamins, post-COVID conditions 433
VZV *see* varicella zoster virus

W

Whitehouse.gov
  publications
    approaching a possible outbreak in the future 621n
    U.S. economy and global pandemic 505n
working remotely, supporting employees with long COVID 441
workplace flexibility, long COVID support 441

X

x-ray
  post-COVID conditions 46, 427
  SARS-CoV-2 240
  telehealth and telemedicine during COVID-19 337

Y

yellow fever, epidemic patterns 459

Z

zoonotic spillover, human-animal interface 8